CW00708763

Distributors

AcuMedic CENTRE
101-103 CAMDEN HIGH STREET
LONDON NW1 7JN
Tel: 071-388 5783/6704
Catalogue on Request

TEXTBOOK OF ACUPUNCTURE

By the same author:

ATLAS OF ACUPUNCTURE. Points and Meridians in relation to surface anatomy. This is the companion volume to "Textbook of Acupuncture"

ACUPUNCTURE: CURE OF MANY DISEASES
This is for the non-medical reader who wants a grasp of the essentials of acupuncture in a few hours.

TEXTBOOK
OF
ACUPUNCTURE

FELIX MANN
MB, BChir (Cambridge) LMCC
Founder of the Medical Acupuncture Society
President 1959 to 1980

This book is a one volume edition, in full, of the
following four books. Appended is a reduced scale
monochrome version of the Atlas of Acupuncture.

Scientific Aspects of Acupuncture
Acupuncture: The Ancient Chinese Art of Healing
The Meridians of Acupuncture
The Treatment of Disease by Acupuncture

HEINEMANN MEDICAL BOOKS

Heinemann Medical Books
An imprint of Heinemann Professional Publishing Ltd
Halley Court, Jordan Hill, Oxford OX2 8EJ

OXFORD   LONDON   SINGAPORE   NAIROBI   IBADAN   KINGSTON

First published as four individual volumes:

Scientific Aspects of Acupuncture 1977, 1983
Acupuncture: The Ancient Chinese Art of Healing 1962 (twice),
1965, 1970, 1971, 1973, 1974, 1978, 1980
The Meridians of Acupuncture 1964, 1971, 1972 (twice), 1974, 1976,
1981
The Treatment of Disease by Acupuncture 1963, 1967, 1972, 1974,
1975, 1976, 1980, 1985

This edition first published 1987
Reprinted 1990

ISBN 0 433 20312 9

© Felix Mann 1987

All rights reserved

Printed and bound in Great Britain by
Redwood Press Limited, Melksham, Wiltshire

CONTENTS

This book is dedicated to my wife Ruth

PREFACE AND ACKNOWLEDGMENTS

EVOLUTION OF THIS BOOK

After having studied orthodox medicine at Cambridge University and Westminster Hospital, I travelled round various parts of the world, Canada, Switzerland, France, Germany, and Austria, working in hospitals and as assistant to general practitioners.

Whilst in Strasbourg a friend had lower abdominal pain which, at the time, we thought was due to appendicitis, though this was probably not the case. Whatever it was, she called in an acupuncturist and the pain was gone in ten minutes. In orthodox medicine and in the majority of diseases, instant responses are a rarity. I was impressed and the seed was sown for my future study of acupuncture, a subject of whose very existence I had previously been unaware.

At the time there was only one doctor practising acupuncture in Strasbourg, who happened to work quite near where I lived above a small family grocer's shop. In those more leisured days customers in small shops would stay and chat for a few minutes, as in a pub, before leaving, and so it was very easy for the grocer and his wife to question their customers on my behalf about this new doctor who practised acupuncture. My 'spies' then informed me that he did have failures, but that he also achieved miraculous results with patients who had been to many doctors previously to no avail.

Nowadays when a new treatment is advocated, a clinical trial is performed and then published in the medical press lauding the beneficial effects of the therapy in question. I personally think that the empirical investigations or 'clinical trial' performed by the grocer and his wife were no more open to error than the more usual sophisticated articles.

The same friend had also for several years suffered from dysmenorrhoea, severe enough to confine her to bed for two days a month despite appropriate treatment. I obtained a book on acupuncture in German by Stiefvater, followed the instructions and needled her at Liver 8 on the medial side of the knee. She has never had dysmenorrhoea since this single treatment, though it is true to say that most patients require several treatments.

After all this the study of acupuncture was of course an absolute must.

It was quite easy for me to embrace unorthodox medicine as my mother had brought me up to accept and even appreciate the unconventional, in medicine as in other things. Being herself one of those people who react badly to drugs, even small doses on occasion producing alarming side-effects, she was drawn to homeopathy and herbal medicine, both of which I had in turn studied to some extent before encountering acupuncture. My mother's very active and intense intellectual life was deeply influenced by the writings of Rudolf Steiner, the philosopher and mystic, and, to a lesser extent, by the similar ideas of Goethe and Paracelsus. Her driving force and enthusiasm had already made me conscious of new intellectual and spiritual horizons and so I took to the metaphysical ideas of traditional Chinese medicine like a duck to water. At the time, the metaphysical concepts underlying Chinese acupuncture were very important for my initial understanding of the subject. Moreover, in Strasbourg I had been the assistant of Dr Jean Schoch who practised medicine with a similar philosophical background.

Later as I learned more and gained clinical experience I very largely revised my views. As can be seen in the first chapter of *Scientific Aspects of Acupuncture*, I now think that 'acupuncture points do not exist, meridians do not exist, and that most of the laws of acupuncture are laws about non-existent entities'. I now believe that the problems of acupuncture can be more clearly understood and effectively resolved if we approach them neurophysiologically.

It should never be forgotten that a knowledge of medicine is required to practise acupuncture satisfactorily: it is not the only prerequisite, but it is an important keystone. A doctor who has studied physiology and pathology, who knows the natural course of a disease, and who has, during his studies and practice, accumulated a wealth of clinical experience, may tackle a large variety of mild and serious disease, for he knows what to expect if a given organ is stimulated.

The numerous practitioners of acupuncture who are not doctors and who do not know the basic principles of medicine, unfortunately, all too often achieve results commensurate with their lack of knowledge.

I first studied acupuncture with Dr Anton Strobl of Munich. Thereafter, I realised that a delicate touch is an advantage in the practice of acupuncture, so at the next acupuncture conference I attended in Germany I looked at the hands of the participants and found one whose hands I thought were particularly sensitive. They belonged to Professor Johannes Bischko, now president of the Austrian Acupuncture Society and head of the Ludwig Bolzman Acupuncture Institute. I went to study with him in Vienna and he taught me more than anyone else. Later studies took me to Dr Van Nha of Montpellier.

At that time in 1958 there were very few books on acupuncture in a non-Oriental language. Probably the most outstanding were the translations of Soulié de Morant (who worked with Ferreyrolles) assembled in a massive tome called *L'Acuponcture Chinoise*. From this, and to a lesser extent, from Hübotter's book *Die Chinesische Medizin* published in 1929, I gained a good initial foundation. However, I realised that my study of traditional Chinese medicine was hampered by the paucity of good textbooks in a Western language. Therefore I did the only possible thing and learnt to read Chinese well enough to be able to read their acupuncture texts in the original language, together with my teachers. My first teacher was Charles Curwen, later I also studied with David Owen and finally for several years with Frank Liu.

At this stage of my career, when I was still particularly interested in the traditional Chinese ideas, I also went to China and studied in Peking, Nanking, and Shanghai.

ACUPUNCTURE: THE ANCIENT CHINESE ART OF HEALING

During my stay in Canada I read several American textbooks on various scientific subjects and was impressed and refreshed by the clarity and simplicity of their language. I was able to assimilate a great deal of information without the extenuating mental effort needed to grapple with English textbooks which at that time were couched in a rather more baroque and rebarbative style. I have, therefore, in writing these books, tried to model myself on the American manner as regards simplicity of expression, though not as regards spelling or the use of unnecessary and inappropriate technical jargon; I prefer to speak of eating rather than of enteral nutrition, for instance. I hope that my readers will be refreshed as I was by reading technical and scientific matter expressed in simple straightforward English.

The original concept of this book owed much to Soulié de Morant, Hübotter, Chamfrault, Veith, and the other authors mentioned in the bibliography. Later reprints and also the *Meridians of Acupuncture* were increasingly based on the Zhingyixue Gailun of the Nanking

Academy of Chinese Medicine published in 1959, and the Zhenjiuxue Jiangyi of the Acupuncture Research Section of the Shanghai Academy of Chinese Medicine published in 1960. In 1971 I added my neurophysiological ideas and research to this book and later in 1977 it was published as a separate book, *Scientific Aspects of Acupuncture*.

THE MERIDIANS OF ACUPUNCTURE

The aim of this book is to describe in words and pictures the fifty-nine meridians that constitute acupuncture. This is the first book in the Western World to do so.

Most Chinese books describe the meridians under the following five headings: *main meridian, connecting meridian, muscle meridian, divergent meridian* and *extra meridian*. Each of the five groups is sub-divided into about twelve sections for each category of meridian.

In this book I have used the reverse classification, having as main headings each of the twelve organ-meridians: lung, large intestine, stomach, spleen, heart, small intestine, bladder, kidney, pericardium, triple warmer, gall bladder, liver. Each of these twelve sections is sub-divided into four groups: main meridian, connecting meridian, muscle meridian, and divergent meridian—the last being paired and described only under the Yang meridian. The extra meridians and their two connecting meridians have been retained as a separate group for reasons mentioned in the first chapter.

I have applied this system of classification as I considered the twelve main meridians of prime importance, and the five types of meridians as specialisations only. From a practical point of view this system of classification is more convenient, since a patient with cardiac disease may have symptoms along the course of the main, connecting, muscle or divergent heart meridians. In this system, the types of diseases or symptoms which occur together may be found in the same section.

The first part of each section entitled, 'Traditional Chinese and Western Scientific Conceptions', has been taken initially from Chinese sources which have many conceptions alien to our accustomed mode of thinking.

In an attempt to correlate all this with Western medicine, I have, after stating the traditional Chinese point of view, added a few scientific interpretations. These are mainly in terms of embryology, comparative anatomy, and physiology, which I must admit is inadequate. It should be remembered that this book is one of the first attempts to link traditional Chinese and Western scientific medicine, that the whole subject is inordinately large, and that, due to my practice, I have only a limited amount of time available for research and writing books. Many of the interpretations are those of embryology and comparative anatomy in part because these subjects interest me, in part because they give a clearer overall picture than the minutiae of body chemistry, and in part because a fuller physiological explanation would require more research. I have not added a scientific explanation to those Chinese concepts which are similar to our own in the West, for this would be superfluous: the stomach, for example, is considered to have a digestive function in both Chinese and Western medicine.

The first section of the lung includes the subdivision into mucous, sobbing, autumn, dryness, etc. This is described more clearly in diagramatic form in *Acupuncture, The Ancient Chinese Art of Healing*. It has only been mentioned in this book in the one section, as this was considered all that was necessary for the practising doctor to be able to apply it to all sections.

The case histories have all been taken from my own practice. Mostly they are typical of a large number of patients, as it has been my aim to discuss failures as well as successes, the difficult as well as the easy cases. The overall picture can be gained from the statistics in *Acupuncture, The Ancient Chinese Act of Healing*.

The second part of each section entitled 'Symptomatology' describes the symptoms and signs of dysfunction of the organ, or the main, connecting, muscle, or divergent meridian.

The system may seem unnecessarily complicated and even contradictory. However, it is the Chinese system and I have left it as such.

The third part of each section, entitled 'Course of Meridians', describes the course of the main, connecting, muscle, and divergent meridians.

The last part of each section, entitled 'Important Points' summarises the most commonly used acupuncture points.

THE TREATMENT OF DISEASE BY ACUPUNCTURE

This book is largely based on Chinese tradition, interlaced with my own experience and that of other European doctors practising acupuncture.

Part I
This section describes those diseases or symptoms which may be alleviated or cured by stimulating a specific acupuncture point.

If a doctor has a patient with, say, dyspnoea, and he looks up in this section a point where the word dyspnoea is mentioned and then stimulates this point with a needle he will be extremely lucky if the patient is any the better. Of primary importance is an understanding and an ability to assess and use the basic principles of diagnosis and therapy in acupuncture. The encyclopaedic data mentioned in this book are only of real value when applied according to the basic principles.

The individual symptoms or diseases mentioned, such as dyspnoea, bronchitis, etc. should not be taken too literally and out of context. The general picture given by the summation of all the individual symptoms or signs of a particular point is of prime importance. It is this general picture of what a specific acupunture point is capable of curing or alleviating that the doctor practising acupuncture should keep in mind. Obviously it is impossible to remember all the facts mentioned in this section. Even if it could be done, it would be of far greater importance to have a vivid, living, general picture of what a specific acupuncture point does—something that can best be gained by long experience coupled with an artistic feeling.

The major part of the description of each point is taken directly from the Chinese books mentioned in the bibliography—mainly the first few. These I read, or at least partly read, while learning to read the largely archaic Chinese in which the acupuncture books are written. Not the whole of this section was covered in this way, the remainder being translated by David Owen.

A few of the diseases or symptoms mentioned by the Chinese cannot in my experience be successfully treated—or at least only rarely. I have therefore reduced, not omitted, as I may be wrong, the frequency with which these diseases or symptoms are mentioned in my text.

I have tended to oscillate between a literal translation of the Chinese and the nearest Western medical term which is applicable. Often the literal translation of the Chinese is more graphic and therefore easier to remember, i.e. 'intestine make sound like thunder', instead of 'borborygmi'; or 'thumping and lurching of the heart' instead of 'palpitations'. Sometimes the Chinese express symptoms in a way which we, by custom, do not; 'heart feels hot' or 'Qi (life energy) rushing madly up and down causing pain': these have often been left literally translated.

In addition to the Chinese description of a point I have added a few diseases and symptoms based on my own practical experience.

Before writing down a single disease or symptom I cross-referenced it with at least two other books and added any extra information thus obtained. Of the European books I am most indebted to those of A. Chamfrault and Soulié de Morant, although to a certain extent, all European books and some of the Chinese mentioned in the bibliography were used.

The various categories of acupuncture point to which an individual point belongs are mentioned under each point to give a concise description. The translation of the name of a particular category of point is somewhat arbitrary. I have tended to adhere to the French translation (the Latin root being the same), particularly that of J. E. H. Niboyet, to maintain at least some uniformity. It will be noticed that in a few places the classification clashes. This is unavoidable in a subject that is not completely and systematically classified. Some of the categories of points are, in my opinion, a natural classification; much as the living world may be classified, with only a few exceptions, into the animal and vegetable kingdoms. Other categories are, in my opinion, artificial. I have, however, retained them as a useful aide memoire in the labyrinth of acupuncture.

Chinese books normally give an anatomical description of the position of a point. I have not done this as I think it is easier to remember a picture than an intricate collection of words. For this reason I have produced the large-scale *Atlas of Acupuncture: Points and Meridians in Relation to Surface Anatomy*.

Part II
This is the reverse of Part I, being the description of acupuncture points that may be used in a specific disease.

There are of course many more variations than those mentioned, which the experienced acupuncturist tucks away in his subconscious mind and is able to use when he sees an individual patient with his individual characteristics and individual subtle variations. Doctors who have been to the courses of lecture–demonstrations which I give to doctors who wish to study acupuncture, will notice that I have certain preferences and tend to use one technique more than another, as I find that certain techniques give better results.

Section 1

This is a translation of Changjian Jibing Zhenjiu Zhiliao Bianlan (*A General Survey of Common Diseases and their Treatment by Acupuncture*), made by David Owen. To this he has written his own preface overleaf on the difficulties of translating this subject.

Whilst studying medical Chinese I read through part of this book elucidating most of the practical medical difficulties. This translation was good enough for my own purposes but not precise enough for anyone else to understand. Therefore David Owen has translated it, trying to make nebulosities that one understands oneself, clear to the reader.

It is divided into five columns:

Cause of disease—in the Chinese sense.
Symptoms.
Diagnostic features.
Main acupuncture points that may be used.
Secondary acupuncture points that may be used.

Section 2

I have written this section as an addition to Section 1, in an abbreviated style, mentioning only the name of the disease or symptom. Generally I think that Section 1 is of considerably more value than Section 2. In this section I have classified diseases in a Western way and have put them under the most suitable Chinese heading that I could find, to facilitate reference, even though, without the Chinese, I would have classified them differently.

In a later edition two new sections have been added:

The first is a translation of a book by Ye Siu-ting. The original Chinese contains a long description of each disease, similar to that in a textbook of medicine. Western doctors will of course already know all this or, if they have forgotten it, may refer to their favourite textbook. For this reason we have only translated the name of the disease and the acupuncture points that may be used in its treatment. I have found the combinations of acupuncture points mentioned in this book better than in most and have therefore added it to my book to make it available to Western readers.

The second new section concerns periosteal acupuncture which I have gradually developed since about 1965. I now practise as much periosteal acupuncture as ordinary acupuncture.

Preface to translation of Part II Section 1

Chinese is never an easy language to translate, however well one may understand the original. In this case the fact that the bulk of the terminology has remained standardised for anything up to three thousand years, while the language itself has, obviously, developed, means that there may be a considerable difference between what a given word means in modern Chinese and what it means as a technical term in acupuncture, defined as it was, some thousands or hundreds of years ago in the great classics of Chinese medicine from the Nei Jing down. Although an increasing number of modern works on acupuncture are appearing in Chinese, the number of quotations from much earlier works is still considerable, and there is no attempt to revise the terminology or indeed to define it in modern terms. Where definitions exist they are invariably given in archaic terms which are themselves not clear; and they are generally supported by a classical quotation which is by no means always helpful, since the classical language was an extremely terse, epigrammatic and to us who think differently, not a clearly defined vehicle of communication.

Another technical difficulty with this particular work is that it is written, as it has been translated, in an abbreviated style, almost in note form. Since Chinese is an almost totally uninflected language, the indications of what part of speech a particular word plays in a given context are fewer here than usual. Normally one relies, as one does very largely in English, but more so, on word order, but in so shortened a style the syntactical structures largely disappear. Most Chinese words are capable of fulfilling more than one grammatical function, and at times it has been a question of choosing a translation which offers the greatest chance of being understood.

By far the greatest obstacle to an acceptable translation, however, has been the relative lack of precedent in English or in other European languages. This is particularly true of the theoretical aspects of the subject, and has meant that generally few accepted equivalents have been available. Words with a capital letter are mostly mentioned in the Glossary. In some cases it has been found to be quite impossible to find an English equivalent and the Chinese word has been retained in romanised form, using the Han-yu Pin-yin system.

There are certain unusual phrases which recur throughout the 'symptoms' column. 'Chest melancholy', 'heart troubled', 'abdomen full and melancholy' etc., are common, and I have refrained from writing each with a capital letter since this would leave very few words uncapitalised. The most common, however, have been included in the Glossary. In fact these phrases become clearer if one is actually feeling what is described or if that feeling can be remembered. The description of various sensations, which one cannot call 'pain' is by no means easy, and in the West they are usually ignored. They are considered of great importance by the Chinese, however. These descriptions have therefore been translated almost literally, rather than as more generalised terms such as 'lethargy', 'general fatigue' etc. They probably appear all the more strange since the sensation is attributed directly to the particular organ or area of the body: e.g. 'heart melancholy' may be less acceptable than 'a melancholic feeling in the heart' but what the Chinese in fact say is 'heart (is) melancholy'.

Sources
Zhongyi Changyong Mingci Jianshi (A brief explanation of common terms in Chinese medicine), compiled by the Academy of Chinese Medicine of Chengdu, published by the Sichuan People's Publishing House, Chengdu 1959 (abbreviated throughout as JIANSHI).

D. T. Owen

SCIENTIFIC ASPECTS OF ACUPUNCTURE

This book is an *attempt* to explain certain aspects of acupuncture in terms of science. It is not a scientific textbook of acupuncture because at the moment I do not think it possible to write one.

In the past few years research into acupuncture and related subjects has increased and may be read in a large number of journals. Perhaps not surprisingly it contains many contradictions which do not necessarily agree with the clinician's experience. This book, as the title implies, discusses only certain aspects.

At a later date I may expand *Scientific Aspects of Acupuncture*. This will depend to a large extent on the investigations of other doctors and researchers and thus might become a multiple-author type of book. My main task has been to initiate the neurophysiological approach to acupuncture, the essentials of which were published as three chapters of the 1971 edition of *Acupuncture: The Ancient Chinese Art of Healing*. I will be glad if my investigations have sown a seed that others may tend further.

In this book I have quoted extensively from the research of others. My friends and colleagues have helped considerably by drawing my attention to articles which they thought would help my neurophysiological investigations of acupuncture and by sending me relevant reprints. I would like to mention David Sinclair, Professor of anatomy at Aberdeen, John Bakody, neurosurgeon of Iowa, Gerald Looney, Lecturer at UCLA, Ken Lingingston, neurosurgeon of Toronto, but these are just a few from a list of names which could go on for one or two pages.

More recently I have been greatly helped by Dr Alexander Macdonald. He is one of the handful of doctors in this country who practise mainly acupuncture and he also does a great deal of research on the subject—a small part of which is mentioned in Chapter VII. He has unhesitatingly and generously shared with me and others the fruits of his researches, experience, and erudition, and has also prepared the more modern scientific section of the bibliography at the end of this book.

Once a year I organise a meeting at my house at which the neurologist Peter Nathan has spoken every year on such neurophysiological and allied research as has been published in the previous year and has some relevance to acupuncture. This neurophysiological survey has greatly helped me and I think also many other doctors in this country.

The papers I have quoted contain research which in many instances has been repeated by a large number of different teams, though usually differing in certain details. On some occasions I could have quoted from ten similar papers, leaving me the somewhat arbitrary choice of mentioning only one.

As a clinician, I have on the whole only quoted papers which fit in with my everyday clinical experience. It is therefore my patients whom I primarily thank.

The three original chapters of this book which were written in 1971 still contain some traditional concepts. This is deliberate so that it may be used as a bridge between the traditional and scientific ideas.

Those of us who practise or conduct research into acupuncture are painfully aware of the endless contradictions which arise. I hope that this book sheds light on a few of them.

ATLAS OF ACUPUNCTURE

The acupuncture points and meridians are shown in relation to the bones and skeletal musculature, stressing those anatomical features which are necessary for quick and accurate anatomical location. The format has been designed to facilitate easy reference to a book of manageable size. It is in two colours.

A considerably smaller monochrome version of this atlas is reproduced with this book. The full-scale version is sold separately.

I have of necessity included more personal information in this Preface than I would otherwise have done because the initiation and development of acupuncture in this country and, to a lesser extent, in other countries where English is a viable language, has largely rested on my shoulders.

Acupuncture first came to Britain at about the beginning of the nineteenth century but soon died out as not enough was known about the subject. Thereafter apparently only a handful of doctors practised acupuncture and did so only part time. When I returned to this country in 1958, to the best of my knowledge, I was the only qualified doctor to practise acupuncture exclusively. The publication between 1962 and 1964 of four out of the five sections of this textbook formed likewise the first relatively comprehensive textbook on acupuncture published here. At the same time since 1962 I have given the first regular acupuncture courses, solely for doctors. I also founded the Medical Acupuncture Society of which I was president for over 20 years. I was one of the first doctors to discard the traditional idea of acupuncture points and meridians. I replaced this with a partly empirical approach and partly one which regards the nervous system as the main system of transmission used in acupuncture.

Now of course acupuncture blossoms: perhaps a thousand doctors practise it to a greater or lesser extent in this country though still only a handful do so full time; there are several acupuncture conferences a year, and several hundred books published on the subject in the English language.

The above-mentioned development of acupuncture would have been slower and on a smaller scale without my publishers Heinemann Medical. Due to their efforts the various constituent books have been published in up to eight languages, with a total sale of about a third of a million copies, a remarkable record for any medical book. The initial manuscript was accepted for publication by the veteran managing director J. Johnston Abraham. Publication was continued under Owen Evans who lived to see the initial blossoming of the subject. This was continued by Richard Emery. This present combined textbook has been accepted by the present publishing director Dr Richard Barling. For most of this long period the production of the books was managed by Ninetta Martyn whose conscientiousness and attention to detail are legendary. The sales of the books was for some years the enthusiastic province of Jean Eales and then of the likewise enthusiastic Michael Pearman. The idea that this book should be published in a single volume is due to Michael Pearman who has gleefully prodded me along. The large production task of bringing all the material together in one book has been that of Christopher Jarvis.

Frederick Metcalf made the drawings for the *Meridians of Acupuncture*. All the other, in my opinion excellent drawings have been made by the well-known medical artist Sylvia Treadgold.

The five books which form the constituent parts of this textbook were originally published separately as this facilitated making changes, additions, or deletions, with each succeeding edition. Now, after 25 years, fewer changes are required and four of the books have been published as a single volume which is also cheaper. However, the *Atlas of Acupuncture* is being published as a separate book due to its larger size.

Doctors who wish to study acupuncture are welcome to write to me. From time to time I give courses, largely of a practical nature, during which I concentrate on those aspects of the subject that are difficult to describe in a book. During these courses the scientific and empirical approach is stressed, with emphasis on periosteal acupuncture. I explain and demonstrate a method of needling a patient at one or only a few places, which requires in total relatively few treatments. These courses are only open to fully qualified and registered doctors who have practised orthodox medicine for at least one year. This is because the way I practise acupuncture requires just as great a knowledge of orthodox medicine as that required by a doctor practising Western medicine.

Felix Mann
London W1
1987

AIDS

(Acquired Immune Deficiency Syndrome)

AIDS has made the general public and the medical profession increasingly aware of the absolute necessity of using sterile needles, whether they be hypodermic needles used in ordinary medicine or acupuncture needles.

The public's fear of contracting AIDS, fed to saturation point by daily reports in newspapers, on television and radio, is so great that some patients, I think quite justifiably, demand disposable needles. Scientifically this may not be necessary, but to ignore patients' psychology and wishes would be cruel and unwise.

It is for these reasons that I and the majority of my colleagues determined at a meeting held at my house that in future we should use only disposable needles, which are used on one patient and then thrown away after each treatment. In 1985 the Department of Health and Social Security sent a circular letter to all doctors urging them whenever possible to use only disposable hypodermic or acupuncture needles.

FM
1987

SECTION 1

Scientific Aspects of Acupuncture

CONTENTS

I

GENERAL CONSIDERATIONS

When I first studied acupuncture in 1958, I did so in the traditional Chinese manner. A scientific approach to acupuncture hardly existed at that time. Thus I trod the pathway of Yin and Yang, the five elements, and the other accoutrements of this effective, yet fairy-tale world. I even spent ten years learning to read medical Chinese, so as to be able to read with my Chinese teacher the ancient and modern books in their original language; and what is more to be able to soak myself in the mentality and thought of this traditional medical art.

After some years, I felt I had to a certain extent mastered the subject: I knew what the ancients said, and also what was preached in this century in the East and the West. It was only then that I seriously examined the validity of all I had learnt, only to discover that most of it was phantasy,

In this book I will show that acupuncture points do not exist, meridians do not exist, and that most of the laws of acupuncture are laws about non-existent entities.

Yet acupuncture works; indeed I practise it nearly 100 per cent of my time. I hope in the ensuing pages to explain, at least partially, how acupuncture works from a neurophysiological point of view, and hence how a Western doctor may practise acupuncture and, as a corollary, why the ancients had good results by acupuncture for the wrong reasons.

I will show that an acupuncture point is like McBurney's point which can vary in size and position to a considerable extent. When the appendicitis is cured, McBurney's point disappears. The reflex pain one has in lumbago or sciatica similar to the pain in the neck, shoulder and arm in cervical disease would in traditional Chinese terms be explained as the pain in an acupuncture point (if only a small area is painful) or as the pain along a meridian (in sciatica or brachial neuralgia).

Clearly it is more appropriate for a scientific doctor to say there is a reflex tenderness in the renal angle in renal disease, than for him to say there is an acupuncture point there. Likewise one should describe the tenderness of the arm in angina pectoris as a reflex rather than as a meridian.

In this book, I not infrequently mention acupuncture points and meridians, even though they have no physical reality. I do this so that those doctors who already know acupuncture may more easily integrate tradition with the scientific.

NEURAL THEORY OF THE ACTION OF ACUPUNCTURE

In acupuncture, the needle is frequently placed at the opposite end, and possibly opposite side, of the body from that of the diseased organ or site of symptoms. Under certain conditions one of these distant and contralateral pricks can have an effect in one or two seconds. This speed of conduction excludes the blood and lymphatic systems (at least in this type of response) and leaves to my way of thinking, the nervous system as the only contender.

There are other, though non-neural, theories:

Kim Bong Han* described a special conducting system of Bong Han ducts and corpuscles, corresponding to the course of acupuncture meridians. Kellner† has shown that some of the above theory is based on artefacts occurring in the preparation of histological slides. Some have thought that the meridians look like the lines of force round a magnet and postulate a magnetic theory. Others somehow manage to bring in quantum mechanics. A Japanese researcher thinks that there is a contraction wave following the course of meridians, along the surface of the skeletal muscles. Some liken

* Kim Bong Han. On the kyungrak system. 1964, Foreign languages publishing house, Pyongyang.

† International acupuncture conference in Vienna and German acupuncture conference in Wiesbaden.

the pinprick in the body to the electrical discharge of a condenser. A few say the pinprick releases cortisone or histamine or adrenaline but fail to explain the specific action of the acupuncture points. I once had a theory concerning the lateral line system in fish, *which I have since discarded. I am now fairly convinced that the nervous system is the transmission system used in acupuncture. The remainder of this chapter discusses this neural acupuncture theory: part is based on well-known anatomy and physiology, part is conjecture, and part requires experimental proof.

Cutaneo-Visceral Reflex

Acupuncture is based on the fact that stimulating the skin has an effect on the internal organs and on other parts of the body, a relatively simple reflex whose therapeutic application is largely ignored in the West. Various experiments demonstrate the existence of this cutaneo-visceral reflex:

Kuntz, Haselwood; Kuntz; Richins, Brizzee†, in several series of experiments stimulated the skin on the back of rabbits or rats and found changes in the duodenum or other parts of the intestinal tract corresponding to the dermatome stimulated.

By employing a quick freeze-drying technique, it was shown that when a cold beaker of ice was applied to the back in the lower thoracic region, the arterioles in the subserosa and submucosa of the duodenum were constricted and the capillary beds in the villi were ischaemic. The vascular changes in the subserosa could also be observed *in vivo* photographically and by plethysmographic recording.

Reflex responses of the gastric musculature and the pyloric

---

* See chapter XII of the 1st edition of *Acupuncture: The Ancient Chinese Art of Healing*.

† Kuntz, A., and Haselwood, L. A. Circulatory reactions in the gastro-intestinal tract elicited by local cutaneous stimulation. American Heart Journal, 1940, 20: 743–749.

Kuntz, A. Anatomic and physiologic properties of cutaneo-visceral vasomotor reflex arcs. Journal of Neurophysiology, 1945, 8: 421–429.

Richins, C. A., and Brizzee, K. Effect of localized cutaneous stimulation on circulation in duodenal arterioles and capillary beds. Journal of Neurophysiology, 1949, 12: 131–136.

sphincter in man have been described by Freude and Ruhmann*
using a fluoroscope by means of warm, cold, chemical or mechanical
stimulation of the skin of the epigastrium. They also produced
hyperaemia of the ascending colon after it had been exposed at
operation, by applying heat to the skin of the lower abdominal wall.

Nine patients with angina pectoris or acute myocardial infarction
were investigated by Travell and Rinzler.† They found that if the
trigger areas on the front of the chest were infiltrated with procaine
or cooled with ethyl chloride, complete and prolonged relief of pain
usually ensued.

Of the first series of experiments mentioned above using rats and
rabbits, some were performed on animals with an intact nervous
system under general anaesthesia, while others were performed on
animals where the spinal cord had been transected in the lower
cervical region. There was no difference in the two types of experiment, suggesting that the cutaneo-visceral reflex is mediated on a
segmental and intersegmental level and not influenced suprasegmen-
tally.

Wernøe‡ has made similar experiments on fishes and amphibians.
In the pithed eel (with its segmental structure), stimulation of 1 sq.
cm. of skin with silver nitrate caused, after a delay of two minutes,
vasoconstriction of the (from the dermatome point of view) appropriate part of the intestine, followed by a concentric contraction
of the intestinal segment, and finally peristalsis, after which bowel
movements ceased. If a more proximal or distal part of the skin was
stimulated the corresponding sharply defined part of the gut
showed the above cycle of events. In the cod electrical stimulation of
the skin just distal to the pectoral girdle caused ischaemia of the

* Freude, E., and Ruhmann, W. Das thermoreflektorische Verhalten von Tonus
and Kinetik am Magen. Zeitschrift für die gesamte experimentelle Medizin, 1926,
52: 338.

Ruhmann, W., Viscerale Schmerzlinderung durch Wärme als Segment-reflex.
Zeitschrift für die gesamte experimentelle Medizin, 1927, 57: 740.

Ruhmann, W. Ortliche Hautreizbehandlung des Magens und Ihre physiologis-
chen Grundlagen. Archiv für Verdaungskrankheiten, 1927, 41: 336.

† Travell, J., and Rinzler, S. H. Relief of cardiac pain by local block of somatic
trigger areas. Proceedings of the Society for Experimental Biology and Medicine,
1946, 63: 480–482.

‡ Wernøe, T. B. Viscero-cutane Reflexe. Pflügers Archiv für die Gesamte
Physiologie, 1925, 210: 1–34.

stomach, whilst stimulation of the skin 5 cm. distal produced ischaemia in a section of the intestine.

Three eels were taken and their brains destroyed. In addition, in the first the entire spinal cord was destroyed, in the second the distal half was destroyed and in the third the spinal cord was left intact. All the skin of the three eels was stimulated with silver nitrate. After a latent period of 2 to 4 minutes the intestine of the first eel showed vasoconstriction, that of the third eel vasodilation, while the second showed vasodilation in the proximal half and vasoconstriction in the distal half. That is: in those sections where the spinal cord is intact there was vasodilation, while in those where it was destroyed, vasoconstriction. In another eel the spinal cord was divided into several segments, of which alternating segments of the spinal cord were destroyed. On stimulating all the skin with silver nitrate, it was again found that the segments with an intact spinal cord had vasodilation whilst the others had vasoconstriction.

From the above Wernøe deduced that the vasodilation was mediated by a spinal reflex, whilst the vasoconstriction by a post-ganglionic sympathetic reflex.

Sato, Sato, Shimada and Torigata* have investigated in greater detail the cutaneo-visceral reflex:

The experiments were performed on rats: some had an intact CNS but were anaesthetized, others were decerebrate and non-anaesthetized, and yet others were spinal preparations with the cord divided at C2 and non-anaesthetized. A small water filled balloon was inserted into the pyloric area of the stomach and alterations of pressure recorded. A sympathetic postganglionic nerve branch coming from the coeliac ganglion and going to the stomach, and likewise a vagal nerve branch going to the stomach were both dissected under a binocular microscope, attached to electrodes and their discharge activities recorded.

Stimulation of the abdominal wall along either the left or right mammary line reduced the pyloric pressure, more or less equally in all three types of preparation (see Fig. 1). In the intact animal the blood pressure was slightly depressed, whilst with the decerebrate and spinal animals it was slightly raised, showing that this is not an

---

* Sato, A., Sato, Y., Shimada, F., Torigata, Y. Changes in gastric motility produced by nociceptive stimulation of the skin in rats. Brain Research, 1975, 87: 151–159.

important factor. Likewise adrenalectomy left the results unaltered. The inhibitory pyloric response though was completely abolished by destroying the spinal cord between T5 and T11.

Transection of both vagi in the neck did not influence the cutaneo-gastric reflex. On the other hand dividing both splanchinic nerves or crushing both coeliac ganglia abolished the reflex (see Fig. 2).

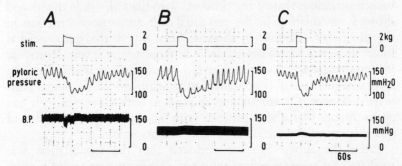

FIG. 1 *A* is CNS intact rat, *B* decerebrate, *C* spinal. Abdominal skin pinched with a pressure of about 2 kg. for 20 seconds. Pyloric pressure from 100–150 mm H_2O and 5–6 contractions per minute.

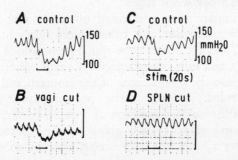

FIG. 2 *A B C D* rats with intact CNS. *A* and *C* control. *B* vagi cut. *D* splanchnics cut.

It was shown that when the abdominal skin was stimulated there was increased activity in the sympathetic splanchnic fibres in the CNS intact animals and also in the spinal animals, whilst there was no alteration in the recording from the vagus (see Fig. 3).

The skin of the rats was stimulated from the cervical area to the groin (see 1 to 7 in Fig. 4) along the mammary line and its extensions, in both CNS intact and spinal rats. It was found that cervical and upper thoracic stimulation had little or no depressor effect on gastric tone (1, 2 and 3), whilst upper and lower abdonimal stimulation had the full effect (4, 5, 6, 7). Various other investigators have found that the cutaneo-gastric reflex is also influenced by stimulating the sciatic and femoral nerves.*

Thus it seems that this gastric inhibitory reflex is initiated by stimulating the appropriate spinal segment or any segment below it. In all these experiments of Sato *et al.* the increased sympathetic activity was observed about 1 second after stimulating the skin, whilst the reduced pyloric pressure required some 2 seconds. The maximum response was reached in about 20 seconds (hence 20 seconds was adopted as the standard time for stimulating the skin).

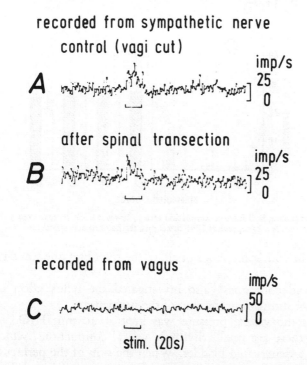

Fig. 3 *A* and *B* recording of gastric sympathetic nerve branch with vagi divided. *B* spinal transection also. *C* recording from vagus

* Babkin, B. P., and Kite, W. R. Jr. Central and reflex regulation of motility of pyloric antrum. Journal of Neurophysiology, 1950, 13: 321–334.

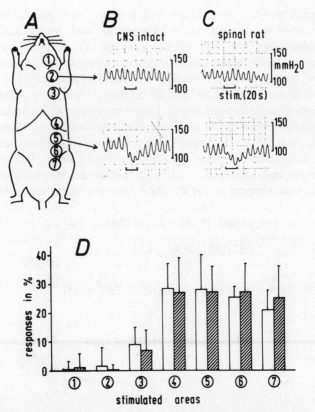

FIG. 4 Upper tracing in *B* is from stimulation area 2, lower tracing *B* from area 5. In *D* the white area represents CNS intact rats, the hatched area spinal rats

This fits in with some, but not all, of the responses one sees clinically in man.

Sato and colleagues* also investigated the reflex effect on the bladder of stimulating the skin of the perineum.

In rats the vesical pressure was kept at 40 mm H_2O. At this pressure there are small, rhythmic vesical contractions, which also occur in a denervated bladder. When the skin of the perineum was stroked or pinched, the intravesical pressure was doubled. Stimulation of the skin of the abdomen or chest had no effect. This reflex

* Sato, A., Sato, Y., Shimada, F., and Torigata, Y. Changes in vesical function produced by cutaneous stimulation in rats. Brain Research, 1975, 94: 465–474.

was observed in CNS intact animals which were anaesthetized, in decerebrate non-anaesthetized animals, and also in animals where the spinal cord had been divided in the upper cervical or mid-thoracic region. The reflex was abolished by destroying the sacral cord or by dividing the pelvic nerve branches to the bladder, which are parasympathetic. Dividing the vesical branches of the hypo-gastric nerves, which are sympathetic, had either no effect or a small equivocal effect. Direct recording of the vesical branches of the pelvic nerve, showed that whenever the perineal skin was irritated there was increased efferent discharge activity.

When the vesical pressure was instead raised to some 200 mm H_2O by injecting more water into an intravesical balloon, the vesical contractions became stronger but less frequent—micturition con-tractions. These contractions were inhibited by pinching the perin-eum, but not by pinching the abdomen or chest. This reflex occurred in animals with an intact CNS who were anaesthetized, and also in decerebrate or spinal unanaesthetized animals. The reflex was abolished if the vesical branches of the pelvic nerve were divided. Recording of the activity of the vesical branches of the pelvic nerve, showed an increase concomittant with the increase in vesical pressure during a micturition contraction.

A reflex between the abdominal skin and the duodenum has also been described by Sato and Terui*, using similar experimental methods to those used in his previous experiments.

The small rhythmic (40 per minute) waves, which correspond to the pendular movements of the duodenum, were inhibited by pinching the abdominal skin. The reflex remained intact in spinal preparations if the vagi were divided. The reflex was abolished if the splanchnics were divided.

The duodenum has also slow waves, corresponding to peristalisis (0.5 per minute). These are likewise inhibited by pinching the abdominal skin. This reflex, as that of the small waves is abolished when the splanchnics are divided.

Pastinszky, Kenedi and Fábert have shown that stimulation of

---

* Sato, Y., Terui, N. Changes in duodenal motility produced by noxious mechanical stimulation of the skin in rats. Neuroscience Letters, 1976, 2: 189–193.

† Pastinszky, I., Kenedi, J., Fáber, U. Experimental studies of the dermato-cardiac reflex effect. Acta Physiologica Academiae Scientiarum Hungariae, 1964, 25: 89–95.

the chest wall in cats produced temporary or even permanent changes in the heart and lungs.

They shaved the left chest wall of cats, which was then painted daily with a strong irritant solution. This produced erythema and oedema of the skin and subcutaneous tissues, which often progressed to ulceration and partial microscopic necrosis. It is thus apparent that this stimulation which was applied for some four weeks, is stronger and more continuous than that in most of the experiments cited in this chapter.

The majority of the cats show E.C.G. changes such as negative T waves, partial atrio-ventricular block, sinus bradycardia, accessory rhythm, complete atrio-ventricular block or bundle branch block. Many of the cats had punctate haemorrhages of the pericardium, likewise of the lungs and pleura bilaterally. Histologically the cardiac muscle showed capillary dilation and likewise dilation of the major branches of the coronary arteries and veins. A few fibres of the cardiac muscle showed micronecrosis with disappearance of the transverse strictions.

In those cats where the skin reaction to painting with the irritant was mild, the E.C.G. changes mentioned above were likewise of a milder nature or temporary. If the skin was painted only once, a smaller proportion of cats developed E.C.G. changes, which were then of only a very temporary nature. If the right buttock instead of the left chest wall was painted, there were no E.C.G. changes whatsoever, except possibly in one equivocal case.

Viscero–Cutaneous Reflex

The cutaneo–visceral reflex mentioned in the preceding section is of prime importance in acupuncture, for it is by its mediation that an acupuncture needle placed in the correct part of the skin is able to affect the appropriate organ or diseased part of the body.

The viscero–cutaneous reflex to be discussed in this section is of importance (1) in diagnosis and (2) in lowering the threshold of stimulation required in treatment by acupuncture.

It is often noticed clinically that a disease of an internal organ will produce in some part of the skin (not infrequently of the same derma-tome) pain, tenderness, hyperaesthesia, hypoaesthesia etc. This can also be seen experimentally:

Wernøe stimulated the rectum of a decapitated plaice electrically, or with copper sulphate or barium chloride. In each case the skin became pale, due to retraction of the melanophores, extending to 3 or 4 spinal segments of the appropriate dermatomes. Likewise in the eel and cod, the stomach, intestines, gall bladder or spleen were stimulated mechanically or by the intramural injection of 10 per cent adrenalin; in each case the skin becoming lighter over an area of several segments, again in the expected dermatomes.

In the decapitated cod, if the spinal cord is in addition destroyed, the viscero-cutaneous reflex is not abolished. If, on the other hand, the cord is intact but the sympathetic chain is excised the reflex is abolished. This suggests that it is not a spinal reflex, but that it is mediated along unknown paths of the sympathetic chain.

The viscero-cutaneous reflex discussed here and the viscero-motor reflex to be discussed later are presumably the mechanism whereby diseases of internal organs produce pain or tenderness of certain acupuncture points, areas of skin, or muscle spasm. Presumably other, though similar reflexes are involved when diseases other than those of internal organs likewise cause pain, tenderness, muscle spasm etc.

In acupuncture a somewhat smaller stimulus is needed if the acupuncture needle is put directly into one of these tender or painful areas or into a meridian that crosses or is related in some other way to the tender area. Presumably facilitation is taking place. This facilitation is also a safeguard, for if the acupuncture needle is put in the wrong place it has little effect, as it is easier to affect a diseased or disease related area than a healthy one.

Viscero-Motor and Viscero-Visceral Reflexes

These reflexes are in many instances similar to the viscero-cutaneous reflexes mentioned above, occurring mostly at the same time, though requiring an intact spinal cord.

Miller, Simpson* and many others stimulated the viscera and obtained muscle contractions in the expected appropriate dermatomes (and distant dermatomes—see later). Distension of the stomach by air, traction on the stomach, mustard oil on the gastric mucosa, squeezing the small intestine, mechanical stimulation of the kidney

* Miller, F. R., and Simpson, H. M. Transactions of the Royal Society of Canada, sec V, 1924, XVIII, 147.

or spleen all elicited the reflex, which could be abolished by dividing the appropriate dorsal root. The reflex from the stomach was stopped by dividing the splanchnic nerves, while stimulation of the central ends of the divided nerve restored it; similar results were obtained with the superior mesenteric nerves for the small intestine, the hypogastric nerve for the kidney, and the splenic nerve for the spleen.

Brown-Sequard* relates an experiment with a dog which had a tube tied into its ureter. When the internal abdominal wall was pricked within the distribution of the 1st lumbar nerve, the secretion of urine was considerably diminished.

Brown-Sequard* also quotes the case of a colleague, Sir Benjamin Brodie, who had a patient with a stricture of the urethra causing pain and lameness of the foot. All symptoms were relieved after a bougie had been passed up the urethra. The urethra and foot symptoms were probably in the same or neighbouring dermatome. I have on several occasions observed in a patient with multiple sclerosis that when the heel is pricked with a needle the patient micturates.

Cannon and Murphy† compared two series of cats who had been given ether anaesthesia. The one group had their testicles crushed whilst the others were not molested. Afterwards both groups were given food mixed with barium and its passage in the ileum followed roentgenologically. In the emasculated group there was no movement of the ileum for 4 hours, after which it started sluggishly; whilst in the control group there was movement from the very beginning. The testicles are usually given as T10 to L3 (varying according to the author) and the small intestine as T6 to T11, so that this is possibly a segmental reflex.

Dermatomes and Acupuncture Points

Some of the acupuncture points, particularly those on the back, having an effect on a specific organ, are in the appropriate dermatomes as a glance at Fig. 5‡ and 6 will show. Account should be

* Brown-Sequard, C. E., Course of lectures on the physiology and pathology of the central nervous system. 1860, Lippincott, Philadelphia, p. 170 and 167.

† Cannon, W. B., and Murphy, F. T. Physiologic Observations in experimentally produced ileus. Journal of the American Medical Association, 1907, 49: 840.

‡ Dermatomes derived from Hansen, K. and Schliak, H. Segmentale innervation, ihre bedeutung für Klinik und Praxis, 1962, Georg Thieme, Stuttgart; and other sources.

taken though that the Chinese do not always mean the same as we do when they say heart, liver, etc. as described in greater detail in 'The Meridians of Acupuncture'.

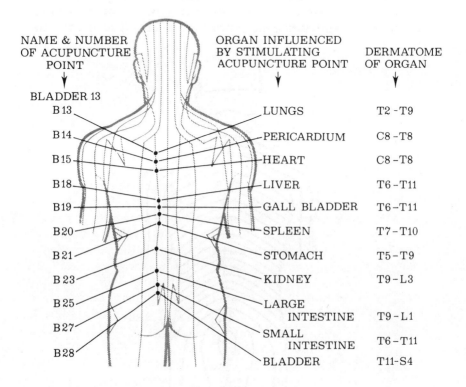

NAME & NUMBER OF ACUPUNCTURE POINT	ORGAN INFLUENCED BY STIMULATING ACUPUNCTURE POINT	DERMATOME OF ORGAN
BLADDER 13		
B 13	LUNGS	T2 - T9
B 14	PERICARDIUM	C8 - T8
B 15	HEART	C8 - T8
B 18	LIVER	T6 - T11
B 19	GALL BLADDER	T6 - T11
B 20	SPLEEN	T7 - T10
B 21	STOMACH	T5 - T9
B 23	KIDNEY	T9 - L3
B 25	LARGE INTESTINE	T9 - L1
B 27	SMALL INTESTINE	T6 - T11
B 28	BLADDER	T11 - S4

FIG. 5 Hyperaesthetic zones in internal disease

The majority of reflexes mentioned in the previous section (cutaneo-visceral, viscero-cutaneous, viscero-motor) are segmental in nature, and hence fit in with the dermatome pattern of acupuncture points described in this section. Some of the reflexes can also be intersegmental, not following the dermatomes. These are described in the next section.

There is often considerable variation in the dermatome pattern according to the method of investigation: hyposensitivity from loss of function of a single nerve root (Keegan and Garrett);* electrical skin resistance in sympathectomised patients; electrical skin resistance on stimulation of anterior spinal roots; pain distribution after hypertonic saline injection of interspinous ligaments (Kellgren).

There is also variation between individuals: Sixteen patients were examined to determine the electrical skin resistance of the arm at operation,† by stimulating the anterior spinal roots. The upper limit

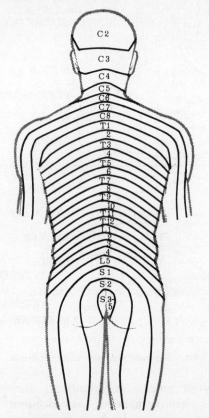

FIG. 6 Dermatomes, after Keegan and Garrett

* Keegan, J. J., and Garrett, F. D. The segmental distribution of the cutaneous nerves in the limbs of man. Anatomical Record, 1948, 102: 409–439. Also Fig. 6.

† Ray, B. S., Hinsey, J. C., Geohegan, W. A. Observations on the distribution of the sympathetic nerves to the pupil and upper extremity as determined by stimulation of the anterior roots in man. Annals of Surgery, 1943, 118, No. 4: 647–655.

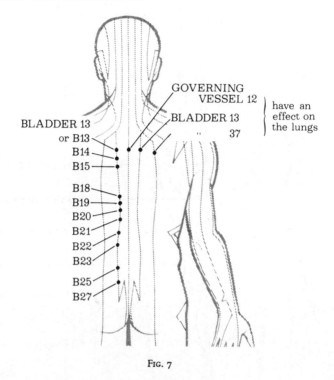

FIG. 7

varied from T1 to T3, whilst the lower limit varied from T7 to T10. The usual range is T2 to T9.

Normally the dermatome of the arm is given as C5 to T1, whilst the sympathetic dermatome obtained by stimulating the anterior spinal root is T2 to T9. When the skin and deeper tissues are pierced by an acupuncture needle both the spinal nerves and the sympathetic nerves of the blood vessels are affected, that of the sympathetic nerves having no effect unless one believes in antidromic stimulation, or as more recently in autonomic afferents.

The series of acupuncture points on the black lateral to the associated points shown in Fig. 7 have an effect on the same organ as its sister point at the same level, e.g. both B13 and B37 influence the lungs (likewise the points on the governing vessel).

The abdomen and front of the chest are traversed by the spleen, stomach, kidney and conception meridians (Fig. 8), which despite their names have, I find, an effect mainly on the region of the body

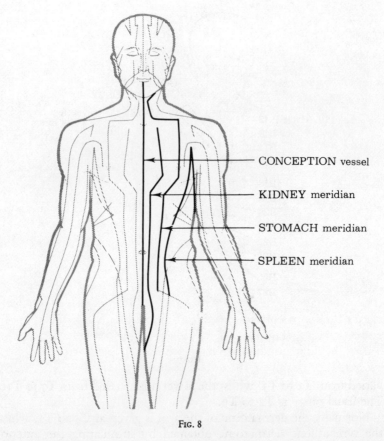

CONCEPTION vessel

KIDNEY meridian

STOMACH meridian

SPLEEN meridian

FIG. 8

traversed. All four meridians where they cross the chest may be used to treat the lungs and heart, yet their abdominal course influences the abdominal viscera. Thus as with the acupuncture points on the back a rough dermatomal pattern is preserved.

It is interesting to note that the majority of acupuncture points on the abdomen, thorax and back are near the mid-ventral and mid-dorsal lines. This corresponds to the segmental reference of deep pain obtained by Kellgren* when injecting hypertonic saline into the interspinous ligaments (Fig. 9).

* Kellgren, J. H. On the distribution of pain arising from deep somatic structures with charts of segmental pain. Clinical Science, 1939–42, 4: 35–46. Also Fig. 9.

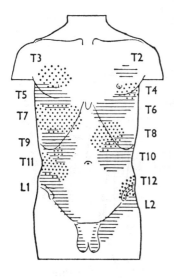 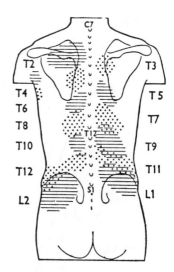

FIG. 9

The meridians of the lung, pericardium and heart on the anterior surface of the arm correspond at least approximately to the appropriate dermatome (Fig. 10). The meridians on the posterior surface of the arm: the large intestine, small intestine and triple warmer, do not correspond to the appropriate dermatome (Fig. 11).

In actual practice the situation is somewhat different, even for those meridians that follow a roughly dermatomal pattern.

If a patient has angina pectoris he may have pain or tenderness in the region of the heart meridian on the medial side of the arm. Just as frequently he may have pain or tenderness in the region of the lung meridian on the lateral side of the arm. Indeed the pain may appear in any part of the arm, along the course of (or in between) any of the six meridians of the arm, or even in the chest, neck or jaw.

Thus clearly the heart meridian cannot exist. It would be true though to say that pain from the heart, pericardium and lung, may be in the arm (and elsewhere), but the essential is that it may be *anywhere in the arm*.

In this section we have discussed the acupuncture points that more or less fit in with a dermatological pattern (Fig. 12),* namely—the

* From Ranson, S. W. and Clark, S. L. The anatomy of the nervous system, 1966, Saunders, Philadelphia.

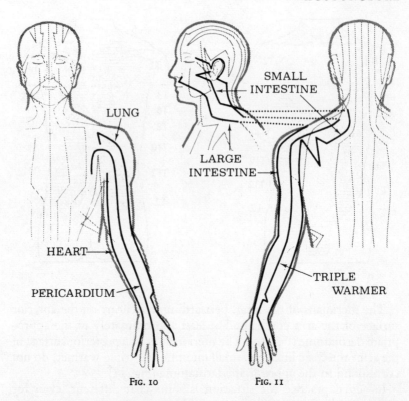

LUNG

SMALL
INTESTINE

LARGE
INTESTINE

HEART

PERICARDIUM

TRIPLE
WARMER

FIG. 10   FIG. 11

whole of the back, the abdomen, the front of the chest and the arms. The acupuncture points of the legs and head do not fit in with what is known of dermatomes and are therefore described in relation to other neurological concepts below:

Intersegmental Reflexes and Acupuncture Points

The acupuncture points on the legs are those of the liver, gall bladder, kidney, bladder, spleen and stomach. In all cases (except the bladder) the dermatomes of these organs are on the trunk and not on the legs. It is however an undoubted fact, observed every day by any doctor who practises acupuncture (for the leg acupuncture points are commonly used), that stimulation of a leg acupuncture point does have an effect on the appropriate organ, even though it may be ten dermatomes away. A possible explanation is via intersegmental

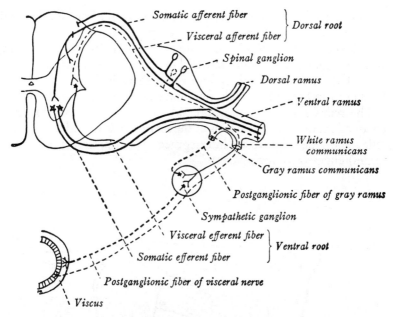

Somatic afferent fiber

Visceral afferent fiber } *Dorsal root*

Spinal ganglion

Dorsal ramus

Ventral ramus

White ramus communicans

Gray ramus communicans

Postganglionic fiber of gray ramus

Sympathetic ganglion

Visceral efferent fiber }
Somatic efferent fiber } *Ventral root*

Postganglionic fiber of visceral nerve

Viscus

FIG. 12 The peripheral nerves and spinal cord

reflexes, called by Sherrington long reflexes, whilst those effects of acupuncture that fit in with the dermatomes are segmental reflexes—Sherrington's short reflexes.

Sherrington* described the *scratch reflex* in the spinal dog (Fig. 13) in which stimulation anywhere in a saddle-shaped area extending from the pectoral to the pelvic girdle caused rapid scratching movements in the ipselateral hind leg and rigidity in the contralateral limb. If the stimulus is moved but slightly to the opposite side of the back the hind legs reverse their roles. Ipselateral hemisection of the spinal cord abolishes the reflex, contralateral hemisection leaves it unaffected.

Sherrington also experimented with decerebrate cats in which the nervous axis is divided at the level of the mid-brain. In the resultant decerebrate rigidity, the cats exhibit *reflex figures* (Fig. 14).

(*a*) In normal decerebrate rigidity all limbs are extended.

* Sherrington, C. S. The integrative action of the nervous system, 1906, Scribner, New York. Also Fig. 13 and 14.

(b) If the left pinna is stimulated there is flexion of the left fore and right hind limbs, with increased extension of the others.

(c) If the left fore limb is stimulated there is flexion of the left fore and right hind limbs, with increased extension of the others.

(d) If the left hind limb is stimulated there is flexion of the left hind limb and right fore limb, with increased extension of the others.

The reflex figures require both sides of the spinal cord for their conduction, not only the one as in the scratch reflex. Both the scratch reflex and reflex figures are intersegmental (jumping several dermatomes) cutaneo-motor reflexes.

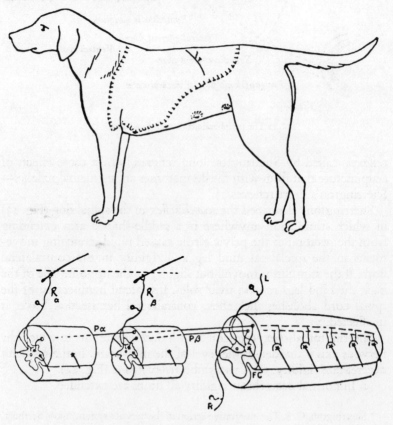

FIG. 13

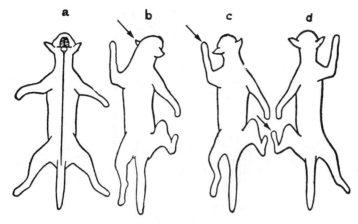

FIG. 14

Downman* investigated long viscero-motor and long cutaneo-motor reflexes in the cat with a spinal transection at T1. The splanchnic nerve serving the viscera, intercostal nerves T3-T13, lumbar nerves L1-L3 and the tibial nerve at the knee were all exteriorised.

Maximal single-shock stimulation of the central end of the splanchnic nerve evoked reflex volleys in all body wall nerves and the tibial nerve (Fig. 15). Even at threshold stimulation several intercostal nerves were involved. If an intercostal nerve was stimulated the response was in some cases as large as with splanchnic stimulation.

Downman showed that splanchnic excitation can spread up the cord by (1) a fast extraspinal route in the sympathetic chain of the same side and (2) a slower intraspinal route of limited ascent. Intercostal excitation can ascend only by a slow intraspinal route. This was demonstrated by the following experiments: Reflex discharges into the lower intercostal nerves on both sides were elicited by stimulating the left splanchnic nerve. Cutting the left sympathetic chain limited the upward spread of the excitation to the

---

* Downman, C. B. B. Skeletal muscle reflexes of splanchnic and intercostal nerve origin in acute spinal and decerebrate cats. Journal of Neurophysiology, 1955, 18: 217-235. Also Fig. 15.

Downman, C. B. B., and McSwiney, B. A. Reflexes elicited by visceral stimulation in the acute spinal animal. Journal of Physiology, 1946, 105: 80-94.

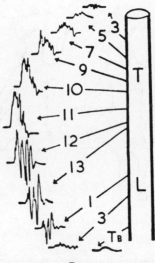

FIG. 15

next 3 to 5 segments of the cord. The discharges in the nerves were now of decreasing size and of longer latency in these segments. Spread of activity on stimulating a lower left intercostal nerve was unaffected. Where the chain had been left intact and the cord transected, splanchnic excitation spread freely into segments above the transection, but spread of intercostal excitation stopped at this level. In those instances where there is a contralateral response, experiments involving unilateral section of the dorsal nerve roots were performed. It was concluded that the splanchnic afferent volleys enter the cord by the dorsal root, traverse the spinal cord and leave by the contralateral intercostal nerves. Similar research has been done by Miller, Ward,* and Duda.†

The movements of the intercostals and tibialis anterior on stimulation of the splanchnics are considerably increased if a spinal instead of a decerebrate cat is used.

* Miller, F. R., and Ward, R. A. Viscero-motor reflexes. American Journal of Physiology, 1925, 73: 329–340.
† Duda, P. Facilitatory and inhibitory effects of splanchnic afferentation on somatic reflexes. Physiologia Bohemoslovenica, 1964, 13: 137–141.
Duda, P. Localization of the splanchnic effect on somatic reflexes in the spinal cord. Physiologia Bohemoslovenica, 1964, 13: 142–147.

Downmann and Hussain* showed that the main descending inhibitory tract is in the dorsal third of the lateral funiculus of the same side. This was demonstrated by sectioning various parts of the cord (most of which had a slight effect) and finding which had the major inhibitory influence (Fig. 16). Likewise deep cuts in the lower medulla, at the level of the middle of the cuneate tubercles, caused full release. Shen Eh† and colleagues have more recently performed similar experiments.

Harrison, Calhoun and Harrison‡ have shown that movement of the hind leg in a dog causes increased respiration—another example of an intersegmental reflex.

In their experiments, the hind leg of a dog was completely severed from the rest of the body at the hip joint, with preservation of only the sciatic nerve and femoral artery and vein. Passive movement of the hind leg produced within seconds an increased volume of

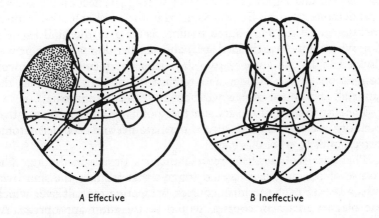

A Effective   B Ineffective

FIG. 16

* Downmann, C. B. B., Hussain, A. Spinal tracts and supraspinal centres influencing visceromotor and allied reflexes in cats. Journal of Physiology, 1958, 141: 489–499. Also Fig. 16.

† Shen Eh, Ts'ai T'i-tao, Lan Ch'ing. Supraspinal participation in the inhibitory effect of acupuncture on viscero-somatic reflex discharges. Chinese Medical Journal, 1975; 1 (6): 431–440.

‡ Harrison, W. G., Calhourn, J. A., Harrison, T. R. Afferent impulses as a cause of increased ventilation during muscular exercise. American Journal of Physiology, 1932, 100: 68–73.

respiration whether the femoral artery and vein were occluded with clamps or not. The respiration returned to normal only two minutes after movement of the leg was stopped. When the sciatic nerve was divided the reflex was abolished.

There are also long intersegmental viscero-visceral reflexes. The gastric-colic reflex is invoked when food entering the stomach causes mass contractions of the colon. Likewise in travel sickness where the afferent fibres are the trigeminal, glossopharygneal or vagus and the efferents are the phrenics and intercostal nerves.

I have thus been able to show in this section that the leg muscles contract if, under the correct conditions, one stimulates: the abdominal viscera, the splanchnics, the intercostal nerves, the outer ear, the front feet, the skin of the back in the upper thoracic region and other areas many segments away from the dermatomes of the human leg (or hind leg in animals). The reverse of the above namely stimulating the skin of the leg having an effect on the viscera, was demonstrated by Brown-Sequard in the same course of lectures mentioned earlier. He poured boiling water over the hind leg of a dog whose spine was divided at L3 and another dog whose spine was divided at T3. At autopsy two days later the former dog showed congestion of the bladder and rectum (segmental), whilst in the latter all abdominal organs were congested (intersegmental).

The distribution of the acupuncture points on the legs is such that each organ corresponds to several dermatomes and each dermatome corresponds to several organs.

There are six meridians representing six organs in the leg. The course of the meridians would suggest that treating the shin over which the stomach meridian courses, or treating the calf over which the bladder meridian courses, would be the most appropriate. As mentioned previously in connection with the arm, this is not correct. A reflexly tender area may appear in either the shin or the calf in disease of the stomach or bladder or vica versa. Indeed as with the arm, the reflex tenderness associated with the lower six organs may appear almost anywhere on the legs (and the lower abdomen and back), though in certain instances it tends to appear more often in certain areas.

Traditionally the meridians of the small and large intestines are on the arm. In my opinion this is completely wrong, as with a few exceptions, these organs can only be treated by stimulation of the lower half of the body. The triple warmer defies definition—though I have described it in my books on traditional acupuncture.

The problem is not too simple, as investigations by Travell and Bigelow* showed. In patients with pain encompassing several dermatomes it was found that a pinprick to the trigger area might relieve the pain in that dermatome or in several dermatomes or in one dermatome, then miss out a dermatome to relieve pain again in a further dermatome.

Acupuncture Points on the Head — Near and Distant Effects

Most of the acupuncture points on the head have a local effect, which could presumably be explained by local reflex arcs similar to segmental reflexes.

The apportioning of the acupuncture points on the head to the various internal organs is hard to follow both theoretically and in actual clinical acupuncture practice, though distant effects undoubtedly occur.

Koblank† investigated a reflex between the nose and the heart. He found a sharply defined area in the region of the superior concha of the nose, which if stimulated with a probe caused various cardiac arrhythmias in man, dogs and rabbits. When the vagus was cut on one side, the reflex remained intact; when cut on both sides the reflex was abolished for a few days and then returned, but weaker than formerly. When the maxillary nerve was divided on one side the reflex was permanently abolished when the same side of the nose was stimulated, but the reflex persisted normally when the healthy side was stimulated. From this it was deduced that the trigeminal nerve relayed the stimulation of the nasal mucous membrane to the region of the nucleus of the vagus, which then passed it on via the vagus to the heart. It was considered though that there was more than one final pathway as dividing the vagus only partially abolished the reflex.

Koblank also investigated the relation between the lower turbinate of the nose and the reproductive organs of rabbits and dogs. He found that if the lower turbinate was excised in young animals that

---

* Travell, J., and Bigelow, N. H. Referred somatic pain does not follow a simple segmental pattern. Federation Proceedings, 1946, 5: 106.

† Alfred Koblank. Die Nase als Reflexorgan. 1958. Haug. Ulm. Also Fig. 17.

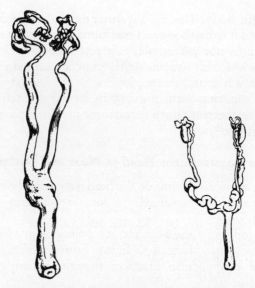

FIG. 17 Left: control. Right: after excision of inferior turnibate

the uterus, fallopian tubes, ovary or testicle failed to develop, even though the adult animal attained the same weight as an unoperated control. The failure of development showed itself both as a considerable reduction in size (Fig. 17) and histologically.

Koblank, Röder and Bickel experimented with dogs who had a Pavlov type exteriorised blind loop, whereby changes in gastric secretion and motility could be observed directly. They found that when the 'stomach area' on the anterior third of the middle turbinate was stimulated that the gastric secretion and movement were increased.

It should be noted that in the above experiments stimulation of the upper turbinate affected the heart, the middle turbinate the stomach, and the lower turbinate the reproductive organs.

Specific Response versus Generalised Response

In the practice of acupuncture it is sometimes found that one (or a small group) of acupuncture points are effective in treating a certain patient. On other occasions, any one of several meridians (encompassing a large number of acupuncture points) can be effective.

In the former case a specific stimulus is mandatory, in the latter nearly any general stimulus is all that is needed.·

The specific response presumably takes place, along the lines of the nervous pathways described in the previous sections.

The generalised hypersensitivity on the other hand seems similar to the pain one can sometimes have with severe toothache when the whole of the same side of the face, arm and upper chest are hypersensitive. In the same way the viscera may sometimes become hypersensitive affecting the nerves in a large area, and hence only require in treatment an acupuncture needle put anywhere in a large area, in any of a large number of acupuncture points, or in any of several meridians.

In other cases a stimulus anywhere in a large area does not depend on hypersensitivity, but on the large number of neurones that have a final common path. Ashkenaz* stimulated the gall bladder of cats by inflating a balloon. This caused contraction of the panniculus carnosus muscle (the cat's equivalent of the platysma, but extending over most of the body). This viscero-pannicular reflex was only abolished when all the dorsal roots T2 to T9 were severed, a single root being sufficient to preserve the reflex, thus demonstrating the convergence that can take place.

Diseased organs seem to have a lowered threshold of response, for only a small stimulus is needed to correct a dysfunction of a diseased organ. On the other hand a very considerable stimulus is needed to alter the function of a healthy organ. For this reason the small prick of an acupuncture needle can cure some of the severest diseases, and yet is normally harmless if the wrong treatment is effected, as the threshold of response of the healthy organ is beyond the stimulus of a mere needle prick.

It should be noted that the Chinese describe the acupuncture points as being quite small—a matter of millimetres. In my experience this is only true to a limited extent, for not infrequently a stimulus anywhere in an area as large as a dermatome (or several dermatomes if there has been spread of hypersensitivity) is sufficient. If this largish area is carefully examined by hand a few small areas

* Ashkenaz, D. M. An experimental analysis of centripetal visceral pathways based upon the viscero-pannicular reflex. American Journal of Physiology, 1937. 120: 587–595.

of maximal tenderness, with possibly small fibrositic-like nodules, will be found (similar to the small areas of maximal tenderness found when a large area such as the neck and shoulders are 'rheumatic'). If these small areas of maximal tenderness, or the 'fibrositic' nodules are stimulated by an acupuncture needle the response is normally greater than when the surrounding less tender area is needled. If the dysfunction of a diseased organ is mild, a reflex tenderness may not be produced over the whole of a dermatome, being demonstrable only in a few small tender areas—the same areas as mentioned a few lines above. These small tender areas of 'fibrositic' nodules are relatively constant in position, whether the remaining surrounding part of the dermatome is tender or not. This constancy in position applies from one individual to another, and is likewise the same for any variety of diseases producing a reflex tenderness in that area. It is these small tender areas of constant position, which are termed the acupuncture points; although, as mentioned above, a stimulus anywhere in the appropriate dermatome (or sometimes even larger area) may work, albeit frequently not so well. Sometimes stimulation anywhere in the correct quarter of the body is sufficient.

Some years ago David Sinclair, professor of anatomy at Aberdeen University, wrote an as yet unpublished paper, which he has kindly let me read, concerning the reflexes between the skin and viscera defined as viscero-somatic, somato-somatic, viscero-visceral, somato-visceral. In this article Sinclair quotes a hundred papers (several of which are mentioned in this chapter) concerning these reflexes which are the presumed mechanism of acupuncture—though probably most of the authors know nothing or little of acupuncture. At the time of writing and in other papers* Sinclair advanced a branched axon theory partially to explain the observed phenomena, but since then he thinks the more conventional nervous pathways are the mediator.

It is remarkable that the stimulation of the skin for a few seconds, should activate a nerve reflex in such a manner, that the dysfunction

* Sinclair, D. C. The remote reference of pain aroused in the skin. Brain, 1949, 72: 364.
Sinclair, D. C., Weddell, G., and Feindel, W. Referred pain and associated phenomena. Brain, 1948, 71: 184.

of the diseased area should be alleviated for a long time or even permanently.

The same phenomenon is observed when the dorsal columns of the spinal cord, or a peripheral nerve, are electrically stimulated in patients with permanent intractable pain. Before the implantation of a stimulator these patients require the *continuous* administration of analgesics. After implantation stimulation for a *short while*, will in the more responsive patients produce analgesia for half a day to one week.

In acupuncture, after the appropriate skin area has been stimulated a few times, the resultant relief of symptoms may be permanent, i.e. there is a cure. This does not happen in dorsal column or peripheral nerve stimulation, for the type of patient to whom this is normally applied has an irreversible pathological process. In acupuncture on the other hand, most patients have diseases which are physiologically reversible.

II

NEEDLE TECHNIQUE

The only thing of importance in acupuncture is to stimulate the right place. What the stimulus is, is of secondary importance.

Normally a needle is used, and this, in my experience, is the most effective. Massage, various types of electrical stimuli, mechanical vibrators, heating, magnetic oscillators have all been tried but are not quite as effective. In the Far East the pith of Artemesia Japonica (moxa) is dried and rolled into balls about two millimetres in diameter; one is placed on the acupuncture point of choice and lit so that it glows like the lighted end of a cigarette. This is an effective stimulus, but it may cause burns and even scars which do not necessarily disappear. This method, called moxibustion is supposed to be more effective in diseases due to cold and dampness, but in my experience this is not the case; and as it is no more effective than a needle I rarely use it. Another type of heating treatment, used in diseases due to cold and damp is to use the long handled type of Chinese needle. About an inch is cut off a moxa stick which is shaped like a cigar, and pushed over the exposed part of the needle. The moxa is lit and the heat is conducted down the shaft of the needle to the surrounding skin and flesh. As I find this no more effective than simple needling, I rarely use it. There are many old and modern variations to the above, but none are as simple and effective as a needle.

The needles may be made of any material. Silver alloys have the advantage of having some self-sterilising properties, which is an additional secondary safeguard. Stainless steel is best for thin needles as silver is too soft. Stainless steel needles have to be thrown away when they become blunt as they are difficult to resharpen. Silver needles can be resharpened on a very fine carborundum or other stone. The silver needles are best sharpened on several surfaces so that the tip is a cross between the cone of an ordinary sewing needle and the pyramid of a leather cutting needle. In this way they pierce the skin more easily yet do not cause bleeding as easily as a leather cutting or surgical needle. The much finer stainless steel needles should be sharpened like a cone, as is usual for ordinary needles. Injection needles may be used, but they easily cause bleeding and theoretically could harbour some dirt in the hollow of the needle; while a solid acupuncture needle, is, as it were, wiped clean on all its surfaces in its passage through the skin. If it is intended to leave the needle in place, it will be found that the head of an injection needle is rather heavy and pulls the needle out of place. I use a hot air steriliser. Small, cheap, automatic ones are sold in dental equipment shops.

Some European doctors differentiate between silver and gold needles founded on a misconception of tonification and sedation (see below). This may have arisen as a translating error as in Chinese the characters for gold and metal are the same. I have found no reference to it in the Chinese literature, though possibly it exists. Whilst in China, several doctors asked me what this new invention concerning silver and gold needles as used in Europe was all about!

Traditional Chinese works on acupuncture describe at great length about fifty different ways of inserting acupuncture needles, with names such as: 'burning mountain fire technique' or 'green dragon wagging tail technique'. These techniques involve the following: Inserting the needle 3 or 9 or 81 times; pointing the needle with or against the direction of flow of Qi along a meridian; twisting the needle clockwise or anticlockwise; inserting the needle fast and taking it out slowly as opposed to slowly in and fast out; inserting the needle in three stages and pulling it out in one as opposed to insertion in one stage and pulling out in three—and many more refinements. I have tried assiduously to find a difference between these methods, but have come to the conclusion that basically there is no difference except insofar as it includes what is said in the ensuing lines.

The size of the stimulus increases with:

1. A fat needle.
2. The deeper the insertion.
3. The more the needle is pushed up and down or twisted, so that the tip causes greater localised trauma.
4. A blunt needle or one with a hook on the end (both undesirable).
5. The more acupuncture points are used having a similar effect (sometimes has severe effect).
6. Leaving the needle in longer (extremely doubtful).
7. Repeating the treatment at frequent intervals.

Many doctors think that the bigger the stimulus, the greater the effect; but just as often it is the very reverse. I have many patients who respond best to only one or two shallow pricks with thin, sharp needles, with the needle not left in place and the treatment repeated only infrequently. Certain constitutional types respond best to light treatment, others to heavy treatment, just as certain patients respond best to small and sometimes even microscopic doses of ordinary drugs while average doses of drugs may have no effect or make them feel ill. Because I recognise this great variation in individual sensitivity I have on occasions been able to successfully treat a patient by giving them a half to a tenth of the same medicine as their general practitioner was unsuccessfully giving them. Most chronic conditions I treat only fortnightly and finish the treatment at even longer intervals, for sometimes the effect of a treatment is only apparent after a week or more and if the second treatment is done before the effect of the first one is apparent, the two treatments may antagonise one another with either no result or a temporary worsening of the patient's condition. Acute conditions may be treated more frequently. Patients whom I see from abroad I of course treat at more frequent intervals; but it requires greater clinical experience and judgement on the doctor's part.

Chinese and European acupuncturists differentiate between tonification and sedation. Diagnostically one can say certain conditions represent underactivity whilst others represent overactivity. If for example the pulse is fine and weak one says it is underactive and requires tonification; if the pulse is strong and full one says it is overactive and the appropriate organ requires sedation. The Chinese and many Europeans also say that if the needle is inserted in a certain way, or one uses a silver needle, or one uses a point of sedation, that the appropriate organ is sedated; likewise if one inserts the needle in a different way, uses a gold needle, or a point of tonification, the same organ is tonified. I find on the contrary that whatever is done, as diagnosed on the pulse, the organ is brought nearer normality. If for example the pulse in the position of the heart is overactive (pulse full and strong) then whichever needle technique one uses, whatever the needle is made from and whichever point of the heart meridian one uses, the effect is the same: namely that the pulse becomes nearer that of a fine and weak pulse. Likewise if the pulse had been underactive (pulse fine and weak) and one had done exactly the same as above, the pulse would have become stronger. In other words the needle seems to exert a normalising influence: sedating the overactive, and tonifying the underactive; and if the doctor wishes it or not, he cannot (except under a few rare conditions) do the reverse. This normalising influence could fit in with the way the autonomic nervous system functions. It is interesting, at least philosophically, that overactivity and underactivity can be diagnosed, but that the treatment does not differentiate the two. Whether or not overactivity and underactivity are important from the point of view of Chinese traditional herbal medicine I do not know. In their theory it is important but perhaps not in reality.

The above jeopardises the whole idea of polarity, of Yin and Yang, coupled organs, hot and cold diseases, full and empty diseases, tonification and sedation, the five element theory, the mother-son law, the husband-wife law, the midday-midnight law. In fact this clearly demonstrates that nearly all the traditional theoretical background of acupuncture is open to doubt.

III

SCIENTIFIC VERSUS TRADITIONAL ACUPUNCTURE - SOME CONCLUSIONS

Acupuncture Points

In my neurophysiological theory I have explained the areas used for stimulation in acupuncture. They are partially on a roughly dermatome basis; partially involving 'long' reflexes to distant parts of the body, which implicates a distribution by specific spinal segments or nerves; and partially via unknown connections.

This theory would transform the classical small specific acupuncture point into an area as large as that of a dermatome, or to the distribution of a specific nerve, or even to an area of several dermatomes if the area has previously been hypersensitised (see chapter I). If only a few neurones are involved the skin area could be considerably smaller than a dermatome.

In most instances no doctor, even if he be an expert in acupuncture, can find an acupuncture point in those areas where there is a big expanse, such as the abdomen, back and thorax. If a group of doctors are asked to locate a specific acupuncture point in such an area, their positions will quite often vary by a considerable amount, and yet all these doctors are able to help or cure a large proportion of their patients provided they have a disease amenable to acupuncture. This suggests to me that small specific acupuncture points rarely exist, and that those researchers who have found specific types of specialised nerve endings or other structures at acupuncture points are mistaken. The structures found by these histological investigations may well be there, but they do not correspond to acupuncture points, for they do not exist. Stimulation of any layer can be effective, whether it be skin, subcutaneous tissue, muscle or periosteum. Hence one should not speak of a dermatome, but rather of a dermo-myo-sclerotome. This poses some problems, for the different layers do not always have the same segmental innervation.

In a disease of the viscera or other parts of the body there is often a reflex tenderness in the associated part of the surface. This tenderness may include muscle spasm or circulatory changes. It also presumably affects most histological structures throughout the entire depth of the appropriate area, due to their similar innervation.

As far as I know there are no specific histological elements in McBurney's point, which becomes tender in appendicitis. I think nearly every single part of the body can become reflexly tender, in a way similar to that of McBurney's point. Hence the number of acupuncture points would become infinite—indeed some books mention so many acupuncture points, that one wonders if there is any normal skin left.

McBurney's point is not a small discrete 'point', but quite a large area, whose position is somewhat variable. McBurney's point lies in the appropriate dermatome. The remainder of the dermatome is not tender or only mildly so, for as Kellgren (Fig. 9) and others have shown, certain areas within a dermatome show greater changes than others.

Some acupuncture points seem to have a constant position and may be tender even in a completely healthy person:—

G21 is situated where the trapezius arches over the first rib and hence is presumably under greater tension than other parts of the muscle.

Sp9 is located below the medial condyle, over the lower part of the medial ligament of the knee, where many women have a tender oedematous area. As this occurs nearly only in women, apart from those who have injured their knee, it is presumably hormonal. In some women this area becomes an oedematous pad of fat the size of a hand.

G20 is next to the greater occipital nerve where it arches over the occiput, just as B2 is adjacent to the supratrochlear nerve where it passes over the supraorbital ridge.

All the above and a certain number of other acupuncture points are nearly always tender, even in the healthy subject. This is probably often due to compressing a nerve trunk against the bone. Other places may be tender due to muscular tension sensitising the area and thus requiring a smaller stimulus from the acupuncture needle to be effective.

H7 is a more effective point than H3, as stimulation of H7 involves the needle piercing thicker skin and a hard ligament. This causes greater pain than needling the fatty tissue around H3 and thus obviously has stimulated more nerve fibres. For a similar reason acupuncture points which involve stimulation of the periosteum have usually a greater effect than those involving only subcutaneous fat, unless the needle is strongly twisted in the skin.

Stimulating a nerve trunk, which produces a lightning pain, is by no means more effective. In patients who have the so called cervical disc syndrome and allied conditions, stimulation of the transverse process of the 6th cervical vertebra is more effective than trying to needle the adjacent nerves of the brachial plexus.

In my experience, contrary to classical theory, the type of stimulus used in acupuncture is of little importance whether it be a needle, a thorn, an electric current, heat, a vibrator or injections. This would agree with the 'all or nothing' response of nerve fibres, which either respond or do not respond to stimulation, there being no qualitative difference. The stronger the stimulus, the greater is the effect due to activation of a larger number of neurones or their repetitive stimulation. The traditional theory that there is a qualitative difference between a hot or a cold needle, or the manner in which it is twisted or inserted, does not concur with my experience and would be harder to explain neurologically. Sometimes if the periosteum is stimulated in the region of a joint the effect is greater than if the overlying skin is needled. Possibly this is due to activation of a local reflex.

Some researchers claim there is a reduced electrical skin resistance at small discrete places, they call acupuncture points. For several years I have diligently tried to confirm this observation both in patients and cadavers. I found there are thousands of smaller or larger skin areas of reduced resistance, some of which might correspond to acupuncture, whilst most did not.

A doctor who knows acupuncture, will be able to find acupuncture points electrically, by passing the searching electrode a few times over the desired acupuncture point. Each time an active electrode is passed over the skin, it is depolarised and its electrical resistance is reduced, and if this is repeated a few times one creates, de novo, one's own electrical acupuncture point.

According to my neurophysiological theory one would not expect to find discrete acupuncture points by electrical or other means. It is possible though that larger areas, related to the distribution of groups of neurones, may be found, whilst in an abnormal state.

Meridians

In some places the course of meridians follows the pathways of nerves or the position of dermatomes, in others it does not. I have shown in chapter 1 that in most (but by no means all) instances a neurological explanation fits in with more of the observed facts than with the hypothetical meridians.

Sometimes a needle in the leg produces a sensation (not a lightning pain) along the stomach meridian where it goes over the abdomen and thorax. This does not fit in with the route taken by a nerve trunk. The connections within the spinal cord are so numerous, that further research might elucidate this and similar problems.

The experiments in chapter 1 have shown that most of the reflexes involved in acupuncture are spinal. It is possible though that some reflexes, especially those which are not instantaneous, might involve higher centres. The experiments of Downman and Koblank illustrate that more than one neural path is excited by a single stimulus. Quite possibly a single pin prick in the leg may invoke two or three separate intraspinal pathways, and also a path along the sympathetic chain. Both the intraspinal and sympathetic routes having quick responses on the target area via a spinal reflex and possibly delayed responses via suprasegmental pathways, which secondarily cause the release of hormones or vascular and other phenomena. I maintain however that the primary transmission system used in acupuncture is neural.

The fifty-nine or more meridians* described by the Chinese seem to link interdependent areas of the body, even though they may be at a considerable distance from one another. For example: A mildly stiff neck may be helped by placing a needle in a gall bladder acu-

---

* see The Meridians of Acupuncture.

puncture point on the foot, because the gall bladder meridian goes through the neck. The nervous pathway between the foot and the neck is not obvious. The ancient Chinese however linked them together by a meridian for they found the connection by experience.

The practical conclusion to be drawn from this is, that although the meridians do not exist as such, they illustrate in an almost abstract manner, the presumed neural pathways, which are as yet unknown. In that way the meridians are of paramount importance to the clinician whose main concern is to get his patients better. The meridians of acupuncture might even be compared to the meridians of geography: imaginary but useful. I hope that the investigations of neurophysiologists and others will map out the true neural pathways involved, which would then only partially correspond to meridians.

Categories of Acupuncture Points

Elsewhere it is shown that tonification and sedation, although they form a major part of traditional theory, are a philosophical conception which does not apply to the actual practice of acupuncture. If on pulse diagnosis the liver pulse is wide and hard, it is called over-active and requires sedation. If the point of sedation or tonification or any other point whatsoever on that meridian or related points on other meridians, is stimulated, the pulse on Chinese pulse diagnosis becomes normal or nearly normal. Likewise if the pulse of the liver is narrow and soft, one could call it underactive, requiring tonification. The result would be exactly the same if any of the before-mentioned points were used.

The obvious conclusion is that the twenty or so categories of acupuncture points (some books describe more categories) are superfluous. There is no physiological connection between the metal point on the heart meridian and the metal point on the liver meridian.

The different acupuncture points on the same meridian exert partly similar effects. Hence the tradition of joining them together with a line called a meridian. They have also partly dissimilar effects, for to some extent different neurons are stimulated.

Laws of Acupuncture

The various laws of acupuncture mentioned in my traditional books fall in many instances into disarray once one has discovered that tonification and sedation do not take place. Yin and Yang, coupled organs, full and empty diseases, cold and hot diseases become untenable.

The law of the five elements demonstrates some connections between organs well known to physiology, and some connections which presumably exist, but are not yet known. In clinical practice one finds that certain of the connections happen frequently, whilst the others occur rarely or never. The frequently occurring connections can in most instances be more easily explained in Western terms than via the Chinese pentagram.

If all the laws of acupuncture are taken together it will be seen that every phenomenon occurring in health and disease can be explained and hence it leaves one with little explanation at all.

A traditional Chinese doctor practising acupuncture will achieve good results, albeit for the wrong reasons, which is though of little concern to the patient: A traditional doctor may say that a specific very small acupuncture point should be stimulated; a Western doctor may say that anywhere within a given area is sufficient. Both doctors achieve equal results if the Oriental's acupuncture point lies within the area of hypersensitivity of the Westerner. Again: A Chinese doctor may say that the fire point on the Yin wood meridian should be used; his Occidental counterpart may suggest that any 'point' on the liver meridian below the knee is sufficient. The two colleagues will have equal results, for the fire point is within the Western grouping.

In certain ways the Chinese scholar, as scholars elsewhere, has made acupuncture more complicated than it really is. To this was added ancient tradition, so that the resultant medical system became a paradise of the inscrutable.

The Energy of Life—QI

The Chinese theories related to Qi (the energy of life), Nourishing Qi, Protecting Qi, Blood, Life Essence, Spirit, Fluid and similar connections mentioned in *Acupuncture: The Ancient Chinese Art of Healing*, are most easily understood as a traditional Chinese concept, linked with a view of the world different to that of most Occidentals. Western doctors who practise acupuncture, or neurophysiologists who investigate its mode of action, can do without this traditional idea.

If a patient, even a Western doctor, has been ill and then recovers, he will say 'I feel better, I have more energy'. If this same doctor is then asked what is energy (called in Chinese Qi), he will probably say that such a thing does not exist. A contradiction and at the same time not a contradiction.

From the point of view of Western medicine, disease ensues when the biochemical processes of the body are disturbed. If for example there is a deficiency of potassium, the body chemistry is altered and the patient has amongst other symptoms little energy. The energy cannot be measured directly, only its secondary effect in reducing muscular activity may be measured.

The Oriental doctor considers energy as something primary and 'real', whose deficiency causes secondarily disease. The Occidental doctor thinks the chemistry of the body is primary which only secondarily affects energy. Textbooks of physiology do not mention the conception of a biological energy as something primary.

These two points of view are only partially contradictory. They are only looking at life from a different point of view.

Much of Chinese medical theory describes what the patient feels. The patient feels differences in energy. He often feels something along the course of meridians. The Western doctor often excludes the patient's feelings and measures the serum electrolytes, haemoglobin and faecal fat instead.

Few people would disagree that when they see a meadow it is green. A physicist would say though that the meadow emits a certain wavelength of light which is then *subjectively* interpreted by the eye and brain as the colour green. This is little different from the person who is hit with a sledge hammer and then subjectively interprets it as the taste of onions—something which a Pavlov type dog could probably be trained to do.

If the physicist is asked, what a wavelength of light is, he might explain it in more detail using Einstein's particle theory of photons, which anyway is not considered to be a physical reality. From which it emerges that Chinese metaphysics is hardly less real or unreal than the theoretical background of modern physics, which is the foundation of most modern medicine.

IV

STRONG REACTORS

Certain patients respond better to acupuncture than do others. In some instances these patients are cured or their symptoms are considerably ameliorated within seconds or minutes of treatment. Both the patient and the doctor have witnessed a phenomenon which seems nearly a miracle. This chapter will describe these patients whom I have called *strong reactors* since 1962, a description which in some aspects is exaggerated in an attempt to clarify the conception.

If one looks at a strong reactor with the eye of an artist one has the impression they are *physiologically alive*; one feels as if their individual components can be moved, can be recreated—they are not an immobile statue. They are like a day in Spring, when the plants grow, the flowers blossom, the birds sing and the insects fly —not a winters day when all is static.

These patients often respond quickly or in a strong manner to the normal drugs used in orthodox medicine. They often need half, a quarter or even a tenth of the usual dose of a medicine. And if they take this small dose it works perfectly, as in the average normal patient.

On occasions I have seen a patient with hypertension, as the drug their doctor had prescribed made them feel 'like death'. Since acupuncture is rarely of benefit in hypertension, there is little benefit in trying it. If I noticed the patient was a strong reactor I would then suggest that they take a fraction of the same medicine as their general practitioner had previously prescribed for them; a dose so small that

I did not dare write it on the prescription for fear of the pharmacist's ridicule. Not infrequently this treatment worked.

Some patients who dislike orthodox medicine do so as they are the type of strong reactor for whom the average dose of a drug is an overdose. This does not apply to all drugs for they may react normally to some drugs yet strongly to others. Even the average patient reacts strongly to an occasional drug or may exhibit a rare allergy, but in the strong reactor this is more frequent. Anaesthetists who use quickly acting and powerful drugs are more aware of this problem than perhaps the average doctor.

The strong reactor responds more often than the average patient to treatment within seconds or minutes of the needle being in place. If they had symptoms these will largely or completely disappear—the headache, the painful knee, the aching back. If they came on a day they had no symptoms they may instead, if they were tense, have a feeling of a pleasant, drowsy relaxation, so that they may nearly fall asleep in the consulting room. Normally the technique which I use for stimulation in acupuncture involves twisting the needle to and fro for a minute or two causing the patient a degree of pain not dissimilar to that caused by a dentist. Despite this pain some strong reactors become soporific whilst the needle twisting is in progress. Some strong reactors may at the same time as feeling relaxed, feel more energetic, a sense akin to that of tasting the first few drops of champagne. This is different to the usual effect, of a tranquilizer for the patient is at one and the same time more relaxed and yet with an enhanced energy. Normal patients may have this relaxed feeling—with or without the champagne effect, immediately after the treatment or after a delay of a few hours; but it is not as frequent as in strong reactors.

If a needle is stuck into the foot of an average patient and twisted to and fro he may feel pain for an inch or two around the needle, unless of course a nerve trunk has been stimulated. The strong reactor on the other hand not infrequently may feel a pain going up the leg which may continue over the trunk and head on the same or opposite side. Sometimes a sensation is felt in a part of the body distant from the stimulating needle whilst the intervening section of the body is unaffected. This sensation which travels along certain paths of the body is not like the shooting electric pain felt on stimulating a major nerve trunk. It is usually fairly pleasant—as if something has just happened there. If a distant area of the body alone is affected, there is often a feeling of pleasant warmth, muscle relaxation, if the sinuses a sense of freeing and crackling. The travelling sensation is often confined to fairly narrow paths which may be centrifugal or centripetal. The sensation may travel from one end of the body to the other in one second or may take several seconds to traverse the leg. Sometimes it fits in with the course of peripheral nerves, sometimes with that of meridians (which often differs from the former), but often with neither.

Anaesthetists, acupuncturists and others who have tried to stimulate peripheral nerve trunks with a needle will know how difficult this can be, necessitating not infrequently several attempts till one is rewarded with a lightning-like pain or a muscle twitch. Surprisingly enough this is considerably easier in strong reactors, sometimes the first judicious attempt is successful. I cannot imagine the nerve trunks of strong reactors have a larger diameter. One must rather suppose that they are in a more reactive state and are more easily triggered.

Strong reactors are on the whole more sensitive people, though there are many exceptions as one may be a strong reactor from certain points of view whilst a slow reactor in other aspects. I remember seeing a colonel who had injured his neck in the Second World War. He was parachuted over Africa and spellbound as he slowly floated down to earth, by the beauty of the clouds, the forests beneath him, the intermingling of colour between light and shade. Then with a bang he suddenly hit the ground and injured his neck. Only a strong reactor would be taken in by the beauty of nature to such an extent that he forgot his own safety—the distance to the ground. Slow reactors may also be overcome by emotion, but not infrequently these emotions belong to the more basic varieties such as sex, money, hatred—though this requires very careful and often contradictory interpretation.

Strong reactors may feel it if someone is looking at them from behind, just as they may sense the atmosphere of a room when they enter it. Strong reactors are often more instinctive than the average person, for they can observe and are influenced by subtle factors to which the normal person is impervious. Many successful business people, or indeed those in many walks of life, are strong reactors. They are able to take a decision, indeed the correct decision, when only a few facts concerning the case is known to them. The ordinary person who plods along has to know all the hundred-and-one facts of a business deal before his computer-like mind, which can only digest proven facts, can function. After this long lapse of time, all other members of the business community have of course ascertained the same facts, and the business initiative of an entirely new and exclusive deal will have been lost. It will readily be apparent that some members of the academic professions are slow reactors, always requiring proof. In certain walks of life it is an advantage, even necessary, to be a slow reactor. Dr Jean Schoch of Strasbourg once said when discussing the contradiction of people's temperaments: "a symphony does not consist of equal notes".

If a patient is in favour and believes in acupuncture, it will of course tip the scales towards the strong reactor. As is readily apparent from the chapter 10* on the interplay of the mind and the body, acupuncture which acts primarily on diseases involving an easily reversible physiological process, cannot be but influenced by the mind. This does not mean that being a strong reactor is a mental process, it merely means that it is influenced by the mind.

There is a tendency for strong reactors to be neurotic, though actually only a few are. The slow reactors not infrequently are the very opposite of neurotic—possibly pedestrian machines.

Strong reactors are influenced more easily by the weather and geological conditions. Those who feel heavenly in Aberdeen and lethargic in London (or vice versa) are more likely to be strong reactors. Likewise those who respond strongly to the special winds one has in some countries such as the Föhn in the southern Alps.

There is no definite division between the strong and slow reactor. The proportion of each in the general population depends entirely on the criteria one uses. From a purely practical and clinical point of view one could say that about 5% of the population are hyper-strong reactors. Hyper-strong reactors and strong reactors counted together might form 10% or even 30% of the population if one is generous.

Acupuncture anaesthesia (really analgesia) works only, in my experience (though others who are experts disagree) in the hyper-strong reactor. In 1974 I reported the results of a hundred experiments in acupuncture analgesia and come to the conclusion that it

* of Acupuncture: The Ancient Chinese Art of Healing.

worked reasonably though not perfectly, in 10% of patients. Since then I have come to the conclusion that the criteria I used were a little optimistic and the figure should be revised to a mere 5%. Some experiments* were performed which showed that the acupuncture analgesia was an objective and not a psychosomatic phenomenon, in the few in whom it worked.

On a few occasions I have had the impression that people who have changed from a mixed diet to that of a vegetarian, have started to react more strongly. This of course often goes hand in hand with an altered outlook on life, which includes being more receptive to the finer things of life, and hence this latter reason might be more important than the change in diet.

Despite many years of experience and interest, I still find that I am only right in some three out of four instances when deciding who is a strong reactor—as measured subsequently by the strength of response to treatment.

In the practice of acupuncture I find it quite important to know who is, and who is not a strong reactor. The strong reactor needs a gentle treatment in acupuncture, just as he needs a small dose of medicine when looked after by orthodox means. In the extreme case it may be sufficient to prick in only one place, with a fine needle to a depth of one millimetre, for one second. In the average strong reactor one or two pairs of needles are sufficient, and they should be twisted with about a quarter of the severity normally employed. If one wishes to stimulate a larger number of places this should be done even more gently. One might compare the dose of acupuncture given to the average adult strong reactor, as the same as one might give to a five-year-old child who is a normal reactor. In this connection it should be added that the easiest way to measure the dose of acupuncture is to compare it to the total pain caused to the patient.

If a strong reactor is treated too vigorously either the treatment does not work, or he has a reaction (see Chapter 10†), which usually consists of a temporary worsening of the patient's symptoms. This is unpleasant but passes off in minutes, hours or days, according to the case. In say migraine a reaction is unpleasant but of no import-

* Mann, Felix. Acupuncture Analgesia, report of 100 experiments. British Journal of Anaesthia, 1974, 46: 361–4.

† of Acupuncture: The Ancient Chinese Art of Healing.

ance. In asthma and some other diseases, it would be of importance and hence such patients should at the first consultation be treated very gently and with caution, in case they are strong reactors.

Those doctors who are particularly interested in such matters, might observe that in some hyper-strong reactors the doctor may have a mild prickly sensation over the whole of his body in the presence of a hyper-strong reactor. At least this is my experience.

Women, who as a rule have more intuition than men, are like-wise more often strong reactors. Before a man will do something he has to understand it; whilst a woman will act on a hunch—and be more often right. In the days when I worked as a junior doctor in a hospital I remember how often the intellectual doctor who judged his patient on laboratory results, was not infrequently eclipsed by the Ward Sister who had little technical knowledge but a heart that judged a patient by his smile.

In deciding if a patient is likely to be a strong reactor or not one has to take many contradictory facets into account, for people are made of contradictions. Whatever is decided can only be tentative till one actually sees the result of treatment. It is therefore sometimes advisable to try an initial tentative gentle treatment.

V

SEGMENTAL AND GENERAL
SYMPATHETIC RESPONSE

Sato and Schmidt* have shown that stimulation of a peripheral nerve, as is done in the everyday practice of acupuncture, has two results. There is a quick effect on the sympathetics of the same and neighbouring segments, and a delayed general sympathetic stimulation of the whole body which originates supraspinally from the sympathetic reflex centres.

Seven cats were anaesthetized and the following nerves or dorsal roots were dissected and mounted for stimulation on electrodes: the intercostals T3 and T4, the spinal nerves L1 to L4, the dorsal roots of L7 and S1, and various nerves inervating the skin and muscles of the hind leg. Recording electrodes were placed on the white ramus communicans of T3, T4 and L1, L2 (Fig. 18).

In the experiments the above mentioned intercostal nerves, spinal nerves, dorsal roots or leg peripheral nerves were stimulated differently according to the experiment, ranging from threshold level to fifty times threshold. The recording electrode or the white ramus communicans measured the preganglionic sympathetic outflow in that particular segment.

At threshold stimulation x 50, the following recordings (Fig. 19) were made, representing in each case for clarity the average computerised record of several experiments. The recording was done only from the L1 white ramus communicans.

* Sato, A., and Schmidt, R. F. Spinal and supraspinal components of the reflex discharges into lumbar and thoracic white rami. Journal of Physiology, 1971, 212: 839–850. Also drawings in this chapter.

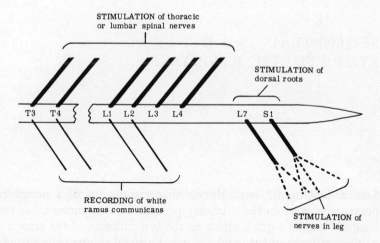

STIMULATION of thoracic
or lumbar spinal nerves

STIMULATION of
dorsal roots

T3 T4   L1 L2 L3 L4   L7 S1

RECORDING of white
ramus communicans

STIMULATION of
nerves in leg

FIG. 18

WHITE RAMI REFLEXES

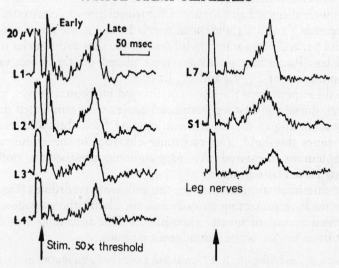

20 µV   Early   Late
                  50 msec

L1

L2

L3

L4

Stim. 50× threshold

L7

S1

Leg nerves

FIG. 19

It will be noticed that in most records the sympathetic reflex discharges fall into two groups: an early and a late, separated by some 50 milliseconds.

The early discharge becomes smaller the further the stimulus is removed from that of the recording segment L1. In contrast, the late component had a rather constant size whether spinal nerves, dorsal roots or cutaneous nerves of the hind limb (the sacral nerve) were stimulated.

The latency of the early discharge increased the further the stimulated segment was from L1. The latency of the late discharge increased only fractionally as the distance to the medullary sympathetic centres was only slightly increased.

The late discharge, which represents the general sympathetic response of the body, is elicited at lower levels of stimulation, for it is activated with a stimulus of 1.5 of the threshold value, whilst the early discharge requires 5, though this can vary according to the state of the animal.

When a recording was made from either the thoracic or lumbar white rami communicans, and then the cervical cord was divided or infiltrated with local anaesthetic at C1, the late discharge disappeared. Thus it is apparent that this is a supraspinal component.

Response in Specific Areas and not in others

If the pulmonary vein-atrial junction in a dog is stimulated there is* :

1. Increased activity in the cardiac sympathetics
2. Decreased activity in the renal sympathetics
3. No alteration in the activity of the abdominal sympathetics below the level of the renal artery.

The above suggests that although there may be a local segmental sympathetic response in addition to a generalised delayed sympathetic response, as described by Sato and Schmidt; there are in addition specific areas that may respond in a positive or negative manner or even remain neutral.

* Karin, F., Kidd, C., Malpas, C. M., Penna, P. E. The Effects of stimulation of the left atrial receptors on sympathetic efferent nerve fibres. Proceedings of the Journal of Physiology, 1971, 213: 38P–39P.

DERMATOMES, MYOTOMES, SCLEROTOMES

Reference of Pain and Tenderness when muscle is Stimulated

J. H. Kellgren has made many experiments* which are confirmed by the everyday practice of acupuncture. As a stimulus he injected 0.1 to 0.3 cc of 6% sodium chloride intramuscularly, which produces a severe pain lasting several minutes. In acupuncture the stimulus is usually less severe, or if severe is due to stimulation of the skin, so that the reference of pain mentioned in the ensuing paragraphs is not so often noticed.

If the gluteus medius in the upper part of the buttock is stimulated, a diffuse pain is felt over the lower part of the buttock and back of the thigh (Fig. 20).

If the upper part of the tibialis anterior is stimulated, there is often a diffuse pain in the whole of the belly of the muscle and also over the instep (Fig. 21).

Kellgren also injected saline into the multifidus opposite the 9th thoracic spine, into the intercostal muscles of the 9th intercostal space in the mid axillary line, and into the rectus abdominus 3 cm above the umbilicus. The pain from all three was referred to roughly the same area near the mid dorsal line and the mid central line (Fig. 22). Interestingly though, the pain from the multifidus was felt

---

* Kellgren, J. H. Observations on referred pain arising from muscle. Clinical Science, 1938–9, 3: 175–190. Also drawings in this chapter.

Ibid. On the distribution of pain arising from deep somatic structures with charts of segmental pain areas. Clinical Science 1939–42, 4: 35–46.

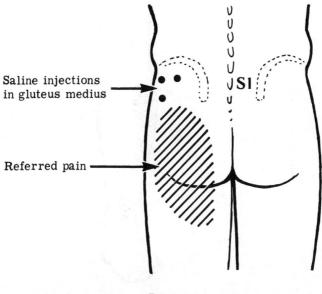

Saline injections
in gluteus medius

Referred pain

FIG. 20

mainly in the back and less ventrally, that from the rectus abdominus mainly ventrally and to a lesser extent posteriorly, whilst the mid axillary line intercostal injection was felt equally in front and at the back.

If the testis is firmly compressed between fingers and thumb, the pain is first felt in the scrotum, the pain radiating to the groin and lower lumbar region only on increased pressure. If saline is injected into the multifidus opposite the space between the 1st and 2nd lumbar spines, there is severe pain in the back which radiates to a lesser extent to the groin and scrotum. When the internal obliques are stimulated near the anterior superior iliac spine, the pain is felt mainly in this region, but is also referred as a slight pain to the lower lumbar area and the testes (Fig. 23).

In most of Kellgren's experiments, the reference of pain remained within the same myotome. If the stimulation was extremely strong the referred pain might spread one segment above and below. When

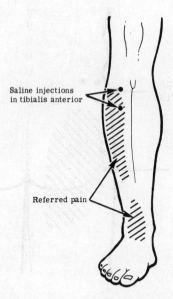

Saline injections
in tibialis anterior

Referred pain

FIG. 21

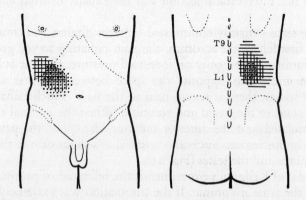

T9

L1

FIG. 22 Multifidus horizontal hatching, intercostals vertical hatching, rectus abdominis stippling

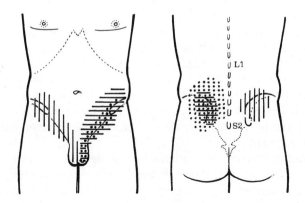

FIG. 23 Testis vertical hatching, abdominal obliques horizontal hatching, multifidus stippling.

long muscles, which span several segments, such as the sacro-spinials or rectus abdominus were stimulated, the pain often spread to several segments.

According to Kellgren the areas of referred pain near the mid ventral and mid dorsal lines, correspond to the area where the anterior and posterior primary divisions of the spinal nerves emerge from the skeletal musculature.

Kellgren differentiated the superficial and deep muscular pain as follows: he injected a muscle belly and obtained distant referred superficial pain and deep tenderness in the same region. If local anaesthetic was injected intradermally, both persisted; when injected deeply, the tenderness on pressure disappeared, whilst the superficial pain remained.

Kellgren came to the conclusion that there are three main layers of the body concerned with pain distribution:

1. When the skin is stimulated, there is normally very accurate localisation of the pain, which is also confined to a small area—unless the stimulus is unusually strong.

2. The middle layer consists of the more superficially placed deep structures: the deep fascia enclosing the limbs and trunk; and any periosteum, ligament or tendon sheath which is situated sub-cutaneously. This layer when stimulated causes pain over a somewhat

larger area, an area which may encompass the site of stimulation or even lie at a small distance from it.

3. Apart from the above there are all the deeper layers which if stimulated give rise to diffuse pain of more or less segmental distribution. This pain is more markedly segmental when arising from the interspinus ligaments, intercostal spaces and deep structures of the trunk and limb girdles. The pain is more local from the extremities and joints. There is a tendency for pain which arises in a limb muscle, to be referred to the joint which the muscle moves, provided it is in the same segment.

The importance to acupuncture of Kellgren's research will be apparent from other sections of the book. If it is possible, when treating a patient to elicit a referred pain, the result is usually better. If in addition it is possible from a distant pin prick, to cause a referred pain in the area of the patients' symptoms or pathology, the result will be even still better.

Many authors such as Janet Travell have written on this subject indeed every doctor who practises acupuncture using a deep needling technique must notice it every day of his practice. It is such a common observation that few I think would deny it.

Comparison of Areas of Reference

The foregoing pages demonstrate the importance to acupuncture of areas of reference, those differing according to the tissue stimulated —dermatome, myotome, sclerotome, vasculartome. The method of investigation is also important: hyposensitivity from loss of function of a single nerve root, electrical skin resistance in sympathectomcised patients, electrical skin resistance on stimulation of anterior spinal roots, pain distribution after hypertomic saline injection of interspinous ligaments. There is also the distribution of the peripheral nerves and also of the sympathetics, though the later probably largely corresponds to the vasculartome.

Once all these areas of reference are taken into account, most of which can be understood from a Western medical point of view, I am sure meridians will be relegated to history.

Many of the books or articles describing reference areas are not too easily accessible to everyone, and hence l am reproducing them here to facilitate use.

The Dermatomes from Keegan and Garrett

Figs. 24, 25 and 26 from: Keegan, J. J. and Garrett, F. D. The segmental distribution of the cutaneous nerves in the limbs of man. *Anatomical Record*, 1948, 102: 409-439.

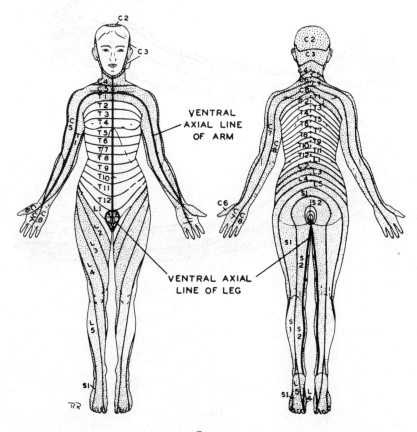

FIG. 24

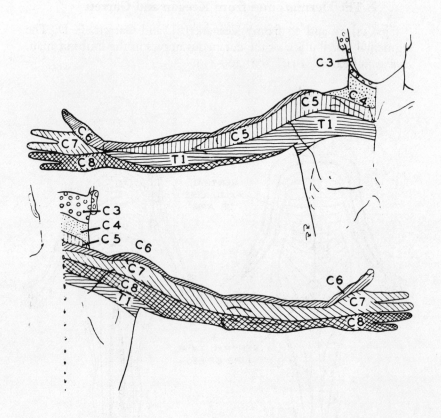

FIG. 25

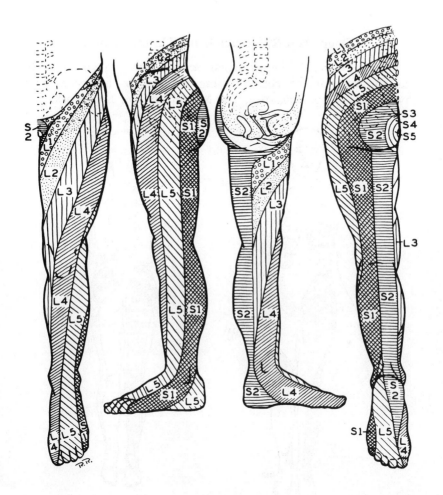

FIG. 26

Deep Pain Reference from Thomas Lewis

Fig. 27. Lewis, T. The segmental areas of deep pain developed by the injection of the corresponding interspinous ligament, with hypertonic saline. *Pain*, 1942, The Macmillan Co., New York.

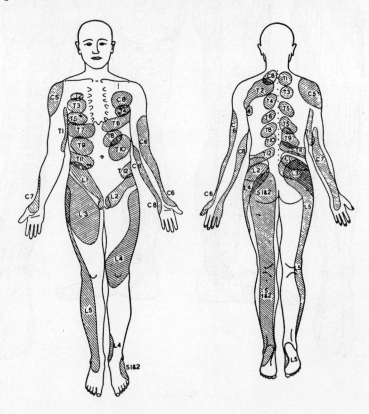

FIG. 27

Dermatomes, Myotomes and Sclerotomes from Inman and Saunders

Figs. 28, 29, 30 and 31. Inmann, V. T. and Saunders, J. B. de C. Referred pain from skeletal structures. *Journal of Nervous Mental Diseases*, 1944, 99: 660-667. Copyright 1944, The Williams and Wilkins Co., Baltimore. Slightly modified by Chusid, J. G.

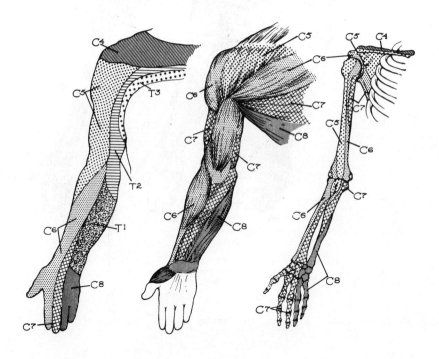

FIG. 28

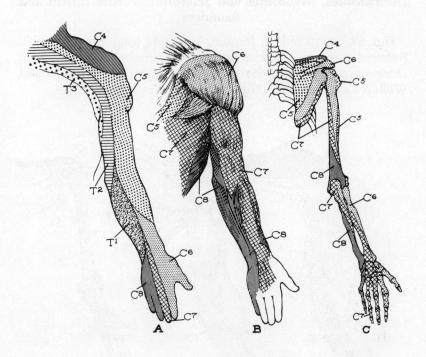

FIG. 29

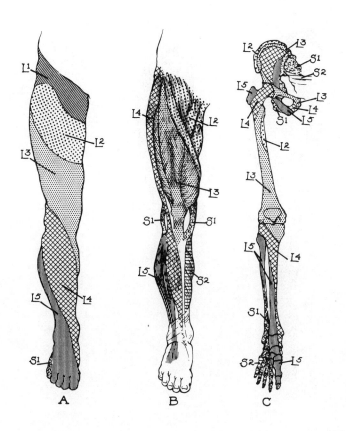

FIG. 30

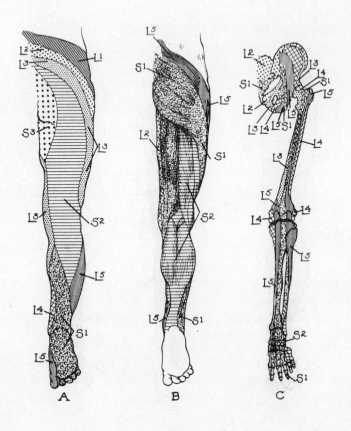

FIG. 31

Trigger Areas and Pain Reference Patterns from Janet Travell

Figs. 32, 33, 34, 35 and 36. Travell, J. Temperomandibular joint pain referred from muscles of the head and neck. *Journal of Prosthetic Dentistry*, 1960, Vol. 10, No. 4: 745-763.

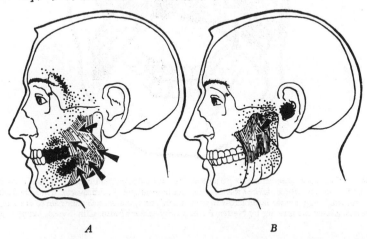

A   B

FIG. 32 Pain reference patterns of the masseter muscle: *A*, Superficial layer. *B*, Deep layer. Trigger areas are indicated by arrows, and their pain reference zones by the stippled and black regions

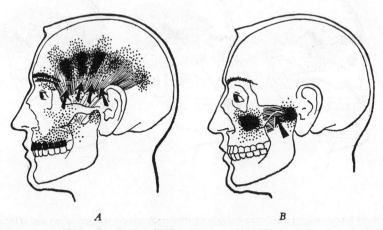

A   B

FIG. 33 *A*. Composite pain reference pattern of the temporalis muscle. Trigger areas are indicated by arrows, and their reference zones by the stippled and black regions. *B*, Composite pain reference pattern of the external pterygoid muscle

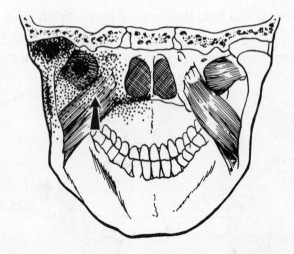

FIG. 34 Composite pain reference pattern of the internal pterygoid muscle. A partial coronal section is shown with a view of the external and internal pterygoid muscles from the back of the mouth. Trigger areas at the arrow in the internal pterygoid muscle refer pain to the stippled regions. (Based on drawing by Netter, F.: Anatomy of the Mouth, Clin. Symp. 10: 76, 1958.)

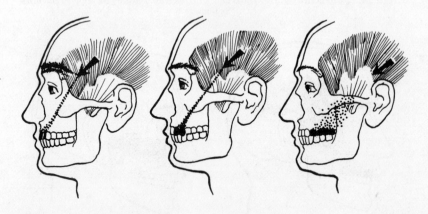

FIG. 35 Specific trigger areas at three sites in the temporalis muscle, as observed in a case of facial neuralgia. Trigger areas were located at arrows, and pain was referred to the black and stippled zones

66

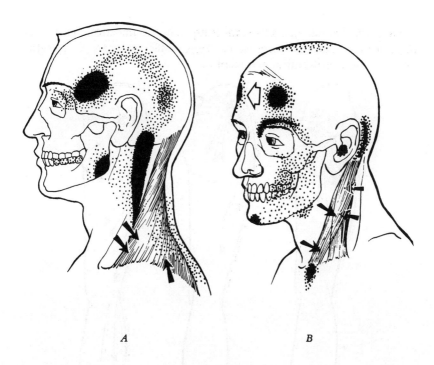

A   B

FIG. 36 *A*, Composite pain reference pattern of the trapezius muscle, suprascapular region. Trigger areas are indicated by arrows, and pain reference zones by the stippled and black regions.

B, Composite pain reference patterns of the clavicular and sternal divisions of the sterno-mastoid. The sternal division refers pain mainly to the cheek, eyebrow, pharynx, tongue, chin, throat, and sternum. The clavicular division refers pain mainly to the forehead bilaterally, to the posterior auricular region and deep in the ear, and infrequently to the teeth. Trigger areas are indicated by arrows, and pain reference zones by the stippled and black regions.

Fig. 37. Travell, J. Factors affecting pain of injection. *Journal of the American Medical Association*, 1955, 158: 368-371. Copyright 1955, American Medical Association.

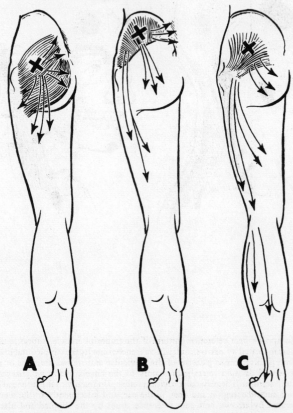

Fig. 37 Distribution of referred pain evoked by needle when inserted into trigger areas (*X*) located at common sites of intramuscular injections. Referred pain is most intense in region of arrowheads. *A*, gluteus maximus muscle. *B*, gluteus medius muscle. *C*, gluteus minimus muscle after removal of gluteus maximus and medius muscles

Fig. 38. Travell, J. Referred pain from skeletal muscle. *New York State Journal of Medicine*, 1955, 55: 331339. Fig. 38 and captions reprinted by permission from the *New York State Journal of Medicine*, copyright by the Medical Society of the State of New York.

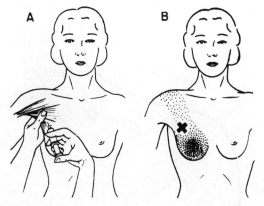

FIG. 38 Breast syndrome of pectoralis major muscle; *A*, manner of holding muscle for local procaine infiltration; *B*, distribution of pain (stippled) from trigger area (X), induced either by compressing it between the fingers or by inserting needle as shown in *A*

Trigger Points and Pain Distribution from Anders Sola

Figs. 39, 40, 41, 42 and 43. Sola, A. E. and Williams, R. L.
Myofasicial pain syndromes. *Neurology*, 1956, Vol. 6, No. 2: 91-95.
Reprinted from *Neurology*, © 1956 by Harcourt Brace Jovanovich,
Inc.

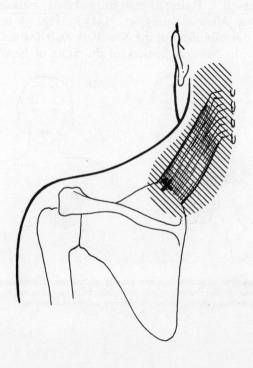

FIG. 39 The attachments of the levator scapulae muscle are shown and the common location of the trigger point is indicated by the cross. The hatched area represents the common distribution of pain in this syndrome

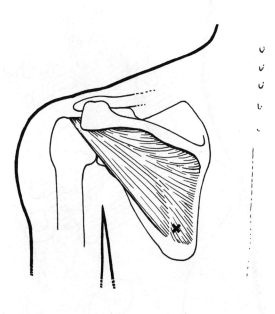

FIG. 40 The attachments of the infraspinatus muscle are shown and the common location of the trigger point is indicated by the cross

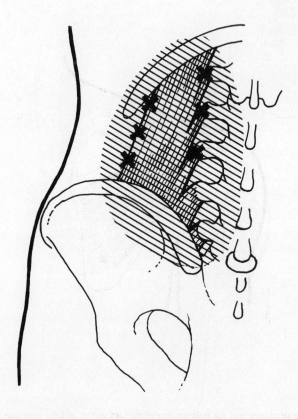

FIG. 41 The attachments and landmarks around the quadratus lumborum are shown. The crosses indicate common locations of trigger points in this syndrome. The hatched area represents the usual area of pain

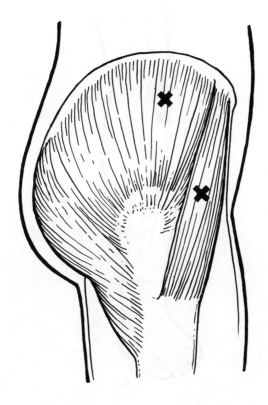

FIG. 42 The attachments of the tensor fascia lata and the gluteus medius are shown. The crosses
indicate the common locations of trigger points

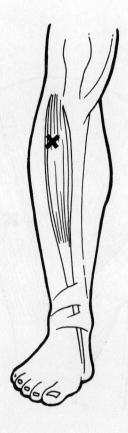

FIG. 43 The attachments of the anterior tibialis and the common location of the trigger point are shown

Dermatomes of Referred Pain from Lumbosacral and Pelvic Joint Ligaments from George Hackett

Fig. 44. Hackett, G. S. Joint ligament relaxation treated by fibro-osseous proliferation, 1956. Charles C. Thomas, Springfield, Illinois. From Homans, John. A textbook of surgery, 6th Ed., 1945. Courtesy of Charles C. Thomas, Springfield, Illinois.

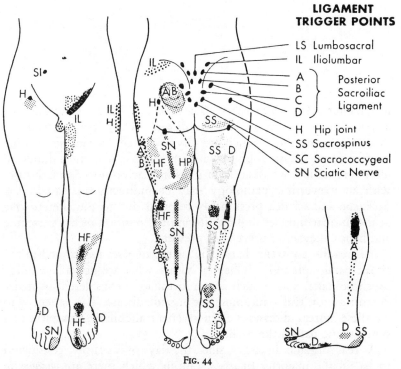

LIGAMENT TRIGGER POINTS

LS Lumbosacral
IL Iliolumbar
A ⎫
B ⎪ Posterior
C ⎬ Sacroiliac
D ⎭ Ligament
H Hip joint
SS Sacrospinus
SC Sacrococcygeal
SN Sciatic Nerve

FIG. 44

IL   Iliolumbar ligament (ilial attachment) abdomen, groin, genitalia, buttock, thigh (inner anterior)
AB   Posterior sacroiliac ligament (upper 2/3rds) buttock, thigh, leg (outer surface)
D   Posterior sacroiliac ligament (lower outer fibers) thigh, leg (outer calf), foot (outer margin and sole to 5-4-3-2 toes accompanied by sciatica, loss of ankle reflex and body list)
HP   Hip articular ligament (posterior superior fibers, pelvic attachment) thigh (posterior medial)
HF   Hip, articular ligament (posterior superior fibers, femoral attachment) thigh, upper half of leg (lateral to calf), lower half of leg (anterior to tibia), top of foot to big toe and half 2nd toe
SS   Sacrospinus and sacrotuberus ligament (sacral attachment) thigh, central calf of leg, heel
SN   'Sciatica'—nerve pain accompanying relaxed ligaments (lower end of sacroiliac joint)

VII

SOME PHILOSOPHICAL CONSIDERATIONS

In Chapter XI of *Acupuncture: The Ancient Chinese Art of Healing*, it was shown that in general the diseases which are amenable to acupuncture are those which are physiologically reversible: asthma may be cured whilst emphysema is irreversible, likewise a duodenal ulcer is reversible whilst an hour glass stomach is not. Some diseases with an irreversible pathology may be indirectly alleviated: low backache and sciatica presumably respond due to the altered tone of the lumbar muscles slightly altering the position of the vertebrae and hence alleviating nerve root pressure.

It is readily apparent that many of the diseases mentioned in the above paragraph and in Chapter XI are what are nowadays called psychosomatic, and as such are unfortunately considered by many doctors as not 'real'—meaning not organic disease. The patient who has these 'unreal' diseases is often given a tranquiliser, an aspirin or a sympathetic pat on the back.

A 'real' organic disease is, since the days of Virchow, considered to be, in the majority of cases, one in which there are *changes in cellular pathology*. More recently gross changes in chemical pathology have been added. If one excludes acute disease (which is barely mentioned in this chapter) this presents a nihilistic dilemma:

'Real' diseases are only recognised as such, if there are accompanying pathological changes when, as a rule the condition is irreversible because the regenerative ability of chronically diseased tissue in man is extremely low—not as in the lower animals. In short: *once a chronic disease is diagnosed it is by definition incurable*.

Orthodox Western medicine is in the same nihilistic dilemma. A surgeon may excise the area of pathological change, but he does not cure. Insulin may alleviate the symptoms of diabetes, but the patient is not cured because the day he does not take insulin he is as ill as before. The achievements of surgery and drugs should not be underestimated, for innumerable lives are saved or disease alleviated, by their use. But, at the same time, it is clear that, in most instances, they do not cure—in the sense that changes in cellular pathology are not usually reversed.

Likewise acupuncture does not cure 'real' diseases. The temporary alleviation which is achieved by taking a medicine every day, cannot be emulated by acupuncture, for acupuncture is normally only applied half a dozen times, followed sometimes by a few single follow-up treatments.

The aim of acupuncture, and I hope that of Western medicine in the future, is to treat disease before it is by definition incurable. But since most 'real' diseases are incurable, what can one do?

I think that most chronic diseases with obvious changes in cellular pathology are preceded by a preclinical phase of perhaps many years duration. I cannot imagine that someone who has diabetes, hypertension or malignant disease one year, was really healthy the year before. In most of these diseases there was probably some mild physiological dysfunction of many years' duration, which only finally culminated in changes in cellular pathology or gross biochemistry.

It is this early stage of a mild physiological dysfunction, still presumably reversible, which doctors should try to treat. Since this preclinical phase of disease cannot be diagnosed by conventional methods, one has to think of a different approach.

A large proportion, if not the majority, of patients seen by a general practitioner have diseases which many doctors consider 'unreal', 'psychosomatic', 'functional', 'supratentorial', 'neuro-vegetative disequilibrium'. The hospital consultant sees less patients with 'unreal' diseases, as the general practitioner tries to refer only 'real' diseases to him. In the final analysis the doctor will insist that his diagnosis of a 'supratentorial' disease was correct for at autopsy a patient who has had symptoms for thirty years and died at eighty will probably show no unexpected pathological changes.

I personally think that most patients who have symptoms have a disease, whether there is any pathology there or not. I find that the proportion of hysterics who should be excluded from the above considerations is exceedingly small—and even they should be cured of their hysteria. I see no reason whatsoever why the average person should invent a disease, why they should invent that they are tired till halfway through the morning, that they do not have the energy to enjoy their work or leisure. Many perfectly normal citizens have vague symptoms such as the above for perhaps half their life. They often do not tell their doctor as they resent his depreciating reception of their psychosomatic symptoms.

Chinese pulse diagnosis* can, not infrequently, find a dysfunction in these patients with 'supratentorial' disease. With the appropriate treatment the 'supratentorial' disease is alleviated or cured and the patient's fatigue, lethargy, restlessness or other symptoms, which he may have had for many years, are dissipated. In these cases acupuncture is sometimes the appropriate treatment, in other cases less food and running a mile before breakfast is the answer.

I think, though I have no proof, that if this preclinical stage of disease is cured it prevents the later development of an obvious disease with pathology. Sometimes a disease may remain at the preclinical stage and develop no further.

In modern medicine, *pathology* is the Queen of Sciences. In the system I am proposing, the *symptoms* of the patient would achieve paramount importance. I believe the human being is more sensitive than a test tube. And a doctor should learn how to evaluate the minutest of symptoms or the slightest change in the bearing or temperament of his patient, making medicine once more an art. Later, when there are chemical and cellular changes, science takes over from that probing, intuitive art.

A not inconsiderable number of doctors, would classify amongst the 'unreal' or 'psychosomatic' diseases, migraine, ulcerative colitis, hay fever and duodenal ulcer. If a method of treatment is able to help these diseases it is often considered little more than hypnosis. Brain tumours and broken bones are the business of 'real' medicine.

The human body though, does not function along purely physical or purely mental paths; usually there will be interaction. If one has had a fright it is normal to have palpitations; those who do not are

* see Chapter IX of Acupuncture: The Ancient Chinese Art of Healing.

considered superhuman or subnormal. If someone vomits at table it is usual for the others present to lose their appetite, with diminished salivary secretion. It is quite normal for young men and women to have not only a mental effect on one another but also some physiological effect—and when this never happens, it is considered abnormal.

It is similar in disease. It is normal for the mind and body to interact. If a disease can no longer be influenced by the mind it is often very advanced with marked pathological changes, making it a 'real' disease which is incurable. In congestive cardiac failure, the cardiac muscle is probably irreparably hypertrophied. Hence this process can no longer be influenced by the mind. Digitalis will help for a day, but the congestive cardiac failure could only have been cured at the preclinical phase, at which stage both the mind, acupuncture and drugs can influence it.

Many consider that a double blind cross over trial can distinguish between a real medicine and a placebo, because the effect of the mind is excluded. This is to a large extent correct in modern medicines with their strong pharmacological actions: pentothal works or it does not work; when it is excreted the effect wears off and more has to be injected. Pentothal presumably temporarily blocks one link in the biochemical chain. Vitamin B_{12} temporarily replaces a deficiency. If normal medicines are to function properly they have to be more or less continuously present in the body.

The opposite holds true with the more biological and pre-clinical type of medicine I am advocating. In acupuncture one only stimulates (via the nervous system) the body a few times, so that afterwards it functions normally and does not require the continuous administration of medicines or acupuncture. As this is a *weak* physiological rather than a *strong* pharmacological effect it probably also requires the synergistic action of the mind and hence a double blind cross over trial has little meaning under these circumstances.

Alexander Macdonald* and colleagues have shown that part of the effect of acupuncture is physiological and part mental. This is of course true of everything in medicine: in surgery and when using modern powerful drugs, the physiological effect usually domin-

*Macdonald, A.J.R., Macrae, K.D., Masters, B.R. Rubin, A.P. Superficial acupuncture in the relief of chronic low back pain: a placebo controlled randomised trial. Annals of the Royal College of Surgeons of England, 1983, 65: 44–46.

Fig. 45 Mean percentage reductions

Patient groups	% pain relief after each treatment	% pain score reduction	% activity pain score reduction	% physical signs reduction	% severity and pain area reduction	Combined average % reduction
(a) Acupuncture (N = 8)	77.35	57.15	52.04	96.78	73.75	71.41
(b) Placebo (N = 9)	30.14	22.74	5.83	29.17	18.89	21.35
	**	—	*	**	**	**

Significance assessed by the Wilcoxon Rank-sum tests

* $p < 0.05$
** $p < 0.01$
—   not significant

ates; whilst in the practice of the average general practitioner, the physiological and mental effects are of probably more equal importance.

Macdonald studied seventeen consecutive patients whose chronic low back pain failed to derive sufficient relief from appropriate conventional methods of treatment. The cases were severe enough to be referred from the orthopaedic or rheumatic departments to a pain relief clinic. They were diagnosed as having: anterior spondylitis, ankylosing spondylitis, degenerative disc lesion, non-articular rheumatism, osteoarthritis, prolapsed intervertebral disc, arachnoiditis, sacro-iliac ligamentous strain, Scheuermann's osteochondritis or ideopathic. There was random allocation of patients with regard to disease, age and sex.

In each patient five measures of treatment efficiency were recorded, subjectively or objectively and the improvement or otherwise in each case, noted by an independent observer.

One group of patients were treated by superficial acupuncture, in which the needle only pierces the skin and subcutaneous fat.

The placebo group were treated by the biggest and most impressive looking machine in the hospital, with many dials and flashing lights, whose cooling system made a whirring sound. Electrodes from this machine were applied to similar parts of the body to those which had been needled by acupuncture. The machine was regulated, though, in such a way, that when it was switched on, no current flowed through the electrodes.

The table (Fig. 45) shows that the acupuncture is some three times as effective as only placebo. Interestingly three patients were temporarily worse after placebo treatment, though this did not happen at subsequent treatments which were deliberately of shorter duration.

VIII

FAILED RESEARCH

When I first studied acupuncture in 1958, many doctors thought that one could locate acupuncture points electrically. It was said that the electrical skin resistance, or impedance, was reduced at an acupuncture point. Hence it was a relatively simple matter of a patient holding an earthed electrode in one hand, whilst the doctor ran a searching electrode over the area of skin where he thought he would find an acupuncture point. It was frequently further postulated, that if an acupuncture point were 'active', that is requiring stimulation, the electrical skin resistance was reduced by an even greater amount than with a 'non-active' acupuncture point. A few doctors, also claimed that the resistance was reduced along the course of the meridians, albeit to a lesser extent than with the active or non-active acupuncture points.

Filled with the enthusiasm of youth, and the uncritical childlike belief that many people have at some time in their lives, I bought what I thought was the best commercially available electrical acupuncture point detector: an apparatus which I bought in the belief that it would work and help to provide some scientific basis for acupuncture.

I found that however diligently I tried using this apparatus, I could detect neither acupuncture points, whether active or inactive, nor meridians. Subsequently I bought two more electrical acupuncture point detectors with the same dismal result. Over the years several dozen different models have been made by various manufacturers, some of which I have tested whilst looking at the manufacturers' displays at acupuncture conferences. But always, to my inexplicable consternation, the acupuncture point proved elusive.

It was only gradually that I realised, as I have described in this book, that acupuncture points and meridians do not exist—at least in the traditionally accepted sense. During the time when this gradual change in my conception of acupuncture was taking place, I met Professor Bernard Watson, Dr Stuart Meldrum and their colleagues many of whom were physicists, at the Department of Medical Electronics at St Bartholomew's Hospital, London. Some of the lines of research mentioned in this chapter evolved through our mutual discussions.

Electrical Skin Resistance Measurements

McCarroll and Rowley* made a grid five units in length and five in width, so that a large square enclosed 25 small squares. This 25 square grid was placed in various positions on the arm where some of the traditional acupuncture points were located. The searching electrode, which was one millimetre in diameter, incorporated a soft spring, so that the electrode, whatever its position, applied a constant force of o. 1 kgm/mm^2 to the skin.

Measurement of the electrical impedance in all 25 squares was made in a random manner, on several occasions, with the grid in various positions. No particular areas of reduced electrical skin impedance were found, except where the electrode impinged on a hard object—bone or tendon.

It was also found that when the electrode was applied to the same place for 20 seconds, the impedance was reduced by some 50%. Beyond this point the impedance was suddenly reduced by 94% of its original value—it was considered that the protein mat of the stratum corneum had been torn.

The above experiment confirms my own experience: If one is searching for an 'acupuncture point', the longer one looks, i.e. the longer one presses the electrode over the same area, the more likely is one to create due to the apparatus, a non-existent acupuncture

*McCarroll, G. Duncan and Rowley, Blair A. An investigation of the existance of electrically located acupuncture points. Transactions on Biomedical Engineering, 1979, 26–3: 177–181.

point. If one passes the electrode over the skin in a regular, but random manner, no obvious correlation exists between the variations in impedance and traditional acupuncture points.

The impedance is sometimes reduced over superficial veins, if an electrode without a spring is pressed harder against the skin, by perspiration, or over a boney prominence. Also some types of skin have a lower impedance. The sudden breakdown in the electrical skin resistance, referred to above, may easily be observed if an electrode is pressed a little harder than usual.

In the case of either a disease of the viscera or spasm of the skeletal muscle, one would expect reflex changes in the skin, due to the viscero-cutaneous or muscular-cutaneous reflexes, mentioned earlier in this book. One would likewise expect these reflex changes to affect various properties of the skin, possibly including the electrical resistance or impedance.

One would however, I think, expect to find quite large areas of skin exhibiting these electrical changes, such as the reflexly tender areas, often the size of a hand, mentioned by Kellgren (see Chapter I, Fig. 9). Possibly the area might even be larger affecting a substantial part of a dermatome, myotome or vasculartome. If a sympathectomy is performed, many nerves have to be divided to produce vascular dilation and a large area of reduced electrical skin impedance. If only a few nerves are divided there is not a correspondingly reduced result, but no result at all.

It is thus apparent, that the researcher should look for *large areas* of skin exhibiting electrical (or other) changes, *which are only present in disease or dysfunction*. Searching for tiny acupuncture points, which are present on both the healthy and diseased body is probably a science-fiction interpretation of certain traditional ideas, which have proved erroneous.

Infra Red Photography

It is often possible to relieve a patient's symptoms within a few seconds or minutes of treatment by acupuncture. It seemed reasonable to suppose that if a patient had headache, pain in the neck and shoulders or pain over the sinuses, and these symptoms were alleviated, that there would be evidence of an altered bloodflow in the affected region and that this could be demonstrated by infra red photography.

Ten friends, patients or members of the department with a variety of symptoms volunteered for the experiment. In some instances the acupuncture alleviated their symptoms, in others it did not. In no instance was there a significant alteration in the infra red photographs, taken before and after the experiment. Even in those patients who had instantaneous relief of symptoms, the changes in the infra red photographs were neither sufficiently significant nor were they consistent.

Other researchers, who have published their results, claim to have found significant changes on their investigation by infra red photography. This is contrary to our experience. It should be remembered though that it is quite easy to have erroneous changes. This may be due to the patient not having reached a stable temperature in a stable environment of sufficient duration. Emotional response easily changes skin temperature as can be demonstrated by bio-feedback techniques. It is also possible to achieve an occasional change, which is difficult to repeat.

Electromyography

Many patients have stiff, tender and painful shoulders. If these are successfully treated by acupuncture, and the shoulders are examined before and after treatment, the doctor may find the shoulders feel softer, giving the impression the muscles are more relaxed.

It seems that many patients suffering from low backache may have spasm of the sacrospinalis, which is relaxed after successful treatment. Such patients may be unable to touch their toes when standing with their knees straight, but are able to do so after treatment; presumably due to muscle relaxation.

It should therefore have been easy to demonstrate the effect of acupuncture by electromyography. In all these experiments the recording was done with surface electrodes over the afflicted area, so that there was little disturbance of the affected musculature or the overlying or adjacent tissue. For the same reason the acupuncture was performed in the hands or feet, as these are at some distance from the site of the symptoms: the shoulders or lumbosacral area.

Twelve friends and patients with the above symptoms were

needled in the appropriate place in the hands or feet, sometimes the feet were used to alleviate the symptoms in the shoulders.

Over 50% of the patients responded within a few seconds of treatment. The symptoms (and presumably the muscle spasm) remained better for a shorter or longer period in each individual. In not one instance was the electromyograph altered by acupuncture.

The electromyograph used was the EMG 100 of Biofeedback Systems Ltd with the setting at mode one. This gives a click feedback, the click rate being proportional to the integrated EMG level shown on the meter. After the electrodes were in place the patient was asked to relax as much as possible the painful shoulder or lumbo-sacral region. This reduced the click rate considerably, but did not alter the pain of the affected part. The patient was then needled in the appropriate part of the hand or foot and again asked to relax the affected part as much as possible. In many instances the pain in the shoulder or lumbo-sacral area disappeared, and the patient if previously unable to touch his toes was then able to do so. The click rate though remained the same (as when the patient consciously relaxed) as did the meter reading. If the clicking was turned off for the duration of the experiment, and the instrument turned in such a way so that the patient could not see the silent meter, the result was the same.

Conclusions

All of the above experiments, were in the nature of a pilot trial. If the pilot trial had been successful the experiments would have continued and involved a larger number of patients.

This, of course, means that each of the experiments was performed only a limited number of times. It is just conceivable, if we had persisted with the experiments, a positive result would have ensued. It is also possible, if we had tried the above experiments in many different ways, we could in the end have demonstrated a positive result.

My main purpose in publishing these experiments, most of which were carried out many years ago and nearly forgotten, is to show that research into acupuncture is far from simple. Many articles have been published in specialist acupuncture journals and also general medical journals, in which the conclusions drawn are opposed to the ones in this chapter.

As acupuncture helps a reasonable proportion of patients with the appropriate type of disease, it should be possible to demonstrate in some objective manner, the effect of treating a patient. The hopefully objective research which several colleagues and I have performed has had no positive result. In the same way, when I have investigated in sufficient detail some of the claims of others, their results could quite possibly be reinterpreted as also negative.

Obviously a considerably greater effort is required. Perhaps if the amount of time, thought and effort which is applied to western medicine, is likewise applied to acupuncture, it will bear fruit. Many doctors and researchers experience difficulty in separating traditional acupuncture, from what *actually happens*: a deficiency which I hope is clarified by this book.

The Mind Versus the Body, or the Mind Plus the Body

At present I believe there are certain aspects of acupuncture which are purely physical: the effect of needling a joint locally seems to be similar to that of a local steroid injection.

Other aspects of acupuncture are probably largely psychosomatic. In this respect it is similar to a reasonable proportion of general practice.

I think quite a substantial part of the success of acupuncture lies somewhere between the mental and the physical aspects: if there is only the mental treatment it does not help; if there is only physical treatment it likewise fails.

Many patients who have headaches or migraine, are treated by doctors practising acupuncture as a reasonable proportion of them are helped by acupuncture, even though they may have had their symptoms for ten, twenty or thirty years. An acupuncture point frequently employed for this purpose is liver 3 (between the 1st and 2nd metatarsals) or bladder 62 (below the lateral malleolus). On several occasions I have needled the ends of toes or the sole of the foot, in a random manner, in positions where there are no acupuncture points – and yet the patient's headache or migraine improved, (though this has not been done often enough to know if the same proportion of patients are helped). Yet patients who stub their toes against a rock or who walk for a few moments with a stone in their shoe, experiencing just as much pain as if they had been needled, have no relief of their headache or migraine.

87

Conversely a psychiatrist is mostly of less benefit in headache or migraine than a doctor practising acupuncture.

It is this peculiar combination of the physical stimulus of a needle prick, together with psychological factors, which seems to produce the results one sees in acupuncture. This is of course a largely new concept in medicine, a concept which should be considered when designing research projects. A rose is a physical object, but a *beautiful* rose is a nonscientific concept as it is a combination of something physical and non-physical. 'Man does not live by bread alone. . . .'

All Roads Lead to Rome

Acupuncture encompasses several phenomena and probably various mechanisms for:

1. On some occasions a needle prick anywhere on the body, is sufficient to produce relief of the patient's symptoms.
2. On other occasions the needle prick may be anywhere in the appropriate quarter of the body.
3. On still other occasions the stimulus has seemingly to be in the correct dermatome, myotome, sclerotome, vasculartome or other area of this magnitude of size.
4. On yet other occasions stimulation of a reflexly tender area, often the size of the palm of the hand, produces the best result. The tender areas mentioned by Kellgren in Chapter I Fig. 9 and in Chapter VI are of this nature.
5. If a trigger point, perhaps a centimetre in diameter can be found, and it is needled, not infrequently the best result ensues.

Often, but by no means always, needling a trigger point of a tender area is more effective than needling anywhere on the body or even in the correct dermatome. If a trigger point or tender area are hypersensitive, or in a 'strong reactor' (see Chapter IV), local needling may aggravate the condition, and hence treatment of a distant area is more appropriate.

Trigger points, or reflexly tender areas are not necessarily relevant to the disease in question. Patients with a painful shoulder not infrequently have a tender area, about two centimetres in diameter, at the insertion of the deltoid, halfway down the lateral side of the humerus. Needling this tender area has no effect.

All Roads Emanate from Rome

The reverse of all the above phenomena may also be observed in at least a limited number of patients:

1. If a patient has, say, a mild pain in the neck, it may be alleviated by needling the appropriate place in the foot (say, liver 3, between the 1st and 2nd metatarsals).
2. If a patient has mild lumbago, it may also be relieved by needling liver 3.
3. If a patient has mild pain in the neck, headache, lumbago and nausea; all four symptoms may likewise benefit when liver 3 is needled. This relief may occur a few seconds after stimulation, thus excluding humoral factors, for the blood or lymphatic flow would be too slow to conduct a chemical substance from one part of the body to another in this short time.

Sensitized Segments of the Cord

One of the few possible explanations for this phenomenon, which I have discussed with the neurologist Peter Nathan, is as follows:

1. If one has a pain in the neck the appropriate part of the cervical cord is sensitized. If one has lumbago certain sections of the lower lumbar or upper sacral cord are sensitized.
2. If a specific part of the skin is needled, the stimulus has a tendency to spread to the rest of the body. This has been shown experimentally by:

   a. Sato and Schmidt (Chapter V) who demonstrated that a stimulus had a primary immediate effect in the same and adjacent segments, and also a delayed general sympathetic response over the whole body mediated by the sympathetic centre in the medulla.

   b. Le Bars, Dickenson and Besson (Chapter XI) have shown that stimulation, nearly anywhere, will inhibit the appreciation of pain in nearly every other part of the body. This is mediated by convergent dorsal neurones, which receive both a noxious and non-noxious input.

Thus a stimulus, applied anywhere in the body, probably often spreads throughout all segments via the above two and probably other means. When this stimulus reaches a sensitized area (such as the neck or lumbar area in our example) it has an effect and hence reduces the pain or muscle spasm. A nonsensitized part of the cord is not influenced, according to this theory, and hence is uninfluenced by the relatively gentle stimulus of ordinary acupuncture.

RADIATION AND REFERRED SENSATION OR PAIN

It is frequently possible, when needling a patient, to obtain radiation or a referred mild pain or sensation. This is most likely to happen if the periosteum is stimulated and more particularly so in certain positions such as the region of the sacro-iliac joint. This phenomenon is less likely to occur if the skin, subcutaneous tissues or muscles are needled.

This radiation is quite different from the sudden, shooting, severe and rapidly moving pain one has if a major nerve trunk is needled or the ulnar nerve is compressed at the elbow.

The radiation sensation is usually gentle and may take several seconds to traverse the length of a limb. It may be so gentle that one is only aware of it when sitting comfortably, without distraction, in relaxed surroundings; the effect being like a gentle breeze blowing on one's foot, or a slight tingling sensation. Usually it is experienced as a mild pain travelling a variable distance along a path a few millimetres to a centimetre wide.

Sometimes the radiation or referred sensation, may start from the site of the needle prick. Sometimes it may only be felt at a distant site. Sometimes it may emanate from the needle prick, travel along a more or less straight course all the way to a distant site. Sometimes en route to the distant site, certain sections of the 'path' may be missing. Sometimes in a distant site it may, particularly in the head, neck and shoulders, produce a feeling of warmth; or if referred to the nose a 'crackling'.

If the region of the sacro-iliac joint is needled and a patient has pain at the back of the thigh, the radiation will most frequently go to the back of the thigh. If instead the patient had pain on the medial side of the thigh and *exactly the same region of the sacro-iliac joint is needled,* the radiation sensation or pain will travel to the medial side of the thigh. If the pain was on the lateral side of the thigh and again the same region of the sacro-iliac joint is needled, the needle pain will radiate to the lateral side of the thigh, in the majority of instances. Likewise with the anterior of the thigh.

It is thus apparent that if a certain specific area of periosteum is needled and a patient has radiation within the possibilities of referred pain from the needled area, the radiation will then go to the patient's painful area.

The course of the radiation, does not follow the path of a major nerve, artery, vein, bone or meridian. This phenomenon of radiation, perhaps gave the ancient Chinese their original conception of meridians, except that if one observes carefully, the pathway of the radiation and its destination, are seen to be infinitely variable. Amongst the infinitely variable possibilities of radiation and its destination there are perhaps, but only perhaps, certain preferred paths which on balance seem to be travelled more frequently than others. But even these preferred paths do not correspond with any obvious anatomical structure or even the meridians.

Radiation may be used clinically in acupuncture. If for example a patient has pain in the thumb, it may be treated, if it is an easily reversible condition, by needling the periosteum of the radius, anywhere along its whole length so as to elicit a radiation of pain into the thumb. If exactly the same place on the radius is needled, but without radiation to the thumb, the treatment may well give ease, but it is less likely to be successful than if there were radiation into the thumb.

If the upper third of the tibialis anterior is needled so that the needle goes through to the periosteum of the lateral side of the tibia (see Fig. 21), there may be radiation down the front of the shin, the front of the ankle and into the toes. If a patient has pain of a mild, easily reversible nature in the ankle, radiation to the ankle may alleviate the condition. If the pain is instead in the transverse arch of the foot radiation has to reach as far as the transverse arch for the most likely optional effect.

In the case of pain in the ankle, it is unlikely (but occasionally possible), for the radiation from the tibialis anterior to go below the ankle, into the transverse arch or toes. It seems as if the site of pain is often the 'end station'. If the pain is in the toes, the radiation is more likely to reach the toes, than if the pain were in the ankle.

It is considerably easier to obtain radiation in a 'strong reactor' (see Chapter IV) than in a normal reactor. Radiation may go from one end of the body to another in a strong reactor, whilst in a normal or slow reactor the distance travelled by the radiation is nearly always less or even considerably less. Sometimes in normal or slow reactors, one has to manipulate the needle for a long time before obtaining radiation, whilst in a strong reactor radiation may occur in the first few seconds.

On a few occasions I have deliberately tried to needle, with a thin acupuncture needle, a major nerve trunk, to obtain the shooting pain well known from compression of the ulnar nerve at the elbow. Interestingly it was much easier to elicit this shooting pain in a strong reactor. Presumably the diameter of the same nerve is the same in a strong and slow reactor. Perhaps the threshold of stimulation is lower in a strong reactor?

It is easier to achieve radiation in the limbs, than in most positions on the trunk and the radiation travels more often centrifugally than centripetally.

Various Chinese authors have stated that inflation of a blood pressure cuff across the path of the radiation, stops the radiation at the level of the inflated cuff. On some occasions I have merely pinched the skin in one place along the path of the radiation, which stopped the radiation going beyond the pinched area.

X

REFLEXES ELICITED BY STRONG STIMULATION

Relevant research has recently been conducted at Goteborg.*
Cholera toxin was placed in the lumen of the jejunum in anaesthe-
tised rats, which produced a large secretion of fluid into the lumen
of the isolated segment of jejunum.

The sciatic nerve was stimulated for 60 minutes, at some 10
times twitch threshold, at 3 Hertz, with a duration of 0.2 milliseconds. The intestinal fluid secretion was considerably reduced in
most rats, for 30 minutes after stimulation had ceased. Thereafter
intestinal secretion slowly returned to normal values.

In a further series of experiments, the sciatic nerve was stimulated in rats whose jejunum had not been subjected to cholera
toxin. In these experiments the intestinal secretion was largely
unaffected.

In another group of rats the tissue surrounding the superior mesenteric artery and vein was divided, thus depriving the jejunum of
its extrinsic autonomic innervation. The jejunum subsequently had
cholera toxin placed in the lumen, which as previously increased
secretion of fluid. Sciatic stimulation did not influence jejunal
secretion in this group, thus demonstrating the importance of the
intestinal innervation.

It is interesting to note that sciatic stimulation had an effect only
in the rats with a diseased jejunum and not in those who did not

*Cassuto, J., Larssen, P., Yao, T., Jodal, M., Thorén, P., Andersson, S., Lund-
gren, O. The effect of stimulating somatic afferents on cholera secretion in the rat
small intestine. Acta Physiologica Scandinavica, 1982, 116: 443–446.

have cholera toxin. This corresponds with the clinical experience of acupuncture: it is possible to affect a region of the body which is not functioning correctly, but it is extremely difficult to alter the function of a region which is completely normal.

It should be noted that the above-mentioned stimulation was continued for an hour (it had less effect when tried for only 30 minutes), whilst one usually only stimulates for a few seconds in acupuncture. Normally by acupuncture, one only treats easily reversible physiological processes. Perhaps the scope of acupuncture could be increased to treat more severe conditions, using long continued stimulation.

The same laboratory* has used the same method of sciatic nerve stimulation in unanaesthetised, spontaneously hypertensive rats. They found that during a 30 minute period of sciatic nerve stimulation: the blood pressure, the heart rate and splanchnic nerve activity remained the same, or even increased. Thereafter, possibly after a delay of one or two hours: the blood pressure was reduced (from 160 mmHg to 140 mmHg), there was reduced splanchnic nerve activity, and mild bradycardia. Interestingly these depressive effects could last up to 12 hours.

All the experiments mentioned in this chapter required a longer period of stimulation and stronger stimulation than is usual in therapeutic acupuncture. It thus resembles the type of stimulation used in acupuncture analgesia.

*Yao, T., Andersson, S., Thorén, P. Long lasting cardiovascular depression induced by acupuncture-like stimulation of the sciatic nerve in unanaesthetised hypertensive rats. Brain Research, 1982: 240, 77–85.

XI

DIFFUSE NOXIOUS INHIBITORY CONTROL

by ANTHONY DICKENSON

An underlying principle of acupuncture is the relief or alleviation of pain somewhere in the body by application of a peripheral stimulus either by needling or electro-acupuncture. In investigating the electro-physiological basis for acupuncture the first criterion is to record the activity of a class of neurone which plays a role in the processes leading to the sensation of pain. It is impossible to extrapolate from neuronal activities to pain sensation but neurones responding to noxious stimuli can be presumed to be involved, to some extent, in nociception. Pain arising from the activation of nociceptors in the skin, muscles, viscera, etc. is transmitted by fine calibre peripheral fibres, the C fibres, which make contact with neurones located in the spinal cord or trigeminal complex. These central neurones responding to noxious inputs fall into two distinct classes. One type of neurone, responding only to noxious pinch and heat, is located in lamina 1 in the superficial layer of the dorsal part of the spinal cord. Despite this selective response to noxious pinch and heat, as most of these neurones extend for only 2–3 segments and do not project up to the brain, and as none responds to muscular or visceral pain, it is unlikely that this class of cell is involved in pain in clinical practice which is rarely from skin origins.

Deeper in the dorsal horn, in lamina 5, another class of neurone can be found, which due to the variety of inputs arriving at the cell body has been designated as a convergent neurone. These cells respond to inputs from the skin, muscles and viscera; many of them project to higher centres of the brain, and the neurones respond in a sustained and powerful manner to noxious heat and pinch. However the cells additionally respond to innocuous peripheral stimuli.

There are two types of peripheral stimuli, both relevant to acupuncture-like procedures, which inhibit the activities of these convergent neurones and which may explain the analgesic effects of these procedures. The independence of these controls suggest that there may be two different bases for acupuncture. The first inhibitory control on these cells is the so called segmental inhibition. Surrounding the excitatory receptive field of these cells, the area of the periphery from which the cells can be activated, is a zone inside which light tactile stimuli can inhibit the pain related activities of these cells. Similarly, electrical activation of the touch fibres can block the activity of these cells. The segmental nature of these controls is critical in that the conditioning stimuli must be applied locally and so acupuncture acting from distant areas of the body must be doing so by a different mechanism. The clinical use of low intensity peripheral stimulation applied locally and known as transcutaneous nerve stimulation (TNS) is derived from these segmental inhibitory effects. So what then is the mechanism of acupuncture effects produced from distant areas of the body and of the acupuncture relief of pain using higher intensities of peripheral stimulation?

Recent electrophysiological studies by Le Bars, Dickenson and Besson seem to provide a basis for the stronger forms of acupuncture acting from far-flung areas of the body. They have found that every convergent neurone either in the spinal cord or the facial equivalent, the trigeminal complex, can be powerfully, and in some cases, completely inhibited by a strong stimulus applied elsewhere on the body. Thus, a convergent neurone with an input from the hindpaw of the animal can be excited by noxious pinch, noxious heat and light touch or electrical stimulation of the incoming peripheral fibres emanating from the defined receptive field of the neurone. If the neurone is steadily activated by one of these inputs, mimicking the state of the neurone in a condition of pain in humans, a strong stimulus applied to the tail, forepaws, ears, nose or elsewhere on the body will inhibit the response of the neurone.

The conditioning stimulus must be at or above the pain threshold and can be natural (mechanical or thermal) chemical or electrical. The inhibitions, so produced, have been described as diffuse noxious inhibitory controls (DNIC) because of their nature. They rely on complex neural loops passing up from the spinal cord and down again from the brain to produce their final effects in the spinal cord. Certain of the neurones modulated by these effects are neurones which project up to the brain via the spinothalmic, the spinoreticular and other tracts, and so their inhibitions can be presumed to alter the quality of the pain sensation. DNIC produce powerful and long-lasting inhibitions of all activities of these neurones whilst other classes of neurones are not influenced. These inhibitions in general outlast the period of application of the peripheral stimulus by several fold and these prolonged post-effects may go towards explaining the long duration of pain relief following acupuncture-like stimulation. But the maximal inhibition still only lasts for four minutes.

Within the limitations of electrophysiological approaches (in that there is the inherent assumption that the activity of neurones represents a functional role) these results demonstrate that both a local and a distant (unrelated either in terms of dermatomes or segments) stimulus can reduce the activity of nociceptive neurones. The local effects seem to depend on innocuous afferent impulses whilst the distant seem to be via high threshold or noxious afferents.

There is now ample clinical and behavioural evidence to support these electrophysiological findings. Early work, originating in the thirties, has amply illustrated the ability of a noxious input to one area of the body to influence the sensation of pain arising from another region. This phenomenon has been illustrated by use of both thermally and mechanically induced pain. In a recent review of the clinical use of peripheral stimulation to reduce the intensity of pain, Andersson has concluded that there are distinct differences, both in terms of causes and effects, between local and distant pain relieving procedures.

The local or segmental mechanisms require low intensity and high frequency stimuli and underlie transcutaneous nerve stimulation (TNS) as used clinically. However, acupuncture-like stimuli require higher intensity and low frequency stimuli and according to Andersson afford a greater relief of pain in terms of both duration and degree of the analgesia.

These conclusions accord well with the neurophysiological evidence for two separate routes of action of peripheral pain relieving stimuli. The distant diffuse acupuncture effects use more complex neural and chemical pathways. This indicates that there are many potentially effective means of influencing pain by tapping into these systems and may explain why attitudes, environment and other psychological variables can interact with acupuncture and pain.

References

Nathan, P. W. The gate control theory of pain. A critical review. Brain, 1976, 99: 123–158.

Le Bars, D., Dickenson, A. & Besson, J. M. Diffuse Noxious Inhibitory Controls (DNIC). I. Effects on dorsal horn convergent neurones in the rat. Pain, 1979, 6: 283–304.

Le Bars, D., Dickenson, A. & Besson, J. M. Diffuse Noxious Inhibitory Controls (DNIC). II. Lack of effect on non-convergent neurones, supraspinal involvement and theoretical implications. Pain, 1979, 6: 305–327.

Andersson, S. A. Pain control by sensory stimulation. Advances in Pain Research and Therapy, Vol. 3, Raven Press, New York, 1979.

Melzack, R. Prolonged relief of pain by brief, intense transcutaneous somatic stimulation. Pain, 1975, 1: 357–373.

Chung, S. H. & Dickenson, A. H. Pain, enkephalin and acupuncture. Nature, 1980, 283–344.

Berlin, S. A., Goodell, B. S. & Wolff, H. G. Studies on pain. A.M.A. Arch. Neurol., 1958, 80: 533–543.

XII

ACUPUNCTURE ANALGESIA:
AN ELUSIVE ENIGMA

Acupuncture was virtually unknown, except in the Far East, before 1971. A small number of doctors were practising therapeutic acupuncture in Europe and Russia; the former had learnt it indirectly via 'colonial' trade, the latter as they were 'fraternal' neighbours.

Most of the doctors practising acupuncture, myself included, were considered part of the lunatic fringe: largely good-natured dreamers, who fooled themselves as much as their patients. We were regarded more as a joke than a pestilence. At that time I gave a certain number of talks at the monthly meetings of local medical societies. Normally these were serious meetings discussing such important topics as surgery of the prostate. Once a year though, there was a ladies' meeting, and it was on this occasion that I gave a lecture—instead of I suppose, a film of Donald Duck.

This was all changed overnight by President Nixon of the United States, who as far as I know was not the slightest bit interested in acupuncture. Unwittingly he transported acupuncture to the West, much as a man may unwittingly carry a flea from one country to another. As far as we are concerned he is the patron saint of acupuncture.

Prior to 1971 there was virtually no contact between the U.S.A. and China. In that year President Nixon inaugerated the 'open doors' policy with China and visited that country. The well-known and respected journalist James Reston went to China at about the same time, had appendicitis which was operated on in China in the normal way with chemical anaesthesia. Postoperatively he had, as is not unusual, some pain which was treated by acupuncture. This was all correctly described by James Reston in a long article in the New York Times and from there spread to the newspapers of the world. I have met many people who read this article with enthusiasm, but somehow they misread it, thinking that the acupuncture had been used for anaesthesia, instead of what was probably only wind pain: the spread of acupuncture to the West was largely brought about by hot air!

At the same time news reached the West that acupuncture was being used in China as an anaesthetic for operations ranging from tonsillectomy to open heart surgery. Most of us in the West, who had been practising acupuncture for several years were surprised, as I doubt if any of us had noticed a patient becoming anaethetised whilst we were treating them for migraine, lumbago or anything else. If one of us had a minor ailment which we had treated ourselves by acupuncture, there was likewise no anaesthesia.

In the early 1960s a comprehensive textbook of acupuncture was published in China which described acupuncture anaethesia for tonsillectomy. After reading all the details carefully I tried this. There was either no anaethesia at all, or so little that it was difficult to recognise.

Then in 1971 the Nixon–Reston bombshell hit us. The acupuncture doctors in the West tried furiously to imitate the 'success' the Chinese had with acupuncture anaethesia. We thought we had been delinquent pupils of acupuncture, the swine who had not noticed the pearls. Some doctors in the West had spectacular success with acupuncture anaesthesia and wrote textbooks on the subject up to 1000 pages long, gave courses on the technique and thought they would make their colleagues the anaesthetists bankrupt. Some anaethetists thought it was 'better to join them than fight them' and the membership of various acupuncture societies increased astronomically.

The early 1970s were the 'boom years' of acupuncture. It was a time when many did not realise there was a difference between therapeutic acupuncture and the fairy tale world of acupuncture anaesthesia. I remember on one occasion Pan American Airways telephoned to say a Boeing 747 had just arrived at Heathrow, full of American tourists. They all wished to experience acupuncture—and would I treat them (in those days there were virtually no acupuncturists in the U.S.A. outside Chinatown). I wished they had telephoned when I started my practice in 1959. Doctors were so keen to learn the miracle from the East that on occasion one week courses were run, attended by 500 doctors at a time. I was treated as an important personality, something that never happened before, or since. I was seated next to astronauts; gave lectures over the whole world; and was honoured to be met at the airport by a young Californian doctor wearing a suit—he had never owned a suit before.

At the same time somewhat more serious investigation of acupuncture anaesthesia was taking place:

Initially I tried to anaesthetise a friend in the tonsillar area, using the technique described at that time in the Chinese literature, by stimulating Li4 (between the 1st and 2nd metacarpals) and S44 (just proximial to the web between the 2nd and 3rd toes). It had no effect. Later I repeated the procedure and afterwards, by chance, pricked the tonsillar area with a needle. With incredulous surprise my friend realised she felt no pain from the pin prick. She could feel the needle going through the flesh. If she moved her tongue round her mouth or if I put my finger in the tonsillar area it felt normal. Temperature sense was likewise normal and the appearance was normal. Hence it was obvious that only pain was affected, no other sensation. Henceforth it was called acupuncture analgesia, not acupuncture anaesthesia, something I think the Chinese had not clarified at that time. I do not think this result was psychological, as the first attempt had failed. In addition my friend and I (due to the vague Chinese descriptions available to us) had expected a sensation similar to a dental nerve block, in which there is absence of all sensation (analgesia) and an unpleasant swollen feeling.

The surprise about this experiment, confirmed by later experiments, was that neither the patient nor the doctor knows if there is analgesia; or if it is present, where it is. To discover if there is analgesia one must prick the patient from head to toe noting if there are, or are not, any areas of partial or complete analgesia.

A simple technique is to use a 23-gauge hypodermic needle. The pricking should be done with equal force over the whole body, or at least that part of the body under consideration. In my experience the pricks should be firm enough to draw a little blood with say half the pricks. If the pricks are too light the result can be confusing.

In 1971 and 1972 I tried acupuncture analgesia 100 times in 35 friends and patients, which were later published in detail.* In essence the results were rather mediocre, and at the same time difficult to interpret.

In the best group of patients there was a relatively uniform analgesia over a specified area. But even within this analgesic area a certain number of pin pricks revealed normal sensation of pain. There was never the complete analgesia one has with a well-given local anaesthetic. In 1972 I considered that some 10% of patients belonged to this rather badly defined 'best' group. Later I thought I had been too enthusiastic and would now rather suggest 5%.

I investigated with the physiologist Tim Horder two patients who belonged to this best group. We knew (though the patients did not), that if acupuncture point T5, on the posterior aspect of the forearm, is stimulated, there may be analgesia in the ipsilateral chest wall, both anteriorly and posteriorly. We told the patients though that the opposite forearm to the one being needled would become analgesic. When the experiment was then finally performed, both patients noticed that there was no analgesia where they had been told to expect it (the contralateral forearm), but that analgesia was present in the correct area (the ipsilateral chest wall).

The above experiment and also the unexpected discovery of analgesia in the tonsillar area mentioned previously, suggests that at least part of the mechanism of acupuncture analgesia is physiological. This of course does not exclude a psychological factor in addition. Nor does it clarify whether the physiological or psychological factor is dominant.

It was found that the 5% or so of patients who respond well to acupuncture analgesia are the 'strong reactors' mentioned in Chapter IV. In therapeutic acupuncture more than 5% of the population are strong reactors. Acupuncture analgesia is effective among only the best of the strong reactors and hence these patients might be called 'hyper-strong reactors'.

Apart from the 5% hyper-strong reactors, there is a variable proportion of people who have a mild or very mild degree of analgesia. This milder analgesia is usually patchy: rather like the Aegean Sea

---

*Mann, F. B. Acupuncture Analgesia. British Journal of Anasthesia, 1974, 46: 361–4.

studded with islands. In the better patients the analgesia corresponds to the all-enveloping sea; whilst in the less responsive patients the analgesia merely corresponds to the small islands.

Acupuncture analgesia is an interesting neurophysiological phenomenon occurring in hyper-strong reactors. It is of little practical use however. It cannot be completely forgotten, as it does exist—but only just. Whether it could ever be further developed is, I think, rather open to doubt. A surprisingly large number of doctors who practise acupuncture disagree with my rather negative attitude to acupuncture analgesia. Some say the effects are better, some even say the effects are very much better.

Some anaesthetists combine chemical anaesthesia with acupuncture anaesthesia, particularly in frail, elderly, rather ill patients who supposedly might have difficulty in withstanding only normal anaesthetics (although this group of patients require less anaesthetic agents anyway). They are usually given normal premedication, and a 50–50 mixture of gas and oxygen. Electro-acupuncture anaesthesia is done in addition.

Other anaesthetists do the same as the above, but in addition curarise and intubate their patients. In this curarised state they are able to pass much larger currents through the acupuncture needles or electrodes, and hence supposedly the acupuncture has a stronger effect. This would not be possible in a non-curarised patient as his muscles would go into tetanic spasm with a current of this magnitude.

The anaesthetists who use the above techniques think they use only about a third of the dose of chemical agents they would use under normal circumstances. I have discussed this with other anaesthetists, who say that if an anaesthetist is particularly interested in using minimal doses of anaesthesic he is usually able to do so, and particularly in frail, elderly and ill patients. These anaesthetists think the acupuncture contributes very little or nothing to the overall anaesthesia.

Once again, however, the process is tedious, and probably even if it works, is not often a practical proposition. An expert, whether in the Far East or the West, can quite often demonstrate anaesthesia, as he knows how to select the hyper-strong reactor.

SECTION 2

Acupuncture: The Ancient Chinese Art of Healing

CONTENTS

I

GENERAL CONSIDERATIONS

Acupuncture is an ancient Chinese system of medicine in the practise of which a fine needle pierces the skin to a depth of a few millimetres and is then withdrawn. The only thing of real importance in the study of acupuncture is to know at what point to pierce the skin in relation to which disease.

The notion that a pinprick, often in a part of the body far removed from the seat of the disease, can cure an illness is alien to conventional thinking. It is unfortunately the case that some doctors, even when faced with one or several patients who have been cured by acupuncture where their own efforts have been fruitless, refuse to believe the evidence.

The oldest records of acupuncture (acus = needle, punctura = puncture) are to be found on bone etchings of 1600 B.C. The first book of acupuncture, which contains a wealth of detail, is the Hungdi Neiging Suwen written about 200 B.C. It is one of the earliest treatises in Chinese on any subject. *

Acupuncture is not the exclusive possession of the Chinese. The papyrus Ebers of 1550 B.C. is the most important of the ancient Egyptian medical treatises. It refers to a book on the subject of *vessels* which could correspond to the 12 meridians of acupuncture. These vessels certainly could not refer to the arteries, veins or

*Hungdi Neiging Suwen—translated by Professor Ilza Veith as "The Yellow Emperors' Classic of Internal Disease". Published by Williams and Wilkins of Baltimore, 2nd edition.

nerves of the four limbs of the human body. However, my enquiries at the Egyptian Department of the British Museum have not been able to make matters clearer as the ancient Egyptian language is not well enough known to distinguish between the words for 'vessel' and 'meridian'.

The Bantu of South Africa sometimes scratch certain parts of the body to cure disease. In the treatment of sciatica some Arabs cauterise with a hot metal probe a part of the ear. This practice probably corresponds to a lesser known form of acupuncture called Ear acupuncture. Some Eskimos practise simple acupuncture with sharp stones. An isolated cannabalistic tribe in Brazil shoot tiny arrows with a blowpipe at specific parts of the body. The only observer ever to have returned from them thinks that, as the tribe show distinct Mongoloid features, this might also be related to acupuncture. Possibly the cautery practised in mediaeval Europe is also related to the tradition though this was mainly applied at congested or painful places and would therefore correspond to the simplest form of acupuncture in which only the *locus dolenti*, and not the distant part, is stimulated.

The great contribution of the Chinese to the primitive, or probably largely local form of acupuncture mentioned above, is that they have developed a fairly complete systematic method. Catalogued and described in numerous text books, it is taught at university and is reproducible at will under experimental conditions.

In China today the intending medical student can enter a university to learn, as in almost all parts of the world, Western medical practice. Or he can choose to study traditional Chinese medicine in another department of the same university. The student who chooses the Western path also studies the rudiments of the Chinese tradition while the other also follows courses in basic anatomy, physiology, pathology and other modern basic disciplines. Both courses take three to five or even seven years. Very few doctors of one school are also experts of the other, but in some hospitals doctors of each medical culture work together: the surgeon performs the operation, the acupuncturist treats the post-operative retention of urine, thus obviating the need for a catheter, and stimulates the lungs to prevent post-operative pneumonia.

Many Chinese are over impressed by Western medicine for they see that everything that has impelled China, or indeed any other non Western civilisation, into the twentieth century originated in the Western world. Quite literally, everything of practical importance: electricity, cars, mass production factories and the like, derives from the applications of Western science. Without Western technology China would still be where she was 100 years ago, that is in conditions relatively little different from those of 1,000 years ago. The impact of the West has been so great that the Chinese have forgotten even those parts of their own culture which, in certain respects at least, is better than that imported from the 'fair haired, big nosed devils'. One of the very few almost exclusively indigenous discoveries that surpasses its Western equivalent in several respects, is acupuncture. There are many diseases, or physiological dysfunctions, which do not yet amount to a disease, that can be cured by acupuncture and not by Western medicine. Naturally, there are also diseases that can be cured by Western medicine which are intractable to the acupuncturist. The Chinese people themselves often do not sufficiently value the traditional skill of the acupuncturist. They take it too much for granted, much as we in the West take for granted the services of electricity, piped water or rubbish collection, only realising their value when a strike or other action interrupts their functioning.

On occasions the viewpoint moves backwards and forwards between traditional acupuncture and scientific medicine. Acupuncture is for the most part based on observed facts which have been woven into a fairly complete system of medicine by a system of theories. The theories themselves are on some occasions accurate at least insofar as concerns clinical treatment. Not infrequently, however, the theory has been based on philosophical and mystical speculation and can then, often, only be useful as a thread which the mind follows as it weaves together the multitudinous and seemingly isolated threads of factual observation..

Much of what is factually observed in acupuncture could be explained in a way completely different from that of the traditional Chinese account. One example might be a different account by way of the discipline of neurophysiology.

In the chapters that follow I have mentioned nearly all the traditional Chinese theories as I think it is important that they should be known in addition to the neurophysiological facts of today. Furthermore, I suspect that much of what seems mystical nonsense to some, in reality portrays many of the laws of nature (even where these are as yet unknown to us) despite the fact that they are expressed in a language that we might call unscientific.

Some doctors or patients may indeed wonder how one can practise a form of medicine where the theories on which that practise is based are possibly suspect. Just as a doctor will prescribe aspirin because he knows what are its effects in the body of a patient, so an acupuncturist will needle a certain acupuncture point because he knows what the consequent reaction of the body will be. It is of secondary importance to the doctor to know just why it is that aspirin has its specific effects, no matter how intellectually interesting such knowledge might be. At the time of writing little is understood of why the known effects of aspirin take place, yet aspirin, with its simple chemical formula, is the most commonly used drug in the world.

The reader will be made aware by various remarks throughout this book, that I believe neither in the major part of the traditional Chinese theoretical explanation of acupuncture nor even in its practical application where this is based *solely* on traditional theory. Doctors who follow my courses in acupuncture will find that this divergence in both theory and practice is no hindrance to the successful treatment of a large number of diseases occurring in their patients.

Doctors who wish to study acupuncture are welcome to write to me. From time to time I give courses, largely of a practical nature, during which I concentrate on those aspects of the subject that would be difficult to describe in a book.

II

THE ACUPUNCTURE POINTS

In all diseases, whether physical or mental, there are tender areas at certain points on the surface of the body, which disappear when the illness is cured.

These are the so-called acupuncture points.*

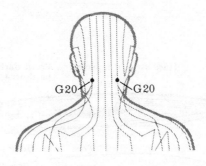

FIG. 2.1

In some cases they will be spontaneously painful. When, for example, a patient suffers from a frontal headache, he will feel pain just lateral to the upper end of the trapezius, a point known as gall bladder 20 (Fig. 2.1). In other cases, however, these points are only tender under pressure, so that there would be no pain at all at, say,

*The anatomical position of the acupuncture points may be seen in my 'Atlas of Acupuncture'.

gall bladder 20 until pressure was applied. To this category belong the many points just above the ankle. Women in particular are unaware how tender this area is unless it is pressed. Thirdly there is the type of acupuncture point where there is no tenderness at all, even under pressure, so that they can only be found by the hand of the experienced physician.

The doctor looking for an acupuncture point will, in the simplest of instances, discover a little nodule, like the fibrositic rheumatic nodules often present at the back of the neck, in the shoulders or in the lumbar area (Fig. 2.2 upper). But in many cases instead of the nodule the examining finger may find a strip of tense muscle within

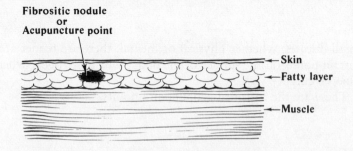

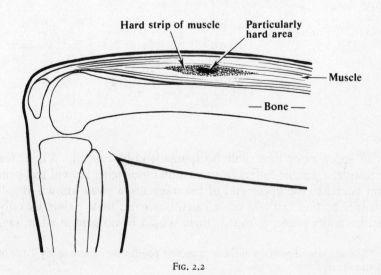

Fig. 2.2

a group of muscles with a particularly hard and indurated area (Fig. 2.2 lower). Sometimes there is an area which is slightly swollen or discoloured. In the most difficult cases the point cannot be found without a knowledge of its exact anatomical position.

Some people use an electrical instrument to measure the electrical

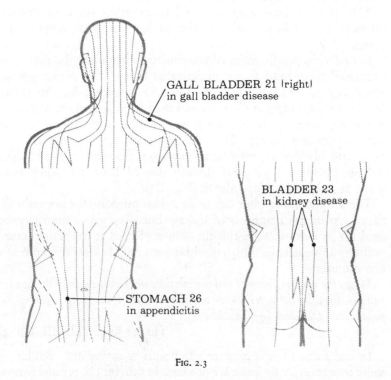

GALL BLADDER 21 (right)
in gall bladder disease

BLADDER 23
in kidney disease

STOMACH 26
in appendicitis

FIG. 2.3

skin resistance or impedance. The theory is that, since the impedance is reduced at the acupuncture points, they can in this way be easily and accurately discovered. I have myself tried several types of experimental apparatus, but have found that the electrical resistance both in living bodies and cadavers varies in so many places, not only at the acupuncture points but thousands of others, that to me this apparatus is not of much use. If the special electrical properties of the nervous system are taken into account, it should be possible to measure some types of electrical variation.

As mentioned above, the pain at those acupuncture points which are either spontaneously tender or tender under pressure vanishes with the cure of the disease. It makes no difference how the cure has been achieved, whether by acupuncture, ordinary drugs, osteopathic manipulation, homeopathy, hypnosis or the mere passage of time: when the illness ends, so also does the pain.

This at once establishes a causal relationship between disease, physical as well as mental, and the tender variety of acupuncture point.

In one very simple form of acupuncture diagnosis, the patient is examined from head to toe in order to find all the tender points, and hence to deduce the internal disease corresponding to them. Some of these points are known and used for diagnosis in orthodox medicine, though of course the average doctor is unaware that these are acupuncture points. Thus the right shoulder, particularly at point gall bladder 21, may be spontaneously tender in gall bladder disease, bladder 23 in renal disease and McBurney's point near point stomach 26 in appendicitis (Fig. 2.3).

The acupuncture points can serve a dual purpose, for not only do they help in the diagnosis of disease but may also conversely be used for its treatment. In this the skin is pierced at the acupuncture point by a fine needle, which is withdrawn usually after the lapse of a few minutes.

When the vision is blurred and the eye does not see, the side of the head is painful, likewise the outer corner of the eye. This is cured by needling the point 'Jaw Detested' (gall bladder 4).

(Jia Yi Jing, Vol. XII, Ch. 4)

In one form of acupuncture the points spontaneously tender or those tender under pressure are needled. In other more refined forms, the acupuncturist needles those points where no pain is felt at all, points which are often remote from the seat of the disease and sometimes even on the opposite side of the body.

Occasionally some wholly accidental stimulus to an acupuncture point may cure a disease. I remember when I was at school seeing a couple of boys fighting together on top of a bed. One of them fell down, hitting his forehead at the root of the nose on the iron bedstead, and was immediately cured of the sinus trouble he had suffered from for two or three years. A parallel case is that of a woman with a dull, though mild, headache accompanied by general malaise, which persisted day after day almost unrelieved for some ten years. During these years she had had several blood tests, which involved pricking the skin to reach a vein at the elbow. She soon noticed that, every time her skin was pricked at this point, the headache and malaise instantly disappeared and for a couple of hours she was free of

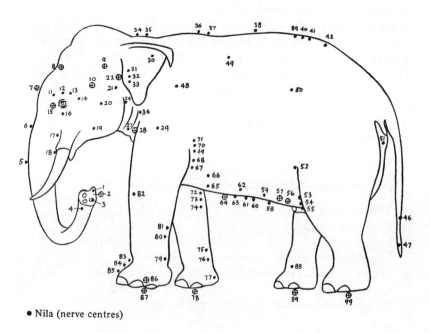

• Nila (nerve centres)

FIG. 2.4

pain. This happened so regularly that she actually began to look forward to her blood tests; but, when she mentioned this to her doctor, tentatively suggesting a connection between the tests and the relief of the headache, he dismissed the idea as nonsensical. When she came to me, I inserted an acupuncture needle into the same place at the elbow. I neither pierced the vein nor drew off any blood; yet the headache at once disappeared, a proof that the cause and effect she had noticed had nothing to do with the loss of blood. She was in time completely cured of her trouble by the additional needling of several other acupuncture points, effective in her particular type of headache.

There are many such apparently accidental correspondences, some of them not generally known. The knock-out points of Judo, for example, are also acupuncture points, which if too strongly stimulated, will cause the subject to collapse in a faint. The Indian points of the Chakras and Nadir similarly correspond to acupuncture points. Deraniyagala, director of the national museums of Ceylon, lists the places which the *mahout*, or Indian elephant boy, prods with a sharp stick to elicit various responses from his elephant* (Fig. 2..4) Having no personal experience here, I do not know if these 'Nila' are really acupuncture points, but at least it seems feasible; and perhaps the reason why the African, unlike the Indian, elephant cannot be adequately trained is because the Nila of the African elephant are unknown.

Some functions of the Nila are as follows:

1. Twists trunk	23. Bends head
2. Straightens trunk	24. Stops animal
3. Frightens	25. Rouses infuriates
4. Frightens and makes trumpet	35. Benumbs
5. Frightens, makes trumpet and stops animal	52. Gets up and runs
	55. Turns round
6. Brings under control	71. Kneels

The drawing of a cow (Fig. 2.5) shows some of the acupuncture points used by Chinese vets in treating animals—cows, horses, pigs and chickens. It will be noted that the points referred to in the cow, as in man, mention diseases, while those on the elephant deal with movements. Possibly the prodding of a sharp stick at the Nila is only a method of training the elephant.

*Some Extinct Elephants, Their Relatives and Two Living Species (Ceylon National Museum Publication).

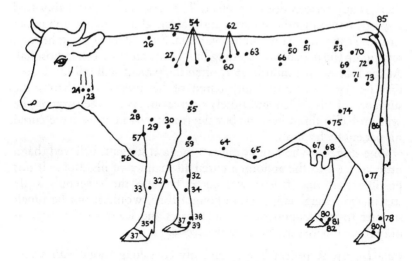

FIG. 2.5 Veterinary acupuncture.

Some acupuncture points on the cow are as follows:

23. 'Hot' disease (Hot, cold, wind, damp are traditional Chinese conceptions)
24. Throat swollen, 'wind' disease of throat
26-29. Disease of front legs due to 'wind' and 'damp'
30. Elbow swollen
32. Front of elbow swollen and painful
33, 34. Knee swollen
38. Heel swollen due to 'wind' and 'damp'
50. Loin swollen

51. Kidney 'cold', disease of lumbar area and back legs
55. Liver and gall bladder disease, spleen swollen
57. Heart and lung disease
59. Pain and discomfort in stomach and abdomen
60. Spleen swollen, lack of appetite
62. Spleen and stomach pain
68. Udder swollen, cannot be milked
70-73. Back leg has disease due to 'wind' and 'damp'

A doctor often has to diagnose mysterious abdominal pains or other symptoms, for which he can find no definite cause. He may therefore suggest to his patient an exploratory operation, in case there is any serious disease present. The surgeon will probably find a spastic colon or mild inflammation of the abdominal lymph nodes or some other not irreversible condition. So he does nothing beyond sewing up the patient and sending him home after a week in hospital. At the follow up a month later, often the patient will tell his doctor that he has been completely cured of his illness, and thanks the surgeon for his skilled and timely operation. As for the surgeon, he will probably think in some bewilderment that he must have cured his patient by hypnosis.

One surgeon who taught me as a medical student, believed that a little air let into the abdomen cured all manner of ills. But is it not possible that the patient was cured because the surgeon's knife stimulated several acupuncture points? If so, would it not be much simpler to try acupuncture in such cases and leave to the surgeon only those where surgery is really necessary?

Case History. A patient limped into my consulting room with severe pain in the lower back and leg due to a slipped disc. Physiotherapy, a corset and traction had been tried to no avail. The next attempt on the agenda was a major operation to fuse several vertebrae.

I tried acupuncture and the patient was soon cured, but he still has to be careful lifting heavy weights. In some cases where the disc is severely prolapsed, an operation may be the only answer, but everything, including acupuncture, should be tried first.

Case History. A lady in her late thirties had severe menorrhagia (called in Chinese 'bursting and leaking disease'). She was anaemic, weak and often had to stay at home. No treatment had helped and her gynaecologist suggested a hysterectomy. Acupuncture cured her—and she still has her womb today.

If the menorrhagia is caused by large fibroids, a growth or certain other conditions, surgery or radiation is often the best treatment. In the majority of instances menorrhagia is due to a mild dysfunction of the uterus or endocrine system, which can often be cured or helped by acupuncture.

III

THE MERIDIANS

The means whereby man is created, the means whereby disease occurs, the means whereby man is cured, the means whereby disease arises: the twelve meridians are the basis of all theory and treatment.

(Ling Shu, jingbie pian)

In Chinese literature there are descriptions of about a thousand acupuncture points, though there may well be even more than this. Books on the subject are full of accounts of illnesses which can be cured or alleviated by stimulating with a needle one or other of these points. The point called bladder 7 (Fig. 3.1) for instance, near the top of the head with the picturesque Chinese name of Penetrating Heaven, has an effect on :-

Headache, heaviness of head, glands swollen in the neck, nose blocked, epistaxis, rhinorrhoea, loss of smell due to catarrh, swelling of the face,

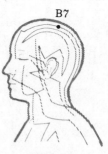

FIG. 3.1

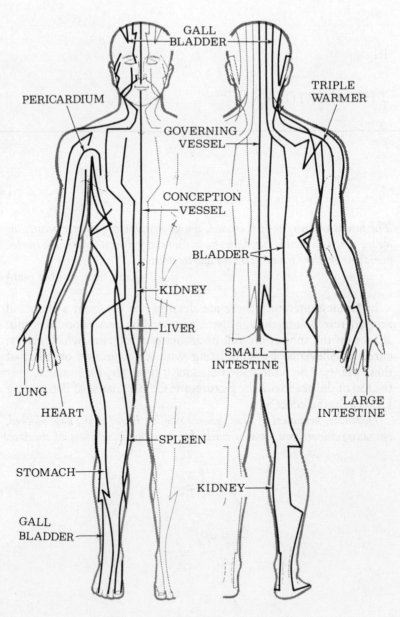

GALL
BLADDER

PERICARDIUM

TRIPLE
WARMER

GOVERNING
VESSEL

CONCEPTION
VESSEL

BLADDER

KIDNEY

LIVER

SMALL
INTESTINE

LUNG

HEART

LARGE
INTESTINE

SPLEEN

STOMACH

KIDNEY

GALL
BLADDER

Fig. 3.2

*neuralgia of the face, breathlessness, chronic bronchitis, dry mouth, thirstiness, epileptic-like convulsions, lack of balance, weak eyesight.**

Since it is obviously difficult to remember the properties of so large a number of acupuncture points, the Chinese classified them into twelve main groups and a few subsidiary ones. All the acupuncture points belonging to any one of these groups are joined by a line, the Chinese word for which (Jing) means a passage, or nowadays forms part of the word for a nerve. In the West it is called a meridian. The meridians on one side of the body are duplicated by those on the other, just as we have a left as well as a right thumb; but there are two extra meridians, which, since they run up the middle of the body cannot of course be thus paired.

The twelve main meridians are those of the (Fig. 3.2):—

lung	bladder
large intestine	kidney
stomach	pericardium
spleen	triple warmer
heart	gall bladder
small intestine	liver

(There is also the governing vessel and conception vessel - see later.)

The number of acupuncture points along each of these meridians varies, the heart meridian, for example, having nine points on each side (Fig. 3.3) while the bladder meridian has sixty seven. All the acupuncture points on a meridian affect the organ after which they are named.

Case History. A patient suffered from recurrent palpitations and a feeling of pressure across the chest, sometimes during periods of slight mental or physical stress, sometimes for no apparent reason. She easily became breathless walking upstairs, had less than her normal energy and was therefore compelled to rest during the daytime, which meant that she found it harder to get through the day's work.

These symptoms were clearly due to a heart condition; so a needle was inserted at the acupuncture point heart 7 (Fig. 3.3all: l ﹐ ﹐ e Chinese the 'gateway of the spirit', since the spirit was thought to live in the heart. Within a few minutes the symptoms were alleviated and, after half a dozen repetitions of the treatment at fortnightly intervals, the patient was cured.

*Taken from: The Treatment of Disease by Acupuncture.

Clearly this system of classifying a thousand acupuncture points into twelve main (and two extra) meridians is in practice very useful, for if, as in the above instance, a patient has a disease of the heart, one immediately knows which group (meridian) of acupuncture

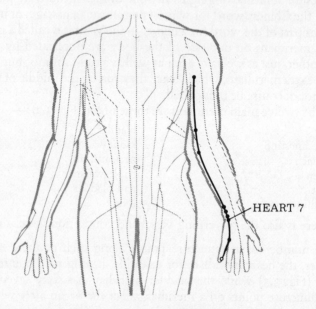

—HEART 7

Fig. 3.3 Heart meridian on left showing its acupuncture points. Heart 1 (under armpit) along the arm to heart 9 (at end of little finger).

points to use. In this case acupuncture point 7 was used, though any of the other eight points on the heart meridian would have helped, but to a lesser extent. The acupuncture point which has the greatest curative effect in a particular disease or on a particular patient is discussed later in the course of this book.

'The kidney meridian starts at the sole of the foot. . . When it is diseased, the face turns black as charcoal, there is loss of appetite, coughing of blood, harsh panting, a wish to get up when sitting down, the eye cannot see clearly, the heart feels as if suspended.'

(Jia Yi Jing, Vol. II, Ch. 1a)

THE TWELVE SPHERES OF INFLUENCE IN THE BODY

The Thunder God said, 'I would like to know about the course and diseases of meridians, and how through them one may cure by acupuncture.'

The Yellow Emperor answered, 'The meridian is that which decides over life and death. Through it the hundred diseases may be treated.'

(Jia Yi Jing, Vol. II, Ch. 1a)

The twelve organs and their associated twelve meridians encompass all parts of the body, with the exceptions of the head and sense organs, the endocrine glands, the reproductive system, and others. Nevertheless, these can all be successfully treated, for (though not directly counted among them) they all belong to one or more than one of the twelve main meridian groups.

The Main Meridian

Anything that happens along or near the course of a main meridian will influence that meridian and the organ which bears its name.

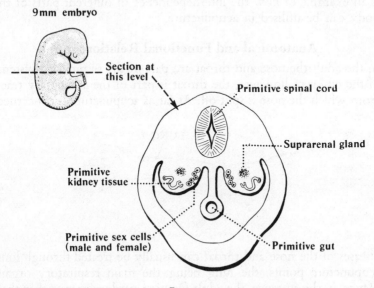

FIG. 3.4

Case History. A patient who had been troubled with palpitations and breathlessness for two months, came to consult me, thinking she had a disease of the heart. In the course of our conversation, she mentioned that two days before the onset of the symptoms she had sprained her wrist, and I found that the place where the tenderness was most acute crossed the heart meridian at acupuncture point 7 (Fig. 3.3). The constant irritation at this point over several days had in turn affected the heart. In this instance the patient was cured of her heart symptoms by treating the sprained wrist rather than by a direct treatment of the heart. The similarity between this case history and that a few pages back, which was concerned with a genuine disease of the heart, should be noted.

Embryological Relationships

When acupuncture points on the kidney meridian are stimulated, they affect not only the kidney but also embryologically related organs, such as the ovary, testicle, uterus, fallopian tube and, to some extent, the adrenal. This is because all these organs are formed in the same region of the embryo—the region of the kidney. This intimate relationship in the embryo is maintained in the adult, at least in so far as kidney acupuncture points are concerned (Fig. 3.4).

This, only one among hundreds of embryological relationships, is an example of how the interdependence of different parts of the body can be utilised in acupuncture.

Anatomical and Functional Relationships

In the adult the nose and throat are part of the respiratory system; in the embryo, however, the throat is part of the alimentary tract, from which the nose is split off. As far as acupuncture is concerned,

LUNG 7

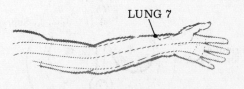

FIG. 3.5

diseases of the nose and throat can usually be treated through lung acupuncture points, the lung being the main respiratory organ. Hence, in this instance, the adult function predominates rather than the embryological relationship described in the previous section. Nasal catarrh, or hay fever, for example, may be treated in this way by using acupuncture point lung 7 (Fig. 3.5), though as a rule a few accessory points are also needed.

Physiological Relationships

The stimulation of one of the fourteen paired acupuncture points on the liver meridian will improve an obvious hepatic disease, like jaundice; but several other ailments less evidently from this source can also be cured or alleviated, such as:—

Migraine, a condition which makes the patient feel nauseated and bilious—and indeed was once known as 'the megrims' or bouts of biliousness.

Cyclic vomiting in children; and what is commonly called 'feeling liverish'.

Certain allergic conditions, such as nettle-rash, asthma and hay fever. Some of the antibodies are manufactured in the liver.

Gout, which is a metabolic disease of the liver.

A tendency to bruise easily, presumably because a weak liver will not produce enough prothrombin, or other clotting agents.

Weak eyesight, pain in, behind or round the eyes and black spots or zig-zags floating in front of them. The traditional Chinese belief in the relationship between eyes and liver may explain this condition.

An inability to wake fresh and alert in the morning, however early one has gone to bed, is often due to the liver.

Some weakness or disorder of the liver is commonly (though not invariably) at the root of all these troubles.

Case History. A photographer had suffered from migraine for about twenty years. The attacks would come on him once or twice a week, sometimes lasting throughout the day, so that, though he often forced himself to carry on with his work, he was equally often compelled to give up and retire to bed in a darkened room. This meant that he could never be sure of fulfilling his obligations.

When he came to me, I treated him by needling acupuncture points liver 8 and a related point, gall bladder 20 (Fig. 3.6). The relationship of these two points illustrates, to the acupuncturist, the known physiological interaction between the liver and the gall bladder.

I treated the patient ten times at these two points. As a result, though he

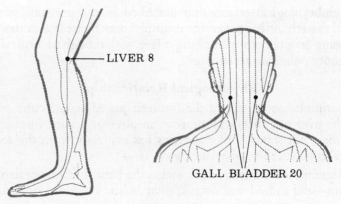

FIG. 3.6

still has an attack of the migraine about four times a year, he is otherwise well.

Branches of the Main Meridian

The main meridian has various subsidiary branches supplying areas of the body adjacent to it. The dotted line in Fig. 3.7 shows how the branch of the heart meridian traverses the lungs, goes to the big blood vessels entering and leaving the heart, penetrates the diaphragm and connects with the small intestine. Another part of this branch travels through the throat to the eye. It is not hard to see how the main meridian's sphere of influence is enlarged by its various branches.

Case History. An elderly woman came to see me some years ago complaining of her eyes, which were red, tender and sensitive to strong light. The stimulation of acupuncture point heart 3 at the elbow cured this condition, presumably because the upper branch of the heart meridian connects with the eye.

Indirect Course of the Main Meridian

Normally the course of the main meridian is taken as the line connecting various acupuncture points along the same meridian. The liver meridian, for example, runs over the inside of the leg and over the abdomen, thus influencing diseases along its course. It also influences not only diseases of the liver itself but those related to the liver by physiology, embryology, anatomy, function etc.

In reality the route taken by the liver meridian is much less direct. It changes its course by joining acupuncture points of other meridians above the ankle and in the lower abdomen, making a detour to the reproductive organs, which the direct course merely bypasses (Fig. 3.8). It can be compared to a traffic diversion on the original London to Brighton road becoming later on the main through route.

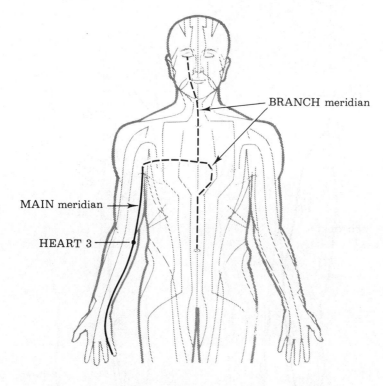

FIG. 3.7

Case History. A patient had painful periods, which caused her to remain in bed two days a month. Being a pharmacist by profession, she had tried various drugs unavailingly. I needled her once a month, halfway between the periods, at liver 8 on the inside of the knee till, after six treatments, she was cured and has been free of pain for the last ten years. From an acupuncture point of view one could say the cure was effected because the indirect course of the liver meridian goes to the reproductive organs.

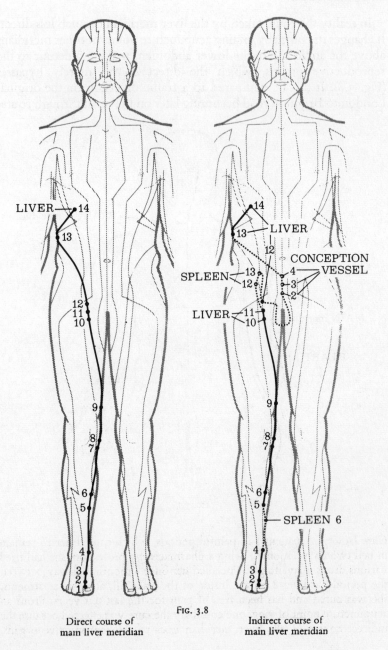

FIG. 3.8

Direct course of
main liver meridian

Indirect course of
main liver meridian

Other Types of Meridians

The other, more specialised, types of meridians (connecting meridians, muscle meridians, divergent meridians, extra meridians) are discussed in my other book—The Meridians of Acupuncture. The main meridian is of incomparably greater importance than the others. In total there are:

The 12 main meridians and their branches.
The 8 extra meridians
The 12 muscle meridians
The 12 divergent meridians
The 15 connecting meridians

IV

THE ENERGY OF LIFE—QI*
including
THE EIGHT BODILY FORCES
OR SUBSTANCES

The ancient Chinese made no precise distinction between arteries veins, lymphatics, nerves, tendons or meridians. They were concerned rather with a system of forces in the body, those forces which enable a man to move, to breathe, to digest his food, to think. As in other so-called primitive systems of medicine, like the Egyptian or the Aztec, the anatomical structures which make these physiological processes possible were not described in detail. They concentrated instead on this elaborate system of forces, whose interplay regulated all the functions of the body.

In Western medicine we have an intricate knowledge of anatomy, microscopic anatomy, the chemistry and biochemistry of the body, but little knowledge of what actually makes it 'tick'. It was this energy at the roots of all life which was the primary interest of the ancient Chinese.

LIFE ENERGY (QI)
Qi (life energy) is one of the fundamental concepts of Chinese thought. The manifestation of any invisible force, whether it be the growth of a plant, the movement of an arm or the deafening

*Pronounced chee as in cheese.

thunder of a storm, is called Qi: though, as we shall see, there are many varieties of it, each with its own specific function. In Hindu terminology the nearest equivalent to Qi is 'Prana'; in Theosophy and Anthroposophy it is called the 'Ether' or 'Etheric Body'.

Qi in the human body is called True Qi, and is created by breathing and eating. The Qi inhaled with the air is extracted by the lungs; the Qi in food and water by the stomach and its associated organ, the spleen.

'*True Qi is a combination of what is received from the heavens and the Qi of water and food. It permeates the whole body.*'

(Ling Shu, cilie zhenxie pian)

Western medicine would explain death from asphyxiation as due to lack of air and death from starvation or dehydration to lack of food or water. The ancient Chinese neither ignored nor denied these obvious physical facts but they did not consider them the complete explanation. That must include the lack of the vital energy of life. The inability of the body to extract Qi from air, food and water is just as much a cause of death as its deprivation of them.

In these particular instances it is clear that the physical and metaphysical phenomena, deriving from the same source, cannot readily be distinguished. In others the difference can be more easily observed.

'*True Qi is the original Qi. Qi from Heaven is received through the nose and controlled by the wind-pipe; Qi from food and water enters the stomach and is controlled by the gullet. That which nourishes the unborn is the Qi of former heaven (pre-natal); that which fills the born is called the Qi of the latter heaven (post-natal)*'.

(Zhangshi leijing)

Qi is universal:—

'*The root of the way of life (Dao or Tao), of birth and change is Qi; the myriad things of heaven and earth all obey this law. Thus Qi in the periphery envelops heaven and earth, Qi in the interior activates them. The source wherefrom the sun, moon and stars derive their light, the thunder, rain, wind and cloud their being, the four seasons and the myriad things their birth, growth, gathering and storing: all this is brought about by Qi. Man's possession of life is completely dependent upon this Qi.*'

(Zhangshi leijing)

Before a mother can conceive and the foetus develop, her body, according to the Chinese, must be in harmony. The two extra meridians called the Vessel of Conception and the Penetrating Vessel should be active and the umbilical cord properly functioning. Only then can the Qi of former heaven be adequately received by the mother. After birth the Qi of Former Heaven is cut off, as the baby begins to take in from the air it breathes and from digestion of food and water the Qi of Latter Heaven.

Qi activates all the processes of the body, '*the unceasing circulation of the blood, the dissemination of fluid in skin and flesh, joints and bone-hollows, the lubrication of the digestive tract, sweating, urination, etc.*' In Chinese treatises on acupuncture the effect of pricking the skin with a needle is called 'obtaining Qi' and if the needle fails to obtain Qi (which is often indicated by various signs and symptoms) the acupuncture treatment will be ineffective.

'*Thus one is able to smell only if Lung Qi penetrates to the nose; one can distinguish the five colours only if Liver Qi penetrates to the eyes; one can taste only if Heart Qi penetrates to the tongue; one can know whether one likes or dislikes food only if Spleen Qi penetrates to the mouth.*'

'*The capabilities of the seven holes (eyes, ears, nose and mouth) depend upon the penetration of the Qi from the five solid organs*' (as mentioned in the preceding paragraph).

(Zhongyixue gailun)

'*That which was from the beginning in heaven is Qi; on earth it becomes visible as form; Qi and form interact, giving birth to the myriad things.*'

(Su Wen, tianyuanji dalun)

The cycle of changes which results from the interaction of Qi and form is what the Chinese meant when they described the 'transformation of air, food and water into Qi, blood and other substances. This is the transformation at work in the rhythms of growth and decay, in the changes from the flower to the fruit or the child to the old man.

The meridians are the tracks along which travel many of the impulses mentioned above—or, as the Chinese put it, '*the meridians are the paths of the transforming action of Qi in the solid and hollow organs.*'

(Yijiang jingyi)

The word Qi in Chinese has, besides 'Life Energy', the further meaning of 'Air'. Only over the last hundred years, since it became possible to weigh air by creating a true vacuum, has it been defined as physical. To the Chinese air was non-material and could therefore only be a vehicle for the forces of energy. Thus they often use the phrase 'bad Qi' for what we, more prosaically, would call a bad smell. This double meaning of air and energy may be an explanation of the breathing exercises in Indian Yoga; the Chinese use a similar system to obtain Qi.

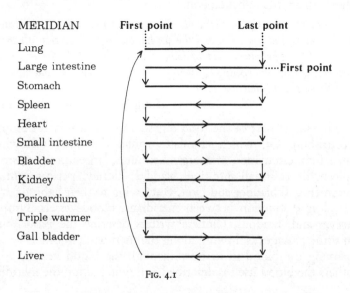

FIG. 4.1

The lungs are principally concerned with the Qi of the whole body. The spleen is concerned with the middle Qi, via its coupled organ the stomach which obtains the Qi from food. The kidney's Qi determines the hereditary constitution, as the production of semen and ova is largely determined by the kidney. (See section on the kidney in The Meridians of Acupuncture).

The meridian cycle begins with that of the lungs as Qi enters there. Also the Qi from the digestion of food and water in the stomach goes via the spleen to the lungs. Thus from the lungs, Qi of both sources is distributed around the body via the meridians in a certain order. Starting with the first point (or point of entry) of the lung meridian, thence to the last point (or point of exit) of the lung meridian, to the first point (or point of entry) of the large intestine meridian etc. (Fig. 4.1).

NOURISHING QI (YING QI)

Qi is not stationary in the body; it circulates much as the blood has since the time of Harvey, been known to circulate. This circulation is of two main types: that of Nourishing Qi, through the meridians and blood-vessels, and that of Protecting Qi, between the skin and the flesh in the subcutaneous tissues.

'*Man receives Qi in his food. Qi, entering the stomach, is transmitted to the lungs, the five solid and the six hollow organs, so that all these may receive Qi. The purer part of food is Nourishing Qi, the less pure part Protecting Qi, Nourishing Qi being within the meridians and blood-vessels and Protecting Qi outside them.*'

(Ling Shu, yingwei shenghui pian)

The purest part of the food digested in the stomach becomes the Nourishing Qi, which circulates round the body following the superficial circulation of energy, i.e. lungs, large intestines, stomach, spleen, heart, small intestine, bladder, kidney, pericardium, triple warmer, gall bladder and liver. But owing to their habit of drawing no clear distinction between meridians, blood-vessels, lymphatics, nerves and tendons, Chinese writers describe the Nourishing Qi in some passages as flowing along the meridians, in others as accompanying the blood in its flow through the blood vessels, while in others the blood itself is described as flowing along the meridians.

PROTECTING QI (WEI QI)

The Protecting Qi complements the Nourishing Qi and, like it, is formed by the digestion of food and water in the stomach (and spleen) and distributed thence to the rest of the body. But while the Nourishing Qi is distilled from the purest elements, the Protecting Qi emerges from the coarser products of digestion, and because of this crude origin has rougher and more aggressive properties. It therefore cannot penetrate the delicate meridians and vessels but instead circulates in the subcutaneous tissues:—

Wei Qi is the fierce Qi of food and water. Trembling, urgent, slippery, sharp, it cannot enter the vessels and meridians but travels between the skin and flesh, vaporises in the diaphragm and scatters in the chest and abdomen.'

(Su Wen, bi lun)

'Wei comes out of a restless urgency of the fierce Qi and at first moves incessantly in the four limbs between the skin and flesh.'

(Ling Shu, xieke pian)

The protecting Qi warms the subcutaneous tissues, moistens the skin, controls the opening and closing of the pores and nourishes the space between the skin and the flesh. But its most important function is the protection of the body from 'outside invading evils'. (See chapter X). If, for example, wind and cold invade the body, it meets the invasion by producing the desire for warmth and the manifestations of fever. Sweat is emitted, the fever subsides and the invading forces are dispersed. If, on the other hand, the invasion is successful, the patient will fall a victim to the disease.

When the Protecting Qi is too weak to permeate the subcutaneous tissues, the meridians will become empty and hollow, the flow of blood sluggish and uneven, the skin and flesh inadequately nourished·

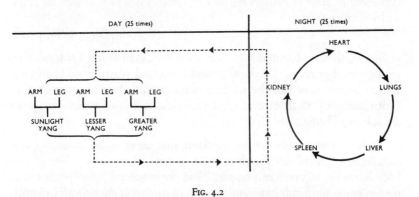

FIG. 4.2

The patient may then become a sufferer from rheumatism; or, if the wind cold and damp remaining in the body affect the meridians, vessels and joints, from an attack of arthritis.

The Nourishing Qi comes into the same category as the Yin, since it is composed of a rarefied substance and circulates with the blood in the interior of the body. The Protecting Qi could be classified under Yang, since it is composed of coarser elements, circulates in the surface of the body and is associated not with the blood-stream but with Qi. (See chapter V).

It is said that the Protecting Qi every 24 hours completes 50 cycles in the body, 25 cycles parallel with the Yang during the day and 25 parallel with the Yin during the night (Fig. 4.2). When it circulates through the Yang meridians in the daytime, it passes through those of the large intestine, the stomach, the triple warmer, the gall bladder, the small intestine and the bladder, in that order. Similarly at night, when it circulates through the Yin meridians, it passes from the kidney to the heart and thence to the lungs, the liver and finally the spleen.

THE BLOOD

'The middle warmer receives Qi, extracts the liquid and turns it red. This is called blood.'

(Ling Shu, juequi pian)

'Nourishing Qi collects fluid and pours it into the vessels, changing it into blood in order to nourish the four extremities and to flow into the solid and hollow organs.'

(Ling Shu, xieke pian)

Blood, then, is formed together with the Nourishing Qi from the process of digestion. To the digested food and water fluid is added, which becomes red in the middle warmer and then flows with the Nourishing Qi in its circuit of the meridians, blood vessels, organs, muscles and bones.

'Only if the vessels are so regulated that there is an uninterrupted circulation of blood can the skin, flesh, muscles, bones and joints of the body be strong, vigorous and supple. Thus the reason why the eyes can see, the feet walk, the hands grasp and the skin sweat is that they are all irrigated by blood.'

(Zhongyixue gailun)

Qi is thought to control the movement of the blood. *'Qi is the general of the blood; if Qi moves, then the blood moves.'* Along the meridians and blood vessels blood and Nourishing Qi travel together.

'If the blood vessels and meridians are empty, so that the flesh cannot

obtain nutriment from blood and Nourishing Qi, symptoms of pain, itching and numbness will result.'

Or again:—

'*If an evil invades the blood vessels, then the movement of the Nourishing Qi is hindered and the blood remains blocked within the flesh, causing symptoms of swelling.'*

It is said that, in addition to Ying Qi, 'blood' also circulates in the meridians, the Ying Qi representing the Yang element, the 'blood' representing the Yin element. Each meridian has a certain proportion of Qi and 'blood' but the proportions differ, as may be seen from the following table:

SUNLIGHT YANG	More	Qi	More	GREATER YIN
	More	Blood	Less	
LESSER YANG	More	Qi	Less	ABSOLUTE YIN
	Less	Blood	More	
GREATER YANG	Less	Qi	More	LESSER YIN
	More	Blood	Less	

Heart – its principal function is blood
Spleen – gathers blood
Liver – stores blood

LIFE ESSENCE: ESSENCE AND SEMEN (JING)

The Chinese distinguished two types of the creative force (Jing) in the human body:—

(1) Jing—Essence

This type of the Life Essence is formed, (as is also the second type, the semen Jing) in the same way as the other bodily substances, by the transforming action of Qi on the food and water in the stomach and spleen. Thereafter it is stored in the kidneys. Whenever Life Essence is required, the kidneys inject it into the body so that it can circulate through the remaining organs. Thus, whenever the 'six evils' or 'seven emotions' (see chapter X) attack the body and injure it, they inevitably also injure this Life Essence.

(2) Jing—Semen

The semen type of Jing is present in both male and female, represented in the male by the spermatozoa, in the female by the ova:

'In the creation of man, appears first the Life Essence.'

(Ling Shu, jinjmo pian)

An embryo is formed by the union of male and female semen Jing. The essence resulting from this union, which nourishes the foetus, is known as the 'life essence of former heaven'. After birth, the child is nourished by the 'life essence of latter heaven' (derived from the food and water digested in the stomach) which also helps in the formation of Qi, Nourishing Qi, Protecting Qi, and blood.

According to the Chinese, the 'semen life essence' becomes mature in girls at the age of 14 (two periods of seven years), in boys at the age of 16 (two eight-year periods). Likewise the menopause occurs in women after seven seven-year periods at the age of 49, while the equivalent happens in man after eight eight-year periods at 64. Thus, ideally, a woman is able to reproduce between the ages of 14 and 49, a man between 16 and 64.

SPIRIT (SHEN)

Shen is usually translated as 'spirit', a word which to the Western mind more often than not suggests the supernatural. But Shen, in common with most other concepts in traditional Chinese thought, is a down-to-earth word. The spirit is created by the normal processes of reproduction: it needs man's heart as a house to live in; it must have food and water to nourish it and, if it is unable to function properly, the result will be actual physical disease.

'The origin of Life is in the Life Essence (the male and female semen). When these two unite to make one, that is called the Spirit.'

(Ling Shu, benshen pian)

'Basically the Spirit is the Life Essence Qi derived from food and water.'

(Ling Shu, pingren juegu)

'The five tastes enter the mouth and are stored in the stomach and intestines, in order to nourish the five Qi. The five Qi then unite creating

fluid, and the Spirit is then formed as a natural consequence of this process.
(Su Wen, liujie zangxiang lun)

Born from the union of male and female semen, sustained in its earthly existence by food and water, the Spirit dwells in the heart, while other human attributes inhabit other organs:—

'The heart houses the Spirit, the lungs the Animal Soul, the liver the Spiritual Soul, the spleen the Mind and the kidneys the Will.'
(Su Wen, xuanming wuqi lun)

It is for this reason that a cardiac disease affects the Spirit to a greater degree than one elsewhere in the body. The physical functions of the Spirit are well documented in Chinese literature:—

'At a hundred years of age the five solid organs are empty, the Spirit and the Qi have gone completely and form alone exists; that is all.'
(Ling Shu, tiannian pian)

'Whoever has the Spirit, flourishes; whoever loses the Spirit, perishes.'
(Su Wen, yijing bianqi lun)

Or (to put it as the Chinese might have done) the seeing of the eyes, the hearing of the ears, the speaking of the mouth, the movement of the limbs and body, the consciousness and activity of the mind, all are manifestations of the Spirit informing the flesh. If the Spirit is weak, the eyes are dull, the vitality exhausted; in severe cases the speech may become abnormal and the mind so affected as to cause hallucinations and delusions, agitation, delirium and unconsciousness.

FLUID

The amount of Fluid in the body chiefly depends on the amount of food and water digested. The liquid in the stomach is metabolised by the action of the Yin Fluid already there and, as a result, takes on a special quality which differentiates it from water outside the body. It is living water; it has 'acquired Life Essence'.

This Chinese doctrine that Fluid is, as it were, a living individual entity means that the amount of Fluid in the body is as important as its quality. Too much or too little upsets the Yin-Yang balance within the system. So Fluid is regulated by various organs. The lungs control the process of energising by the action of Qi, the kidneys the amount of water to be used or rejected, the bladder stores the Fluid and the triple warmer manages the drainage. It is said, too, that the small intestine divides the liquid into 'pure' and 'impure', the 'pure' becoming Fluid and being distributed for the nourishment of the rest of the body, the 'impure' passing into the bladder to be excreted. The seasons also influence the amount of Fluid in the body, for perspiration increases in the hot weather and urination in the cold. Any failure in this system of control and response can lead to illness and it is said that the oedema and diabetes are both diseases of Fluid.

The Chinese distinguish two types of Fluid, the Clear Fluid (Jin), which is of the nature of Yang and circulates with the Protecting Qi, and the Thick Fluid (Ye), which is Yin and circulates with the Nourishing Qi and the blood in the blood vessels.

'*When the pores leak and sweat is emitted, it is called Clear Fluid.*'

'*Thick Fluid is poured into the bones, so that they have the property of bending and stretching; if broken, they leak Thick Fluid.*'

(Ling Shu, juenqi pian)

The Clear Fluid, then, moistens the flesh and skin and exudes as normal sweat; the Thick Fluid keeps the sinews pliant, lubricates the joints, fills the marrow of the bones and the hollows of the brain and exudes on to the surface of the body as the greasy excretion of the sweat glands.

By the action of the middle warmer Fluid and Nourishing Qi become blood and each of the five solid organs likewise has a transforming effect on the Fluid. The liver transforms it to tears, the heart to sweat, the spleen to saliva, the lungs to mucus, the kidneys to urine.

CORRELATIONS OF THE EIGHT BODILY HUMOURS

In harmony with the general nature of Chinese thought, the eight bodily humours are seen as interdependent, not isolated: some of them wax while others are waning, some wax or wane together. The inter-related effects vary according to circumstances.

Qi is the great energiser. It causes the blood to circulate and the Fluid to be disseminated throughout the body and excreted as urine and sweat. It transforms the food we eat into Life Essence, blood, Fluid, etc. and the organs of the body are active only because these elements which transfuse them have been energised by Qi. It activates the process of digestion and regulates the capacity of the intestines to absorb only those substances which the body needs and to excrete the remainder.

In Chinese texts it is often not possible to distinguish between blood and Nourishing Qi, for they both flow along various pathways (blood vessels, meridians, etc.) to nourish the body and, if the flow of the one is interrupted so is that of the other, with the result in each case of symptoms of 'pain, itching and numbness'.

Blood and Nourishing Qi are the basic constitutents of what the Chinese call Jingshen, a combination of Life Essence and Spirit which might be translated as 'Vitality' in both its mental and physical aspects. This is an example of a Vitality disease caused by an excessive loss of blood after childbirth:—

'When a woman has given birth, fluid has been lost, the blood is empty and the mind weak, causing her Vitality to become confused, her speech delirious etc., and, in extreme cases, resulting in madness. This may be treated by tonifying the blood and stimulating the heart, pacifying the heart and stimulating the mind.'

(Guaiji zonglu chanhoumen)

A man whose Vitality is excessive will be prone to violent rages, sometimes so violent that, as the blood and Qi surge upwards, he will actually vomit blood. Moreover, if the Spirit is not at ease then the heart in which it dwells will be uneasy also and the blood and Nourishing Qi weak.

In comparing blood and Nourishing Qi with Qi and Protecting Qi, the Chinese held that the first two nourish the interior of the body, while the second two protect its surface. Each of these pairs assists the other; for nourishment cannot proceed if the surface of the body is unprotected and, without nourishment, the forces protecting the surface cannot do so. It is not wise, in other words, to fight a war on two flanks. Although in this context it is the function of the Qi to protect the exterior and of the blood to nourish the interior of the body, in another sense the functions are not separate but interchanged; for the blood is also nourishing the skin on the surface while the Qi energises the organs within.

'Yin in the interior is the guardian of Yang; Yang in the exterior motivates Yin.'

(Su Wen, yinyang yingxiang dalun)

It is said that blood is created by Qi and that blood is the basis of Qi.

'*If Qi and blood are not evenly balanced, then Yin and Yang will oppose one another; Qi will rebel against Protecting Qi, blood against Nourishing Qi, blood and Qi will be separated, one being full and the other empty.*'

(Su Wen, tiaojing lun)

To the ancient Chinese, Life Essence Qi and Spirit were 'the three precious things', the basis of all being; for Life Essence is formed from food and water, Qi from food, water and air, and both Qi and Life Essence are combined in Spirit. The Spirit, they said, flourishes in one whose Life Essence and Qi are sufficient; if it does not flourish, then the Life Essence is weak.

'*Although the Spirit is produced from Life Essence and Qi, nevertheless that which governs and selects Life Essence and Qi and controls their function, is the Spirit of the heart.*'

(Zhangshi leijing)

Because of their common origin, a deficiency of Fluid entails a corresponding deficiency of Qi and blood, and vice versa. A patient suffering from excessive sweating, vomiting and diarrhoea, with a resultant loss of Fluid, will also have what the Chinese call 'Qi and blood deficiency symptoms'—shortness of breath, shallow breathing, fine pulse, palpitations and coldness of the limbs. Conversely, a loss of blood will produce 'Fluid deficiency symptoms'—dryness of the mouth, constipation and infrequent micturition. Sweat being a transformation of Fluid, a patient who has lost blood or is otherwise dehydrated cannot easily perspire.

V

THE PRINCIPLE OF OPPOSITES

The Chinese believed that in the beginning the world was a formless indivisible whole. There was no distinction between heaven and hell, fire and water, day and night; there was neither birth nor death, growth nor decay; all imaginable things were merged together without definition in an unchanging unity. Had man existed, he would have remained forever incapable of evolution, a static and perfect image.

For life as we know it to be possible with all its richness and variety, its infinite potentialities for good and ill, this world had to be split in two. The Unity had to become a duality; and from this duality arose the idea of the complementary opposites, the negative and the positive, which the Chinese called the Yin and the Yang. These two principles are at the very root of the Chinese way of life; they pervade all their art, literature and philosophy and are therefore also embodied in their theories of traditional medicine.

These principles are of course, up to a point, accepted in the West. We too divide every phenomenon into its two contrary components. Male and female, hard and soft, good and bad, positive and negative electrical charges, laevorotary and dextrorotary chemical compounds —all these are 'opposites'. It is indeed a fact that nothing can happen in the physical world unaccompanied by positive or negative electrical changes. If a man moves his hand or a raindrop falls or a child rolls a marble across the floor, such changes will affect the balance of positive and negative charges in each of these instances. But in Europe we have not formulated this polarity as a universal law as have the Chinese, to whom the perpetual interplay of the Yin and the Yang is the very keystone of their thinking. It is the law operating throughout all existence that the states of Yin and Yang must succeed one another, so that, in a Yin condition, the corresponding Yang state can be precisely foretold. The practical application of this law to acupuncture can be illustrated thus:—

	Yang	*Yin*
In the natural world:	Day	Night
	Clear day	Cloudy day
	Spring/Summer	Autumn/Winter
	East/South	West/North
	Upper	Lower
	Exterior	Interior
	Hot	Cold
	Fire	Water
	Light	Dark
	Sun	Moon
In the body:	Surfaces of the body	Interior of body
	Spine/back	Chest/abdomen
	Male	Female
	Clear or clean body fluid	Cloudy or dirty body fluid
	Energy (Qi)	Blood
	Protecting Qi	Nourishing Qi
In disease:	Acute/virulent	Chronic/non-active
	Powerful/flourishing	Weak/decaying
	Patient feels hot or hot to touch or has temperature	Patient feels cold or cold to touch or has under-temperature
	Dry	Moist
	Advancing	Retiring
	Hasty	Lingering

The twelve basic organs and meridians are similarly divided into the Yang hollow (Fu) organs, which 'transform but do not retain' and the Yin solid (Zang) organs, which 'store but do not transmit':—

Yin	*Yang*
Liver	Gall bladder
Heart	Small intestine
Spleen (Pancreas)	Stomach
Lung	Large intestine
Kidney	Bladder
Pericardium	Triple warmer

The qualities of Yin and Yang are relative, not absolute. For example, the surface of the body is Yang, the interior Yin. But this relation also remains constant within the body, for the surface of every internal organ is always Yang and its interior always Yin, down to the individual cells that compose it. Similarly, a gas is Yang, a solid Yin; but among the gases the more rarefied are Yang, the denser are Yin. Life and death belong to Yang, growth and storage to Yin, so that 'if only Yang exists, there will be no birth: if only Yin exists, there will be no growth.' The life of every organism depends upon the correct balance of its various components.

'*Yin and Yang are the Tao of heaven and earth (the basic law of opposition and unity in the natural world), the fundamental principle of the myriad things (all things can only obey this law and cannot transgress it), the originators (literally parents) of change (change in all things is according to this law), the beginning of birth and death (the birth and creation, death and destruction of all things begins with this law), the storehouse of Shen Ming (the location of all that is mysterious in the natural world). The treatment of disease must be sought for in this basic law (man is one of the living things of nature, so the curing of disease must be sought for in this basic law).*'

(Su Wen, yinyang yingxiang dalun)

Since everything in life can be classified according to its Yin and Yang components, it is said:—

'*Now the Yin/Yang has a name but no form. Thus it can be extended from one to ten, from ten to a hundred, from a hundred to a thousand, from a thousand to ten thousand (i.e. it can embrace all things).*'

(Ling Shu, yingang xi riyue pian)

Each component not only opposes but also contains its opposite, for :-

'*There is Yin within the Yin and Yang within the Yang. From dawn till noon the Yang of Heaven is the Yang within the Yang; from noon till dusk the Yang of heaven is the Yin within the Yang; from dusk till midnight the Yin of heaven is the Yin within the Yin; from midnight till dawn the Yin of heaven is the Yang within the Yin.'*

(Su Wen, jinkui zhenyan lun)

Thus 'functional movement' belongs to Yang, 'nourishing substance' to Yin, nor can the one exist without the other; for, if the intestines and other internal organs do not move, 'nourishing substances' cannot be digested and, if over a long period 'nourishing substances' are not provided, the organs cease to move.

'Yin in the interior is the guardian of Yang; Yang in the exterior is the activator of Yin.'

(Su Wen, yinyang yingxiang dalun)

The opposition of Yin and Yang is not static; it is a perpetually changing rhythm of movement, whose interplay produces growth, transformation and death.

'The relation of Yin and Yang is the means whereby the myriad things are able to come to birth, Yin and Yang react upon each other, producing change.'

(Su Wen, yinyang yingxiang dalun)

This changing rhythm in the balance of Yin and Yang ensures that there is never an excess of either of these polar opposites, for over-activity of Yang is at once adjusted by the yielding passivity of Yin.

'In Winter on the 45th day (the beginning of spring) the Yang Qi is slightly superior and the Yin Qi slightly inferior; in summer on the 45th day (the beginning of autumn) the Yin Qi is slightly superior, the Yang Qi slightly inferior.'

(Su Wen, maiyao jingwei lun)

In the former case, Yang Qi waxed with the upsurge of spring as Yin Qi waned; in the latter, Yin Qi waxed with the decline to winter as Yang Qi waned.

'When speaking of Yin and Yang, the exterior is Yang, the interior is Yin; when speaking of Yin and Yang in the human body, the back is Yang, the abdomen Yin; when speaking of Yin and Yang of the Zang and Fu in the body, then the Zang are Yin, the Fu are Yang; liver, heart, spleen, lungs and kidney are all Yin, the gall bladder, stomach, large intestine, small intestine, bladder and triple warmer are all Yang.'

'*Thus the back is Yang and the Yang within the Yang is the heart.*
The back is Yang and the Yin within the Yang is the lungs.
The abdomen is Yin and the Yin within the Yin is the kidneys,
The abdomen is Yin and the Yang within the Yin is the liver.
The abdomen is Yin and the extreme Yin within the Yin is the spleen.'
(Su Wen, jinkui zhenyan lun)

If this balance of Yin and Yang is upset there is a reaction:—

'*Excess of Yin causes a Yang disease, excess of Yang a Yin disease.*
Yang in excess produces heat and, if the heat is extreme, it will produce
cold; Yin in excess produces cold and, if the cold is extreme, it will produce
heat.'
(Su Wen, yinyang yingxiang dalun)

In diagnosis:

'*The skilled diagnostician examines the countenance and feels the pulse.*
First dividing them into Yin and Yang, he judges the pure (Yang) and the
impure (Yin) and thus knows the diseased part of the body. . . He feels
the pulse to ascertain whether it is floating (Yang), deep (Yin), slippery
(Yang) or rough (Yin) and knows where the disease originated. If there is
no mistake in his diagnosis then nothing 'will be overlooked.'
(Su Wen, yinyang yingxiang dalun)

In the treatment of disease, if Yang is hot and over-abundant, thus injuring the Yin fluid (Yang excess causing a Yin disease), the surplus Yang can be decreased by a method called 'cooling what is hot'. If Yin is cold and over-abundant, thus injuring the Yang Qi (Yin excess causing Yang disease), the surplus Yin can be decreased by the method called 'heating what is cold'. Conversely, if Yin fluid is deficient and so, unable to control the Yang, causes it to become violent; or if Yang Qi is deficient and, unable to control Yin, causes it to become over-abundant, then the deficiency must be tonified. The Neijing describes the method thus:— '*In Yang diseases treat the Yin; in Yin diseases treat the Yang.*'

Ever since the days of the legendary Yellow Emperor, preventive medicine has to some extent depended on keeping the activities of the body in harmony with the rhythm of the changing seasons. Therefore, as the Su Wen shaggutian zhenlun puts it: '*Harmonise with the Yin and Yang, harmonise with the four seasons.*' And again:—

'*The Yin and the Yang of the four seasons are the basis of the myriad things. Therefore a wise man will nourish Yang in spring and summer, Yin in autumn and winter. Follow this fundamental law and you will be on the threshold of birth and growth; rebel against it and you will destroy its root and harm its truth. For Yin and Yang and the four seasons are the beginning and end of the myriad things, the roots of life and death. If you rebel against them you will destroy life, if you follow them disease will not arise. . . He who follows Yin and Yang will have life; he who rebels against them will die. Obey, and you will be cured; rebel and calamity will follow.'*

(Su Wen, siqi tiaoashen dalun)

The Chinese held that the causes of disease come not only from outside, as, in the above quotation, from a disharmony with the seasons, but also from within the body itself. Foremost among these causes of disease are the emotions:—

'Violent anger injures Yin; violent joy injures Yang.'

(Su Wen, yinyang yingxiang dalun)

Man should live in harmony with heaven and earth for, while his feet rest always on the earth, his mind can reach upwards beyond the remotest stars.

'If you understand, above, the writings of heaven (astronomy): below, the principles of earth (geography): and, in between earth and heaven, the affairs of man: then may you have long life.'

(Zhu zhijiao, pian)

'If in curing the sick you do not observe the records of heaven nor use the principles of earth, the result will be calamity.'

(Yin yang, yingxiang dalun)

This interplay of heaven and earth was thought to be the beginning of all life. Before that there was the Great Void, which nothing created, nothing preceded, nothing sustained, till it was brought into movement by the Great Qi of the universe. Then the Qi of heaven began to descend and the Qi of earth to ascend and from their interplay came change, movement and transformation; and thus there was life. With the beginning of movement came the beginning of silence, the rhythms of activity and quiescence producing more life, further changes.

The intercourse of Qi between heaven and earth resulted in the creation of man.

'*In heaven there is wind, in earth there is wood; in heaven there is heat, in earth there is fire; in heaven there is damp, in earth there is earthiness; in heaven there is dryness, in earth there is metal; in heaven there is cold, in earth there is water; in heaven there is Qi, in earth there is form; form and Qi interact, thus creating the myriad things.*'

(Su Wen, tian yuanji dalun)

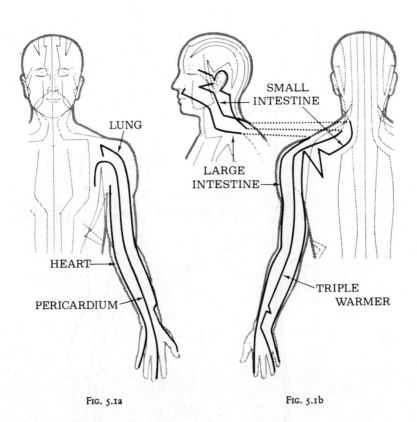

FIG. 5.1a   FIG. 5.1b

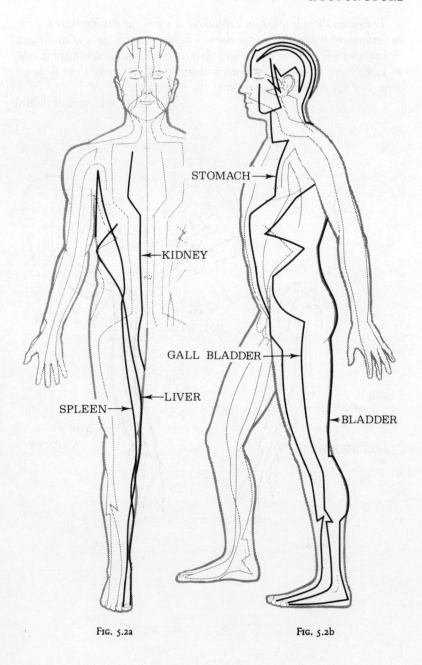

FIG. 5.2a   FIG. 5.2b

YIN-YANG AND THE MERIDIANS

1 (*a*) There are three meridians, the upper Yin (Fig. 5.1a), going from the chest, down the inside of the arm to the tips of the fingers. They are (from inside to outside) the meridians of the heart, pericardium and lung.

(*b*) There are three meridians, the upper Yang (Fig. 5.1b), going from the tips of the fingers, up the external surface of the arm to the face. They are (from the inside to the outside) the meridians of the small intestine, triple-warmer and large intestine.

(*c*) There are three meridians, the lower Yin (Fig. 5.2a), going from the toes, up the inside of the legs, over the abdomen to end on the front of the chest, near the origin of the upper Yin. They are (from the inside to the outside—in adult anatomy) the meridians of the spleen, liver and kidney.

(*d*) There are three meridians, the lower Yang (Fig. 5.2b) going from the head, down the body and the external surface of the legs to the toes. They are (from the inside to the outside—in adult anatomy) the meridians of the stomach, gall bladder and bladder.

2 The Chinese normally speak of the meridians in pairs and they distinguish the members of each pair by reference to the arm or leg, thus indicating the main location of the particular meridian instead of the particular organ to which it is related:

Sunlight Yang	arm—large intestine leg—stomach
Lesser Yang	arm—triple warmer leg—gall bladder
Greater Yang	arm—small intestine leg—bladder
Greater Yin	arm—lung leg—spleen
Absolute Yin	arm—pericardium leg—liver
Lesser Yin	arm—heart leg—kidney

Thus the small intestine meridian is referred to by the Chinese as the Arm Greater Yang, and the bladder meridian as the Leg Greater Yang. Used on its own the term Greater Yang would refer to the two meridians jointly.

3 Other interrelationships are shown in Fig. 5.3. (see also chapter VII and The Meridians of Acupuncture).

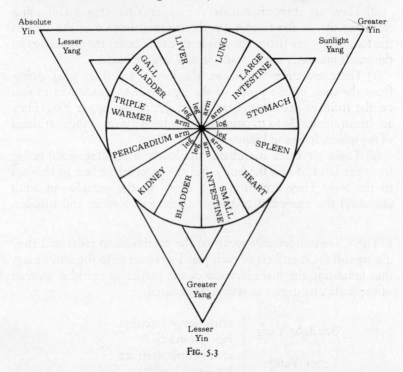

FIG. 5.3

4 If the arms and legs are held in the normal walking position with the thumb and toes anteriorly whilst the little finger and heel are posterior, the following arrangement ensues, whether it be the arm or leg (Fig. 5.4).

5 If the arms and legs are held in the embryological position with the medial surface of the arm and leg turned anteriorly, the positions of the twelve meridians are more easily followed.

152

FIRST MERIDIAN CYCLE (Fig. 5.5).

(*a*) The meridian of the lung starts on the chest and then runs down the *outer* side of the *anterior* surface of the arm to the thumb.

(*b*) This meridian is followed by the meridian of the large intestine, that starts at the end of the index finger and runs up the *outer* side of the *posterior* surface of the arm to end at the nose.

(*c*) This is again followed by the meridian of the stomach, starting

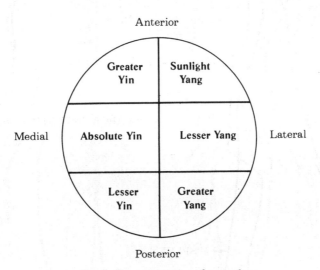

FIG. 5.4 Transverse section of arm or leg

below the eye and running down the *outer* side of the head (relative to bladder and gall bladder meridians), chest and abdomen and the *outside* of the external (embryologically *posterior*) surface of the leg, to end at the end of the second toe.

(*d*) Finally, the meridian of the spleen starts at the big toe, which, although it is apparently the inside of the foot, is in fact embryologically the *outer* side of the foot. This meridian runs up the *outside* of the medial (embryologically *anterior*) side of the leg and the outside of the *anterior* surface of the abdomen and chest to end near the origin of this first meridianal cycle, not far from the starting point of the meridian of the lung.

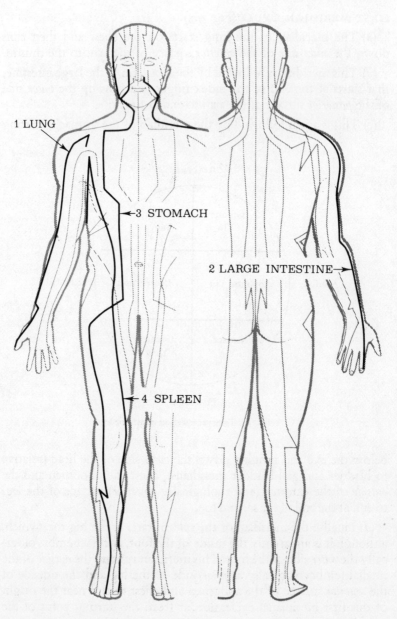

1 LUNG

3 STOMACH

2 LARGE INTESTINE→

4 SPLEEN

FIG. 5.5

Thus following the embryological surfaces of the human body, the first meridian cycle, the outer cycle, consists of:

(*a*)	Outside	anterior surface	arm	lung
(*b*)	Outside	posterior surface	arm	large intestine
(*c*)	Outside	posterior surface	leg	stomach
(*d*)	Outside	anterior surface	leg	spleen

THE SECOND MERIDIAN CYCLE (Fig. 5.6).

The second meridianal cycle takes its origin with the meridian of the heart, which follows the meridian of the spleen in the circulation of energy.

(*a*) The meridian of the heart takes its origin from the anterior surface of the chest and then runs down the *inside* of the *anterior* surface of the arm to end at the little finger.

(*b*) This is followed by the meridian of the small intestine which takes its origin at the end of the little finger and runs up the *inside* of the *posterior* surface of the arm to the cheek.

(*c*) This is followed by the meridian of the bladder that starts at the nose, runs over the *inside* of the skull and down the *inside* of the *posterior* surface of the back and leg to end at the little toe, which embryologically is on the *inside*.

(*d*) Finally, the meridian of the kidney starts on the sole of the foot and runs up the *inside* of the embryologically *anterior* surface of the leg, abdomen and chest, to end the second meridianal cycle near its origin on the *anterior* surface of the chest.

The second meridianal cycle, the inner cycle, is thus made up as follows:

(*a*)	Inside	anterior surface	arm	heart
(*b*)	Inside	posterior surface	arm	small intestine
(*c*)	Inside	posterior surface	leg	bladder
(*d*)	Inside	anterior surface	leg	kidney

THE THIRD MERIDIAN CYCLE (Fig. 5.7).

(*a*) The third and final meridianal cycle, starts as all others on the front of the chest, with the meridian that follows the kidney meridian in the circulation of energy, namely the meridian of the pericardium. This runs down the *middle* of the *anterior* surface of the arm, be-

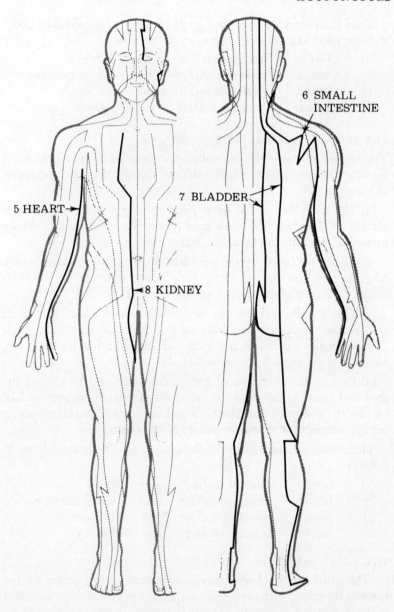

5 HEART→

7 BLADDER

6 SMALL
INTESTINE

←8 KIDNEY

FIG. 5.6

tween the other two Yin meridians of the arm (heart and lung), to end at the middle finger.

(*b*) This is followed by the meridian of the triple-warmer, which starts at the end of the fourth finger and runs up the *middle* of the *posterior* surface of the arm between the other two Yang meridians of the arm (small intestine and large intestine), to end near the ear.

(*c*) This is again followed by the meridian of the gall bladder, starting near the ear and running down the *middle* (between the other two Yang meridians of stomach and bladder) of the *posterior* surface of the trunk and leg to end at the tip of the fourth toe, between the other Yang meridians of the leg, the meridians of the stomach and bladder.

(*d*) Finally the twelfth meridian, that of the liver, takes its origin on the lateral side of the big toe, between the origins of the other Yin meridians of the leg, those of the spleen and kidney. Thereafter the liver meridian goes up the *middle* of the medial (embryologically *anterior*) surface of the leg, over the abdomen to end at the lower end of the chest, near the origin of the first meridian cycle.

The order of the 3rd, middle, meridianal cycle is thus:

(*a*)	Middle	anterior surface	arm	pericardium
(*b*)	Middle	posterior surface	arm	triple warmer
(*c*)	Middle	posterior surface	leg	gall bladder
(*d*)	Middle	anterior surface	leg	liver

These relationships of the outer, inner and middle meridians may be best visualised by regarding each group in a major part of the body:

(*a*) With the upper Yin, (lung, pericardium, heart, from outside to inside) on the anterior surface of the chest and arm, the relationship is obvious.

(*b*) With the upper Yang, (large intestine, triple warmer, small intestine, from outside to inside) on the posterior surface of the arm, the relationship is again obvious. The complicated course on the head is discussed under (*e*).

(*c*) The lower Yang meridians (stomach, gall bladder, bladder, from outside to inside) follow a straightforward course on the neck, trunk and legs if account is taken of:

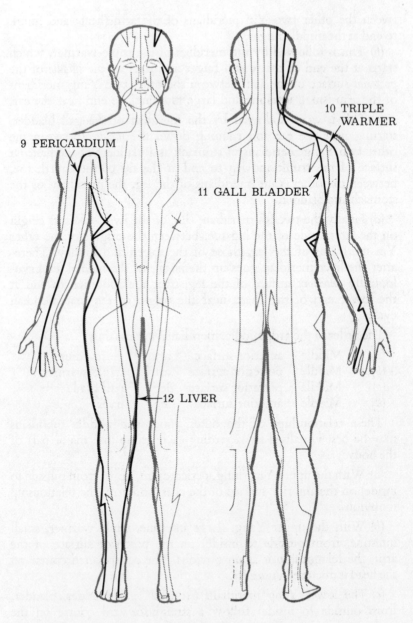

9 PERICARDIUM

10 TRIPLE
WARMER

11 GALL BLADDER

12 LIVER

FIG. 5.7

(i) The lateral surface of the leg is embryologically speaking posterior, while the medical surface is embryologically anterior; and that the foot has twisted in embryonic evolution through 180°. Then on the leg the stomach meridian is posterior-outside, the bladder meridian posterior-inside, and the gall bladder meridian posterior-middle.

(ii) A shift has taken place so that the stomach meridian (outer meridian) has moved right out laterally and then moved in anteriorly so that in the adult it lies within the outer and middle lower Yin meridians (spleen and liver).

(d) The lower Yin meridians (spleen, liver, kidney, from outside to inside) follow the embryological pattern along their whole course except that in the lower leg the liver meridian (middle meridian) moves anterior (embryologically laterally) to the outer position. The kidney meridian takes its origin from the sole of the foot near the base of the third toe which is in agreement with the embryological condition.

(e) On the head the arrangement of the meridians is more complicated:-

The lower Yang meridians (stomach, gall bladder, bladder) follow the correct order: the bladder meridian on the inside, the gall bladder meridian in the middle, and the stomach meridian on the outside, if account is taken of the anterior shift of the stomach meridian as mentioned under (c).

The upper Yang meridians (large intestine, triple warmer, small intestine) follow the correct order except on the head and neck, where the large intestine meridian has moved two meridians anteriorly. This is similar to the anterior movement of the stomach meridian with which the large intestine meridian is coupled as the 'Sunlight Yang'.

There are still some obvious inconsistencies in the course of the adult meridians and the true embryological order.

The above theory may be coincidence, with as little meaning as some of the traditional Chinese ideas, for acupuncture abounds with theories involving numerical relationships, and anyone with a mathematical mind can easily invent new ones.

6 The anterior-posterior, or Yin-Yang relation of the meridians

produces coupled meridians. The Chinese use the term outside and inside meridians (instead of coupled meridians) in reference to say the outer part and the lining of a coat, or in this context to the outer and inner part of the limbs.

Anterior or Yin	Lung	⎫	Coupled meridians
Posterior or Yang	Large intestine	⎬	or organs
„ „	Stomach	⎫	
Anterior or Yin	Spleen	⎬	„
„ „	Heart	⎫	
Posterior or Yang	Small intestine	⎬	„
„ „	Bladder	⎫	
Anterior or Yin	Kidney	⎬	„
„ „	Pericardium	⎫	
Posterior or Yang	Triple warmer	⎬	„
„ „	Gall bladder	⎫	
Anterior or Yin	Liver	⎬	„

Each of the coupled meridians belongs to one of the five elements as discussed in the next chapter.

VI

THE FIVE ELEMENTS

'The five elements: wood, fire, earth, metal, water, encompass all the phenomena of nature. It is a symbolism that applies itself equally to man.'

(Su Wen)

The Chinese divided the world into five elements and everything on the earth was considered to belong, by its nature, to one or several of these five categories. These will recall to mind the

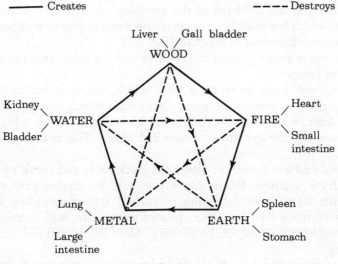

FIG. 6.1

four elements which were a familiar part of western practice up to recent times. These were: earth, water, air, fire; nor is it difficult to see (at least for anyone acquainted with this type of thought) that everything in the world belongs of its essence to one or several of these categories. For example, a brick belongs to the element earth; a glass of wine to the elements earth (glass) and water (wine); a barrage balloon to the elements earth (the balloon) and air (helium), a coal fire to earth (coal), air (carbon dioxide and other gases) and fire.

The above four elements are common to both the European and the Chinese systems. (Air = Metal). The fifth element designated 'wood', is only known to the Chinese and certain other civilizations whose roots extend to prehistoric times.

As mentioned, the five elements are:

Wood

Fire

Earth

Metal (Air in the western tradition)

Water

The macrocosm, of which the human constitutes the microcosm, is considered the resultant of the interplay of these five primeval forces, which are linked in an unvarying pattern, one to another, in the manner illustrated in the chart (Fig. 6.1).

The outer lines represent the creative and the inner ones the destructive forces:

Wood will burn to create a *Fire*, which, when it has finished burning, leaves behind the ashes, *Earth*; from which may be mined the *Metals*; which, if heated, become molten like *Water*; which is necessary for the growth of plants and *Wood*. This is the creative cycle.

Wood destroys *Earth*, i.e. plants can crack rocks and break up the soil. *Earth* destroys *Water*, i.e. a jug with its earthenware sides prevents water from following its natural law of spreading out. *Water* destroys *Fire*, i.e. water, poured over a fire, will extinguish it. *Fire* destroys *Metal*, i.e. by melting. *Metal* destroys *Wood*, i.e. by cutting.

In medicine the law of the five elements is applied as follows:

			Yin	*Yang*
Wood is equivalent to the			Liver	and Gall bladder
Fire	„	„	Heart	and Small intestine
Earth	„	„	Spleen	and Stomach
Metal	„	„	Lung	and Large intestine
Water	„	„	Kidney	and Bladder
Fire	„	„	Pericardium	and Triple warmer

It should be understood that the Chinese when they used the terms 'Wood', 'Fire', etc., did not use the words in the actual restrictive sense of the physical wood, fire, etc., but rather as implying an archetypal idea in the sense in which it is used by the psychologist Jung, who studied Chinese philosophy profoundly. For example, the *idea* of the genus house is opposed to the idea of an *actual* house. Before it is possible to build a house it is necessary to have conceived the idea of 'house', whether this be a bungalow, a skyscraper, a modern glass and concrete affair, or an imitation Tudor perpetration. The general generic idea of 'house' is primary and covers a vast number of possibilities; an actual individual physical house made of bricks, etc. is only secondary to the general idea comprising all houses.

Thus what I have expressed above as '*Metal* destroys *Wood*, i.e., wood may be cut by a metallic saw;' is really a material vulgarisation of what is essentially an idea, an idea which may manifest itself in various physical guises such as wood, or the liver.

In the actual practice of acupuncture this theory of the five elements dictates that when the liver (wood) is tonified, the heart (fire) will automatically be also tonified, while the spleen (earth) is sedated; or, if the kidney (water) is sedated, the liver (wood) will also automatically be sedated, while the heart (fire) will be tonified.

The effect is similar with the related Yang organs. e.g. Tonification of the gall bladder will produce tonification of the small intestine and sedation of the stomach.

This law may seem to Western minds like the fanciful application of a philosophical law. Nevertheless, it operates whether one wishes it or not, provided the conditions of its working are complied with. For example, if the liver and heart are underactive and the spleen is overactive, tonification of only the liver will produce equilibrium between all three. If the heart were overactive or the spleen underactive the conditions for the operation of the law would not be met and there would be no result except for tonification of the liver.

Certain of these relationships are obvious in the practice of ordinary medicine, i.e., tonification of the kidney (water) will produce by its increased excretion of water and solids a tonification (decongestion) of the liver (wood) and also a sedation of the heart (fire) which no longer has to force too much fluid through the body. A fuller explanation, however, will require much more research from the side of ordinary science.

The interplay of the creative and destructive forces in the five elements is, to the Chinese, another aspect of that delicate balance of all life in the polarity of Yin and Yang, which has been mentioned earlier. Only when this balance is upset and an organ cannot correctly react to a stimulus will disease result.

If, for example, the heart were weak and nothing else could be done but to tonify it, the consequences in the body would resemble the pile-up of a traffic jam and the patient might fall seriously ill. For to tonify only the heart would at once increase its pumping action, and therefore also the circulation of the blood. But, in order to pump more vigorously, the muscular wall of the heart requires more oxygen: so the breathing becomes deeper or more rapid. Greater activity of the heart causes the release of more metabolites, which (since these have to be excreted) increases the action of the kidneys. Moreover, since the cardiac muscle needs more glycogen to fuel its energy, the liver too must come into action to release this.

In physics, chemistry, mechanics and all the sciences concerned with the non-living, the Western mind is accustomed to express such interactions in terms of exact laws. We accept, for example, unquestioningly the second law of thermodynamics, that every action has an opposite and equal reaction; or the law that the momentum of an object is proportional to its mass and the square of its velocity. But in the biological sciences, among which is that of medicine, exact laws are, to the Western mind, virtually non-existent. The Chinese, however, aimed at introducing into biology the same precision, at least in a qualitative if not a quantitative manner, as we have into mechanics. The paragraph above shows how the tonification of the heart cannot be considered as an act in itself, unrelated to the many accompanying readjustments it entails. In the West these are seen as physiological events; the Chinese expressed them in laws of almost mathematical precision.

In certain abnormal conditions the balance of the five elements is not maintained. Normally the tonification of the liver sedates the spleen; but sometimes the reverse can happen and the tonification of the spleen will sedate the liver. This process is called 'mutual aid' and 'mutual antagonist'.

'If there is a surplus of Qi, then control that which is already winning and antagonise that which is not winning; if there is a deficiency of Qi, then antagonise and regulate that which is not winning, and bring out and antagonise that which is winning.'

(Su Wen, wuyunxing dalun)

This shows how an excess or deficiency of the five elements can play havoc with the laws which govern normal conditions. For example, a surplus of water Qi may destroy fire Qi (that which is winning) but may also insult earth (the 'not winning'). If water Qi is deficient then earth aids it (the 'not winning') and fire insults it (the 'winning').

This is further elaborated in the Nan Jing, wushisan nan shuo:—

'If a disease has empty evil, full evil, thief evil, minute evil and upright evil, how can they be distinguished? That which comes from behind is empty evil, that which comes from in front is full evil, that which comes from the not-winning is thief evil, that which comes from the winning is minute evil, and autogenous disease is upright evil.'

The quotation indicates the various paths taken by 'invading disease evils'. 'Empty evil' coming from 'behind' is a mother disease affecting the son as, for instance, a liver disease which is transmitted to the heart. 'Full evil' coming from 'in front' is a son disease going back to the mother, like a disease of the spleen which is transmitted to the heart. 'Thief evil' coming from the 'not-winning' can be illustrated by a liver disease being transmitted to the spleen and 'minute evil' coming from the 'winning' by a lung disease transmitted to the heart. 'Upright evil' is an autogenous heart disease, originating in the heart, and is not transmitted to any other organ (Fig. 6.2).

The following pages give some examples of the above laws, taken from the Zhongyixue Gailun with the Chinese phraseology, though it sounds a little strange to our ears, left for the most part intact.

Heart disease—palpitations and insomnia.

(a) If the fire of the heart is vigorous and abundant, the blood in the heart will be deficient, producing the following symptoms: restless sleep, an unquiet spirit, palpitations, constipation and ulcers of the tongue and mouth.

This type of insomnia originates in the heart itself; and, since it neither spreads to other organs nor results from their influence on

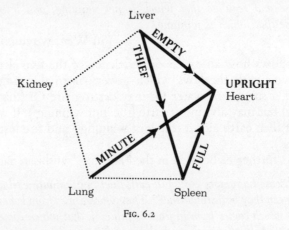

FIG. 6.2

the heart, it is treated directly by sedating the heart fire and tonifying the heart blood.

(b) If the spleen is empty and this emptiness affects the heart (son depriving mother of Qi), there will be a decrease of thirst and appetite, thin and watery stools, lethargy and weakness, palpitations, insomnia, amnesia etc.

In this case treatment of the heart would be ineffectual since the cause lies in the spleen. Therefore *'the spleen earth must be fortified, so that the spleen Qi becomes vigorous and does not deprive its mother of Qi; then the heart blood will be sufficient, the heart's spirit nourished and the illness cured.'*

(c) What in China are called 'empty exhaustion diseases' generally result from a deficiency of kidney Yin, causing 'empty fire' (the heart belongs to the element 'fire') to burn upwards. Fever ensues, with copious and spontaneous sweating, coughing, vomiting of blood etc. and often insomnia. The insomnia is the result of a deficiency of kidney water; true Yin is not ascending and so the violence of the heart fire interferes with sleep.

Here the treatment is to strengthen the water and restrain the Yang, so that, when the kidney Yin becomes sufficient and the empty fire subdued, the disease will pass away.

These three examples show that heart disease, though the primary, is not the only cause of palpitations and insomnia. For a weakness of spleen earth or a deficiency of kidney water, by producing a corresponding deficiency of heart blood or a violence of the heart fire, may also occasion these symptoms.

Liver disease—headache and dizziness.

Among the commonest complaints caused by a dysfunction of the liver are headaches and dizziness. The condition is called 'liver fire ascending', because the patient often feels as if something hot were rising from the region of the liver into his head. In certain circumstances, however, these symptoms may be due to a deficiency of kidney water, a dysfunction of the lungs or inactivity of the spleen.

(a) If the liver Yang rises, wood (the liver belongs to the element 'wood') and fire will increase their activity, causing headache and dizziness, a flushed face, bloodshot eyes, a bowstring, unyielding pulse etc.

Since in this case the disease is in the liver and has not affected other organs, it is sufficient to treat the liver alone by sedating its excessive fire. Thereby the liver Yang will be balanced and the headache and dizziness will disappear.

(b) When headache and dizziness are due to a deficiency of water (kidney) and over-activity of wood (liver), the liver wind will rise and rush around in the head. The condition often occurs in those whose complexions are haggard and who experience the feeling of heat and emptiness. It is described by Shishi milu as one where *'kidney water is deficient and evil fire rushes into the brain'.*

According to the same source, *'if only the wind is treated, then the headache will increase and the dizziness become more pronounced. The appropriate treatment is full tonification of the kidney water, which will cause the symptoms to disappear.'*

In conformity with the teaching of the five elements, this phenomenon is described by the saying, 'Water fails to submerge wood.' The water of the kidney must be nourished so that it is able to sub-merge the wood of the liver; or, as the Chinese put it, 'If weak, then tonify the mother.'

(c) Liver (wood) is under the control of lung (metal). (See Fig. 6.1) In a patient whose lung Qi (the word means either energy or breath) is deficient, the air does not permeate the lungs so that the fluid in the interstices, not being properly diffused and transformed, becomes phlegm. In this condition the lungs are moist, the respiratory passages become partially obstructed, there is coughing up of sputum and a diminution of thirst and appetite. (In Chinese thought, food and drink are associated with the stomach coupled to the spleen, and both spleen and stomach with the element 'earth', which is endangered by dampness and phlegm.) The accumulation of moisture and phlegm causes also dizziness and a feeling of obstruction in the area of the diaphragm. In this connection the Su Wen, xuanji yunbing shi, says:-

'If liver wood is violent, it must be because metal is decayed and cannot regulate it; and wood also creates fire.'

The best cure therefore for this type of dizziness is stimulating earth to create metal, so that the lung Qi may circulate and the liver wood become balanced.

These three examples show that, though headache and dizziness are directly due to a disharmony of liver wood, they may also be the results of a dysfunction of the lung, kidney, spleen and stomach. The treatment is nourishing water to submerge wood, purifying the liver to sedate fire and tonifying the lungs to regulate the liver.

Spleen diseases—diarrhoea.

Commonest among the many causes of diarrhoea is an empty spleen, with its accompanying dampness. It can also result from a deficiency of kidney Yang, where fire does not create earth, or from a liver disease affecting the spleen.

(a) Weakness of the spleen Yang may produce uncontrolled diarrhoea, with associated symptoms of a lack of appetite and thirst, the desire to pass stool after eating, a feeling of obstruction and melancholy in the lower chest and upper abdomen and a weakness in the limbs. This type of diarrhoea may be cured by tonifying the spleen.

Another type is caused by dampness and may be treated via the spleen in order to dry this out, in accordance with the advice of the Su Wen:- 'If dampness is excessive, then sedate.'

(b) One form of diarrhoea, in which the stool is variegated in colour, can occur because the 'fire of the gate of destiny' (see 'The Meridians of Acupuncture', ch. IX) is too weak and cannot create earth. It may be associated with symptoms of uneasiness in the stomach, anorexia and slight abdominal pain. The cause is described in the Yizong bidu thus:—

'*The kidneys, the roots of sealing and storing, control the two excretory passages; and, though they belong to the category 'water', true Yang lodges within them. A little fire creates Qi; and fire is the mother of earth. If this fire is decayed, how can the triple warmer, which belongs to ministerial fire, be activated or nourishment digested?*'

This is treated by tonifying fire to create earth, thereby restoring the kidney Yang; which, in actual practice, means tonifying the kidneys.

(c) If the liver wood is excessive, it may injure the spleen earth, causing abdominal pains, which are relieved by diarrhoea.

The cure will be incomplete if only the spleen is tonified or the liver sedated, for the abdominal pain is caused by the liver Qi rebelling, and the diarrhoea by the spleen Qi being empty.

Lung diseases—coughing and dyspnoea.

Coughing and dyspnoea are the two most characteristic symptoms of a lung disease but they are not in every instance directly attributable to this cause.

(a) If fluid from within the body collects in the lungs at the same time as chilly conditions prevail outside, there will be difficulty in breathing, fever, perhaps urinary trouble and a strong dislike for cold weather. In this instance the origin of the disease is in the lungs, which should be treated directly.

(b) Under the heading 'empty exhaustion disease' the Chinese include pulmonary tuberculosis, the general condition which often precedes this, and other conditions with similar symptoms. The patient will suffer from a chronic cough of long duration. The lungs will be empty and the spleen and stomach inactive, with consequent lack of appetite and watery stools.

The best treatment is to stimulate earth to create metal. Merely to tonify or moisten the lungs will often aggravate these symptoms, for the type of medicine that tonifies the lungs may obstruct the stomach and the type of medicine that moistens them may render the intestines slippery. One should first rectify the spleen and harmonise the stomach, thus restoring the balance in the function of these organs. There will then be an improvement in the appetite and the diarrhoea will cease. At the same time, if the lungs gain sustenance from the 'nourishment Qi' they will be naturally restored to health, and the coughing will be cured. The underlying principle of this treatment is that the spleen belongs to earth and the lungs to metal: so that earth is tonified to create metal.

(c) If the lungs (in the upper part of the body) are full and the kidneys (in the lower part of it) empty, the condition will cause coughing with much phlegm, aching of the loins, a fine pulse and, possibly, spermatorrhoea.

In this case both the lungs and the kidneys must be treated, for to treat only the fullness of the lungs might aggravate the emptiness of the kidneys, while to tonify only the kidneys might increase the fullness of the lungs. The lungs belong to metal, the kidneys to water and, because of their mutual interaction, should both be treated together.

(d) If the kidneys are empty and cannot transmit their Qi to the lungs, the result will be:— coughing, dyspnoea, a weak voice, shortness of breath, insufficient phlegm, breathlessness after exertion and possibly also an ache in the loins and increased urination.

To treat this condition one should tonify the kidneys so that they are able to transmit Qi. As we have seen, kidneys belong to water, lungs to metal. Normally, metal creates water, but in this case kidney water is deficient and thus unable to effect the basic transformation of lung metal. This disease therefore belongs to the category known as 'depriving mother of Qi' and the appropriate treatment is for the 'son to cause the mother to be full.'

(e) In a case where liver wood is violently active, and wood and fire blaze upwards, the inability of lung metal to descend will cause numbness of the throat with coughing and pain in the ribs.

In such a condition one should purify metal to regulate wood. If liver wood is balanced, lung metal is not insulted by it and the disease will disappear. This treatment follows the law known as 'insulting backwards'.

Kidney diseases—spermatorrhoea

Spermatorrhoea, is due to a deficiency of kidney Qi. *'The kidneys receive the Jing (sexual power) from the five solid organs and the six hollow organs, and store it.'*

(Neijing)

Thus the principal treatment of spermatorrhoea is so to tonify the kidneys that they can store and control Jing. There are, however, other causes of the disease.

'Each of the five solid organs has its separate function. As long as Jing is stored, there is health; if one of the solid organs is in severe disorder, it will weaken the control of the heart and kidneys over the Jing'.

(Yixue rumen)

This quotation shows that, apart from an empty kidney causing the Jing gate to be weak, abnormality in some other organ may have the same effect, such as excessive heart fire, dampness and heat in the liver meridian, emptiness of the heart as well as kidneys or failure of the reciprocity of water and fire.

(a) Certain people are weak by nature from birth, sometimes because they were born of elderly parents, and will therefore suffer from a deficiency of true Qi in the kidneys. They will not infrequently have nocturnal emissions, with aching of the loins, dizziness and noises in the ears. This condition, being due to a weakness of the kidneys, is therefore treated by direct stimulation of them.

(b) Spermatorrhoea may occur in patients who suffer from constant anxiety, frustration, worry and dreaming.

The appropriate treatment here is to purify fire in order to pacify water. If heart fire is balanced, kidney water will be restored to tranquillity and the patient cured; but, if mistakenly the kidneys are tonified in order to strengthen the Jing gate, the treatment will not only be ineffective but may even aggravate the condition.

(c) Sadness and depression, associated with over-abundance of liver fire, may cause spermatorrhoea.

This may be treated by purifying and sedating the liver fire. Because the kidneys control 'closing and storing', and the liver manages 'clearing and purging', violence of liver fire will result in excessive clearing and purging, which can affect the closing and storing of the kidneys and so cause spermatorrhoea. Although purifying and sedating the liver fire will not directly cure spermatorrhoea, balancing the liver fire to reduce the clearing and purging will restore the kidneys naturally to their proper function. This is what is meant by: 'If full, sedate the son.'

(d) A general physical weakness will often produce aching of

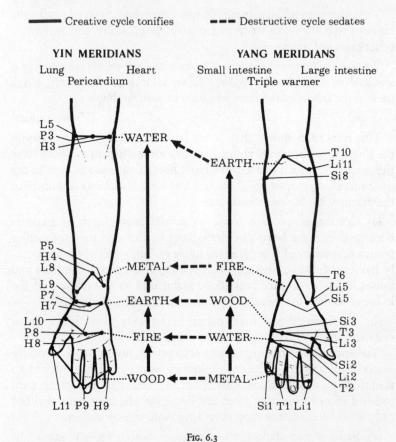

FIG. 6.3

the loins, lack of strength in the legs, dreaming, insomnia and nervousness. This is usually caused by deficiency of the heart and kidneys. Patients will also often suffer from spontaneous sweating and spermatorrhoea because, kidney water being absent and heart fire disquieted, water and fire are not co-operating.

The appropriate treatment is to cause water and fire to assist one another, so as to restore the relation between kidneys and heart.

The Five Element Acupuncture Points

The general classification of the five elements is worked out in greater detail for those acupuncture points that lie between the fingertips and the elbow, and between the tips of the toes and the

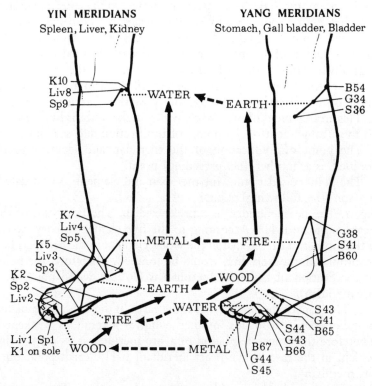

━━━ Creative cycle tonifies   ▬ ▬ ▬ Destructive cycle sedates

YIN MERIDIANS
Spleen, Liver, Kidney

YANG MERIDIANS
Stomach, Gall bladder, Bladder

K10
Liv8
Sp9
WATER
EARTH
B54
G34
S36

K7
Liv4
Sp5
K5
Liv3
Sp3
K2
Sp2
Liv2
METAL
FIRE
G38
S41
B60

WOOD
EARTH
WATER
FIRE

Liv1 Sp1
K1 on sole
WOOD
METAL
S43
G41
B65
S44
B67
G43
G44
B66
S45

FIG. 6.4

knees, a series of points whereby it is possible to treat nearly any disease, wherever it may appear on the body, without having recourse to any other acupuncture points (Fig. 6.3 and 6.4).

173

It will be noted that the direction of movement is centripetal, from the finger or toe tips inwards in accordance with the creative cycle, i.e., from the finger tip, anterior surface, wood, fire, earth, etc. Equivalent positions on the anterior and posterior surfaces are by the law of five elements, antagonistic to one another, i.e., at the finger tip metal and wood are antagonistic in such a manner that the external surface (metal) is the destructive agent. Thus both the creative and the destructive cycles are centripetal, moving from without inwards, i.e. from the tips of fingers or toes to the elbow or knee, (creative cycle); or from the posterior surface, which is embryologically an external surface, to the anterior surface, which is embryologically a more internal surface, (destructive cycle).

It will also be noted that the arrangements of the elements on the anterior surface of the arm is the same as that on the medial (embryologically anterior) surface of the leg, and, similarly, the arrangement of the elements on the posterior surface of the arm are the same as those on the lateral (embryologically posterior) surface of the leg.

This arrangement of the five elements on the limbs is fundamental to the arrangement of the points of tonification and sedation:

The point of tonification of the meridian and element to be tonified, is a 'mother' (i.e. preceding) point.

The point of sedation of the meridian and element to be sedated, is a 'son'. (i.e. following) point.

e.g. 1. The heart meridian is a fire meridian. The fire point of the heart meridian is H8. According to the five element theory, wood is the mother of fire, so that, if the wood element in the fire meridian is stimulated, the 'son' fire, would be tonified. Therefore, the point of tonification of the heart meridian is H9 (the wood point on a fire meridian).

2. The 'son' of the element fire is the earth. If the 'son' is stimulated he takes energy from his 'mother' who, as a result, is weakened. Therefore the point of sedation of a fire meridian is its earth point which, in the case of the heart meridian, is H7 (earth point on a fire meridian).

3. The gall bladder meridian is a wood meridian. The 'mother' of wood is water, so that the point of tonification would be the water point G43. The 'son' of wood is fire, so that the point of sedation would be the fire point on this Yang wood meridian, point G38.

YIN meridians:

Organ	Element	Wood	Fire	Earth	Metal	Water
Lung	Metal	L11	L10	L9	L8	L5
Heart	Fire	H9	H8	H7	H4	H3
Pericardium	Fire	P9	P8	P7	P5	P3
Liver	Wood	Liv1	Liv2	Liv3	Liv4	Liv8
Spleen	Earth	Sp1	Sp2	Sp3	Sp5	Sp9
Kidney	Water	K1	K2	K5	K7	K10

YANG meridians:		*Metal*	*Water*	*Wood*	*Fire*	*Earth*
Large intestine	Metal	Li1	Li2	Li3	Li5	Li11
Small intestine	Fire	Si1	Si2	Si3	Si5	Si8
Triple warmer	Fire	T1	T2	T3	T6	T10
Gall bladder	Wood	G44	G43	G41	G38	G34
Stomach	Earth	S45	S44	S43	S41	S36
Bladder	Water	B67	B66	B65	B60	B54

Treatment via Law of Five Elements

The creative and the destructive cycles of the law of the five elements may be used together or separately in the treatment of disease:

1. If the pulse of the stomach shows an overactivity, as is usually the case with a hypersecretion of acid, with resultant duodenal or stomach ulcers, the following will usually correct it:

(a) The stomach meridian belongs to the element earth which should be sedated after the 'mother-son' law. Metal is the 'son' of earth. The metal point of the earth Yang meridian (stomach) is S45—which is sedated.

Also the metal point of the metal Yang meridian (Large intestine) is sedated (in order to further drain the energy from earth) which is Li1.

(b) The gall bladder is opposed to the stomach by the law of the five elements. This is therefore tonified at its wood point (to destroy earth), which is G41.

Similarly the wood point of the stomach meridian itself is tonified as this destroys the element earth within the stomach meridian itself. This is S43.

2. Likewise, if the pulse of the stomach is underactive:

(a) The 'mother' must be tonified. The 'mother' of the Yang

earth (stomach) is Yang fire (small intestine). Hence the fire point in the stomach meridian itself is tonified, point S41.

Also the fire point in the fire Yang meridian (small intestine) itself is tonified, point Si5.

(b) The opposed element, wood, must be weakened, so that the element (earth, stomach) that it opposes is, as a result, strengthened. Hence the wood point of the stomach meridian itself is sedated, point S43.

Also the wood point of the wood (Yang) meridian (Gall bladder) itself is sedated, point G41.

It will be noted that in this context the law of the five elements only operates within elements belonging to either Yin or Yang, i.e., if an organ is a Yin organ its 'mother', 'son' and opposed element are also Yin. Sometimes this is not the case: a Yin organ may effect a Yang organ, and a Yang organ a Yin organ.

Continuing this line of reasoning, a full table of what should be done in each circumstance is therefore as follows:

Organ	To Tonify, i.e. if organ is underactive				To Sedate i.e., if organ is overactive			
	Tonify		Sedate		Sedate		Tonify	
Lungs	L9	Sp3	L10	H8	L5	K10	L10	H8
Kidney	K7	L8	K5	Sp3	K1	Liv1	K5	Sp3
Liver	Liv8	K10	Liv4	L8	Liv2	H8	Liv4	L8
Heart	H9	Liv1	H3	K10	H7	Sp3	H3	K10
Spleen	Sp2	H8	Sp1	Liv1	Sp5	L8	Sp1	Liv1
Large intestine	Li11	S36	Li5	Si5	Li2	B66	Li5	Si5
Bladder	B67	Li1	B54	S36	B65	G41	B54	S36
Gall bladder	G43	B66	G44	Li1	G38	Si5	G44	Li1
Small intestine	Si3	G41	Si2	B66	Si8	S36	Si2	B66
Stomach	S41	Si5	S43	G41	S45	Li1	S43	G41
Pericardium	P9	Liv1	P3	K10	P7	Sp3	P3	K10
Triple warmer	T3	G41	T2	B66	T10	S36	T2	B66

It will be noticed that amongst the four points that should be used in tonifying an organ, is the point of tonification; likewise amongst the four points that should be used in sedating an organ is the point of sedation.

For this reason the law of the five elements is quite often used if the simple points of tonification or sedation do not work, or only do so partially.

Likewise the law of the five elements may be used if it is noticed that the initial illness has various complications corresponding to the other factors mentioned under each element. e.g., If a patient has predominately a cardiac disease which is due to an under-activity of the heart and has as complications a malfunction of the liver and kidney, the choice of this law is obvious, for underactivity of the heart not only is the heart treated, but also the liver and kidney—as may be seen from the chart, points H9, H3 (heart), Liv1 (Liver), K10 (Kidney).

Extension of the Law of Five Elements

We have already seen that the basis of Chinese traditional medicine is the polarity of Yin and Yang, the negative and the positive, in addition to which is the division of the body in accordance with the twelve primary organs and meridians. But, forming a bridge between these two groups, is a third: that of the five elements.

Six of the twelve organs and meridians are Yin, six are Yang, and each of the five elements controls one Yin organ and meridian and one Yang, except the element 'fire', which in both groups controls two. In the Yin group, the heart belongs to 'princely fire', the pericardium to 'ministerial fire'; in the Yang group, the small intestine belongs to 'princely fire', the triple warmer to 'ministerial fire'.

The six Yin organs are referred to in Chinese literature as the five Zang (or solid) organs; the six Yang organs are called the six Fu (or hollow) organs and are mentioned in the following quotation:—

'What are called the five solid organs store life essence and energy (Jing and Qi) and do not let them leak away; therefore they are filled but cannot be full. The six hollow organs transmit and transform matter but do not store it; thus they are full but cannot be filled.'

(Su Wen, wuzang bielun)

The Chinese consider that each organ has an effect on and interacts with a bodily tissue, sense organ, season etc., as described below.

Element	Wood	Fire	Earth	Metal	Water
Yin organ	Liver	Heart	Spleen	Lungs	Kidney
Yang organ	Gall bladder	Small intestine	Stomach	Large intestine	Bladder
Sense commanded	Sight	Words	Taste	Smell	Hearing
Nourishes the	Muscles	Blood vessels	Fat	Skin	Bones
Expands into the	Nails	Colour	Lips	Body hair	Hair on head
Liquid emitted	Tears	Sweat	Saliva	Mucus	Urine
Bodily smell	Rancid	Scorched	Fragrant	Fleshy	Putrid
Associated temperament	Depressed	Emotions up & down	Obsession	Anguish	Fear
	Anger	Joy	Sympathy	Grief	
Flavour	*Sour	Bitter	Sweet	Hot	Salt
Sound	Shout	Laugh	Sing	Weep	Groan
Dangerous type of weather	Wind	Heat	Humidity	Dryness	Cold
Season	Spring	Summer	Midsummer	Autumn	Winter
Colour	Green	Red	Yellow	White	Black
Direction	East	South	Centre	West	North
Development	Birth	Growth	Transformation	Harvest	Store
Beneficial cereal	Wheat	Millet	Rye	Rice	Beans
Beneficial meat	Chicken	Mutton	Beef	Horse	Pork
Musical note	chio	chih	kung	shang	yu

I myself have not been able to verify all the factors mentioned in the above chart, and I have my doubts about the correctness of a few of them, but that the majority are correct I have no doubt as I use them in diagnosis and treatment with success.

It is known for example that someone who has a liver (wood) weakness is more sensitive than the average person to an East (wood) wind (wood), that his nails (wood) may be blemished and that he may have foggy vision with black spots (wood). That the person who feels cold (water) in his bones (water) is found by the

*Sour like vinegar, bitter like bitter lemon, sweet like sugar, hot like ginger, salt like common salt.

pulse diagnosis to have a weakness of the kidneys (water). That the person with verbal (fire) diarrhoea and a high colour (fire) has an overactivity of the heart (fire). That the frightened (water) child who does not want to sleep in the dark and wets (water) his bed has a weakness of the kidney (water). That the diabetic (earth) who eats too much sugar (earth) will probably end up with a diabetic (earth) coma, or the renal (water) hypertensive who eats too much salt (water) may finish in the grave.

The Zhongyixue Gallun gives the following example of the interdependence of various factors within one element (in this case, wood). In spring, all plants, as they grow and put forth their fresh green shoots, are visible manifestations of the luxuriant Qi of birth. Wood, therefore, represents the season of spring. Of the five developing processes it belongs to birth; of the five climatic conditions, to wind. In the physical body, both wood and spring are represented by the liver, whose nature is happy, straightforward and cheerful. Closely connected to the gall bladder, the liver influences the eyes and controls the muscles, which is why liver diseases are usually revealed by symptoms of disturbed vision and muscular spasm. People with too violent a liver are liable to fits of rage and, conversely, fits of rage are liable to cause injury to the liver. Among the five emotions, therefore, anger is under the control of the liver. The colour green is associated with wood, and it is worth noting that many liver diseases are recognisable by a greenish tinge in the patient's skin.

Indirect effects, which are more rarely found must not be forgotten: Foggy vision (wood) is normally due to an underactivity of the liver (wood), but occasionally it may be caused by an underactive kidney (water) [which is the 'mother' by the law of five elements.]

This system may also be used therapeutically:

In psychology a person who has an endogenous depression (wood) may be cured by treating the liver (wood). Or someone who weeps (metal) a lot may after the destructive cycle of the five elements be told to laugh (fire) more, which quite naturally would stop the weepiness. If just being told to laugh (fire) is not enough, the heart (fire) itself may be stimulated either by acupuncture or by giving the correct cardiac (fire) tonic or by eating bitter (fire) food—though as a rule the more powerful acupuncture works best.

Case History. A patient was seen who was unable to stop talking (words-fire). The pulse diagnosis revealed an overactivity of the pulse of the heart (fire). The 'son' of the fire is the earth. Therefore to sedate the fire the earth point (H7) of the fire (heart) meridian was used. Within a few minutes of the needle being in place the verbal diarrhoea stopped and the patient spoke normally for about a day when the incessant flow of words started again. Similar treatment was repeated to effect a cure.

Case History. A patient had nails (wood) which kept on cracking and were thin and brittle with longitudinal ridges (calcium had been tried to no avail). Her eyes (wood) watered very easily especially in the wind (wood). Her body had a slightly rancid (wood) smell and she easily became angry (wood) when she would shout (wood) a lot. The pulse diagnosis revealed an underactivity of the liver (wood). The 'mother' of wood is water. Therefore the water point (Liv8) on the liver meridian was used. This or similar treatment was repeated to effect a cure.

It is interesting to note that the improvement in the nails started within two weeks of initiating treatment. Yet a nail takes some four months to grow up from its base, suggesting that a little revision is needed in the theory of the physiology of nails. This observation has been made repeatedly with various patients: the time of response may vary, but is always faster than would be expected from the speed of growth of the nail.

Passages from certain Chinese texts discuss in detail the correlation of the five elements shown in the chart a few pages back.

'*The liver creates the muscles, the muscles create the heart. . . the heart creates the blood, the blood creates the spleen. . . the spleen creates the flesh, the flesh creates the lungs. . . the lungs create the skin and body air, the skin and body air create the kidneys. . . the kidneys create the bone marrow, the bone marrow creates the liver.*'

(Su Wen, yingyang yingxiang dalun)

The reciprocal relationship among the five (or six) solid organs is as follows:—

'*The kidneys are the controller of the heart, the heart is the controller of the lungs, the lungs are the controller of the liver, the liver is the controller of the spleen, the spleen is the controller of the kidneys.*'

(Su Wen, wuzang shengcheng lun)

Certain organs, mainly hollow, have the function of transmitting and transforming:—

'*Spleen and stomach, large intestine, small intestine, triple warmer and bladder are the root of the granaries, the dwelling-place of nourishing Qi, and they are called organs. They are able to transform the dregs and transmit tastes so that they can enter and depart.*'

(Su Wen, liujie zangxiang lun)

The alternating function of the organs, so important a principle in Chinese medicine, is thus referred to:—

'*If the stomach is filled, then the intestines are empty; if the intestines are filled, then the stomach is empty; they are alternately filled and emptied, so that energy is able to ascend and descend.*'

(Ling Shu, pingren juegu pian)

Coupled organs, or Yin and Yang organs belonging to the same element are also mentioned:—

'*The bladder and kidney are outside and inside, the gall bladder and liver are outside and inside, the stomach and spleen are outside and inside. These are the Yang and Yin organs and meridians of the leg. The small intestine and heart are outside and inside, the triple warmer and pericardium are outside and inside, the large intestine and lung are outside and inside. These are the Yang and Yin organs and meridians of the arm*'

(Su Wen, xueqi xingzhi pian)

There is also a relationship between the solid organs and the limbs:—

'*If the lungs or heart have an evil, its Qi remains in the two elbows; if the liver has an evil, its Qi remains in the two armpits; if the spleen has an evil, its Qi remains in the two thighs; if the kidneys have an evil, its Qi remains in the knees.*'

(Ling Shu, xiekepian)

Apart from the relationship between what the Chinese called 'the eight hollows' (elbow, armpit, groin, knee) and the solid organs, the spleen has a special function in relation to the limbs:—

'*The Emperor asked, "Why is it that with a disease of the spleen the four limbs are useless?" Qi Bo, the Emperor's physician, replied, 'The four limbs all take Qi from the stomach; but, if it cannot get through, then it must be taken from the spleen."*'

(Su Wen, taiyin yangming lun)

Further interconnections, which may be useful in diagnosis and for an understanding of Chinese physiology, are illustrated below:—

'*That which combines with the heart is the blood vessels, and its flourishing is the colour of the complexion. . . That which combines with the lungs is skin, and its flourishing is the body hair. . . That which combines with liver is muscle, and its flourishing is the nails. . . That which combines with the spleen is flesh, and its flourishing is the lips. . . That which combines with the kidneys is the bones, and its flourishing is the hair on the head.*'

(Su Wen, wuzang shengcheng lun)

The relationship is extended to the orifices of the body:—

'*The liver is related to the holes of the eyes, the heart is related to the holes of the tongue, the spleen is related to the hole of the mouth, the lung is related to the holes of the nose, the kidneys are related to the holes of the ears.*'

(Su Wen, yinyang yingxiang dalun)

The five emotions are also correlated:—

'*Man has five solid organs, which transform the five Qi to create anger, joy, over-concentration, anguish and fear.*'

(Su Wen, yinyang yingxiang dalun)

In detail: the liver is injured by anger, the heart by joy, the spleen by over-concentration, the lungs by anguish and the kidneys by fear.

It is a well-known fact that the colour of the face reflects the inner condition of the body; the alcoholic can be recognised by his florid complexion, the anaemic by his pallor; the skin of the hepatic is dusky or pasty, that of the jaundiced a distinctive yellow. The Chinese classify the colouring of the whole face, including eyes and eyebrows, in a traditional pattern: green indicates a hepatic disease, red a cardiac disease, yellow a splenic disease, white a pulmonary disease and black a renal disease. The colours may, however, be changed by some indirect effect. The patient with a liver disease may be white rather than green, because metal destroys wood; the cardiac patient black rather than red, because water destroys fire.

Clearly this colour system cannot be taken too literally. It should be regarded rather as a guide to very slight differences in colour, so slight that a doctor, aware of them at a first quick glance, might fail to perceive them at all, if he stared too hard at his patient. They are like the subtle variations of colour revealed to the artist when he sees a delicate harmony of reds, yellows and blues in a cloud, which the average man would describe simply as 'white' or 'grey'.

The five tastes (sour, bitter, sweet, hot and salty) are related to their corresponding organs:—

'Each of the five tastes moves to what it likes. If the taste of the nourishment is sour, it moves first to the liver; if bitter, it moves first to the heart; if sweet, it moves first to the spleen; if hot it moves first to the lungs; if salty, it moves first to the kidneys.'

(Ling Shu, wuwei pian)

According to this theory, if food of the same type of flavour is continuously eaten, the corresponding organ will be overloaded and disease will result:—

'Sour injures muscles, bitter injures energy (Qi), sweet injures flesh, hot injures skin and body hair, salt injures blood.'

(Su Wen, yinyang yingxiang dalun)

Health is best maintained by a diet of balanced flavours.

Theoretically it should be possible to tonify or sedate a malfunctioning organ by a one-sided diet, increasing or decreasing one or other of the five flavours so as to stimulate the organ. While I was in China, I enquired of many doctors whether this was in fact their practice, but I never heard of anyone who had tried it. The law seems to be applied only in the positive sense of preserving health by a mixture of the flavours. This theory should be compared with that in chapter X at the end of the section 'excess of food and drink.'

The five elements and organs are also associated with meteorological conditions:—

'The heart communicates with the summer Qi, the lungs with the autumn Qi, the kidneys with the winter Qi, the liver with the spring Qi, the spleen with the earth Qi (i.e. late summer)'

But the meteorological conditions could also be the cause of disease:—

'In spring, if one is injured by wind, the evil Qi remains and causes diarrhoea; in summer, if one is injured by the heat, it causes intermittent fever during the autumn; in autumn, if one is injured by the damp, it rebels upwards and causes coughing and paralysis; in winter, if one is

injured by the cold, warm diseases are inevitable in the spring. Thus the Qi of the four seasons injure the five solid organs.'

(Su Wen, shengqi tongtian lun)

Some inconsistencies can be observed in this quotation.

The evolution of the whole of life was governed not only by the division into the Yin and Yang of birth and death but also by the division into the five elements of creation, growth, change, gathering and storing. In the botanical sense, this would mean that the season of creation, when plants put forth their first shoots, is spring ('wood'); their main period of growth is during the summer ('fire');' they begin to change their colouring in late summer ('earth'); their fruit is gathered in autumn ('metal') and their seeds or bulbs are stored beneath the earth in winter ('water'). The evolution of man and animal traces the same pattern: infancy ('wood'), youth ('fire'), adulthood ('earth'), decline ('metal') and death ('water').

'Thus the Yin and Yang seasons are the beginning and end of the myriad things, the root of birth and death. If they are disobeyed, calamity will result; if they are obeyed, disease will not arise.'

(Su Wen, siqi tiaoshen dalun)

LAWS OF ACUPUNCTURE

The organ-meridians that are made use of in acupuncture are not isolated, nor do they function entirely independently of one another.

It is well known in standard medical practice that if, for example, the heart is tonified, whether it be by medicinal or other means, there are other secondary indirect effects which ensue. These secondary effects, whether they be wished for or not, are a more or less unavoidable sequence of the primary stimulus.

The main law discussing the interrelationship of these primary and secondary effects, is that of the five elements, largely mentioned in the previous chapter. This chapter will deal with other inter-relationships and some applications of the law of five elements.

It is inadvisable to treat patients by acupuncture unless possible secondary effects are clearly visualised and, if necessary, avoided or corrected by secondary treatment, for occasionally in a hyperacute state or in an over-sensitive patient, the reaction obtained may be too acute. In this case the diseased organ is treated indirectly, e.g. for a disease of the heart the gall bladder is treated.

Chinese tradition expressed the interrelations between the various meridians and the methods of treatment designed to take advantage of, and to avoid undesired ill-effects which might result from, the intimate connections between organs, in a series of laws. These, formulated in the symbol imagery characteristic of Chinese thought, are as follows:

The 'Mother-son' law.

The 'Husband-wife' law.
The 'Midday-midnight' law.
etc.

The 'Mother-son' law

The essence of this law is set out in the Chinese text as follows:

'If a meridian is empty, tonify its mother. If it is full, disperse the child.'

(Zhenjiu Yixue)

As the Qi (in the superficial circulation of energy) flows through the meridians in a certain order, the preceding organ (the 'mother') receives the energy first and gives it on to that which follows (the 'son'). In the case of excess or deficiency of one to two such related organs, it is frequently preferable to give treatment via the 'mother' of the affected meridian, rather than directly.

This law has various applications:

A. SUPERFICIAL CIRCULATION OF ENERGY

As mentioned Qi flows through the meridians in a certain established order, i.e. from lung to large intestine, stomach, spleen, heart, etc.

Here the lung functions as the 'mother' of the large intestine; i.e. the large intestine is the 'son'. Or again, the large intestine is the 'mother' of the stomach; i.e. the stomach is, in this case, the 'son'. In this example the large intestine may function either as the 'son' or the 'mother', depending on whether it is related to the preceding or the following meridian respectively.

The flow of Qi to the 'son' is dependent on that of the 'mother'. Therefore, if the large intestine is tonified, so that the large intestine (in this case the 'mother') has more energy, its child, the stomach, will, as the energy flows on, also receive more energy i.e. be tonified. As the 'mother' (large intestine) is full of energy the flow of Qi coming from the preceding meridian (the lung) is dammed back, so that there is also an increase of energy in the lungs. Hence:

Tonification of the 'mother'—(Large intestine)

produces tonification of the 'son'—(Stomach)

and secondarily tonification of the preceding meridian—(Lung)

The effect on the preceding meridian (in this case the lung) is usually less marked than the true 'mother'—'son' effect.

If correspondingly the 'mother' meridian is sedated instead of tonified the result will be:

'Mother' meridian   — sedated
'Son' meridian   — sedated
Preceding meridian   — sedated

The process involved is the same in reverse.

B. DEEP CIRCULATION OF ENERGY

According to the plan of the pulse diagnosis the organs follow one another in a certain order. This order is the same as that used for the pulse diagnosis at the wrist, which will be described in a later chapter.

THE ORDER OF PULSES

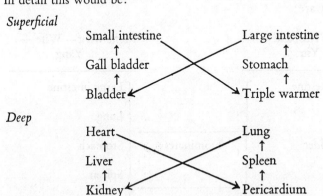

	Left radial artery		*Right radial artery*	
Superficial	*Deep*	*Deep*	*Superficial*
Small intestine	Heart	Lung	Large intestine
	↑		↑
Gall bladder	Liver	Spleen	Stomach
	↑		↑
Bladder	Kidney	Pericardium	Triple warmer

In detail this would be:

Superficial
    Small intestine   Large intestine
    ↑   ↑
    Gall bladder   Stomach
    ↑   ↑
    Bladder   Triple warmer

Deep
    Heart   Lung
    ↑   ↑
    Liver   Spleen
    ↑   ↑
    Kidney   Pericardium

The above circulation of Qi is independent of the circulation of Qi in the better known superficial circulation of energy. The energetics of deep circulation of energy is often noted in the pulse diagnosis when a weakness of the kidney, if it has persisted long enough, is accompanied by a weakness of the liver.

Some examples of the deep circulation of energy and the 'mother' —'son' law:

1. Tonification of the kidney ('mother') produces,
   Tonification of the liver ('son') and,
   Tonification of the lungs (preceding organ).
2. Sedation of the large intestine ('mother') produces,
   Sedation of the bladder ('son') and,
   Sedation of the stomach (preceding organ).

It will be noted that when various laws operate at the same time, certain effects are additive while others cancel each other out, or, on the other hand, the more powerful effect may dominate.

The deep circulation of energy is exactly the same as the creative cycle of the five elements for both the Yang and Yin organs— perhaps an unnecessary complication of saying the same thing in two ways. The only additional information given, is that it shows that the triple warmer is the son of the small intestine, and the peritardium the son of the heart.

The 'Husband-wife' Law

Organs which have equivalent positions on the left or right pulse are related to one another by the law, called in Chinese, 'husband'— 'wife'. They are:

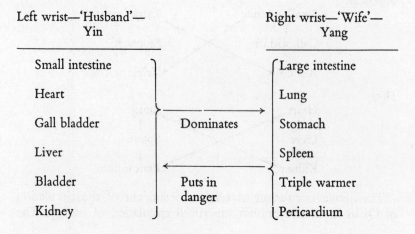

Left wrist—'Husband'— Yin		Right wrist—'Wife'— Yang
Small intestine		Large intestine
Heart		Lung
Gall bladder	Dominates	Stomach
Liver		Spleen
Bladder	Puts in danger	Triple warmer
Kidney		Pericardium

There is thus a relationship, for example, between the heart and lungs.

The pulses on the left wrist are considered Yin while those on the right are Yang. This fits in the general conception that the right hand is the active hand—the hand that holds the bow of the violin, that throws the ball, etc., so it is not surprising that it is the right hand which functions as the Yang.

The pulses on the left are considered the 'husband' while those on the right are the 'wife'. This is the opposite of what one might expect as the 'husband' is the male principle (Yang) and is therefore on the right-hand side of the body, the reverse being true for the 'wife'. This is a conception that is often met: namely, that polar opposites are at the same time opposed to one another in function, and yet constitute a single unit. e.g. In the upper half of the body the right hand is usually the more powerful and is the doing hand, while in the lower half of the body it is the left foot which is more active, setting the rhythm in marching or in beating time to the music. The marching soldier keeps time in the rhythm between his left foot and right hand.

The 'husband' (left wrist), is said to dominate the 'wife', while the 'wife' (right wrist) is said to contribute stability and solidarity.

The pulses on the left ('husband') should be slightly stronger than those on the right ('wife').

'Weak "husband", strong "wife"; then there is destruction. Strong "husband", weak "wife"; then there is security.'

(Zhenjiu Dacheng)

The 'Midday-midnight' law

Qi takes its course through the twelve meridians, as mentioned before, over a period of twenty-four hours.

According to the law based on this daily rhythm there is a relationship between organs which receive their maximal flow at opposed times. e.g. The heart, which has its maximal activity at twelve midday, and the gall bladder, which has its maximal activity at twelve midnight (Fig. 7.1). The relationships of the heart and gall bladder are well known to Western medicine:

1. A patient presenting symptoms of typical angina pectoris with the usual electrocardiographic findings, may in reality have

biliary colic, the cardiac symptoms, although they are more severe, being secondary to the law 'midday—midnight', to the gall bladder.

2. I have noticed that if I have treated a patient's heart by acupuncture rather too powerfully, that he may have biliary colic, lasting for about half an hour round about midnight of the same day.

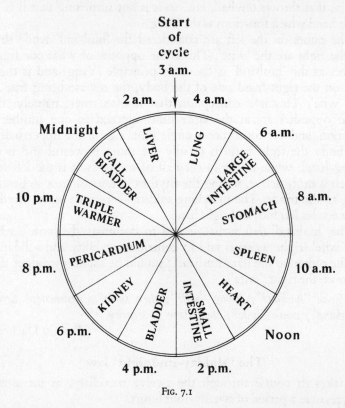

**Start
of
cycle
3 a.m.**

2 a.m.   4 a.m.

Midnight   6 a.m.

LIVER   LUNG

GALL BLADDER   LARGE INTESTINE

10 p.m.   TRIPLE WARMER   8 a.m.

STOMACH

PERICARDIUM   SPLEEN

8 p.m.   10 a.m.

KIDNEY   HEART

6 p.m.   BLADDER   SMALL INTESTINE   **Noon**

4 p.m.   2 p.m.

FIG. 7.1

3. Possibly the relation (if it is true) between angina pectoris and the continual excessive eating of saturated fatty acids or carbohydrates may one day be explained by means of a lipolytic function of bile or the metabolism of the liver.

The 'midday—midnight' law is applied as follows:

If an organ is stimulated by a moderate stimulus only the organ itself is effected. If the same organ is strongly stimulated, the organ with which it is connected by the law 'midday—midnight', is stimulated in the opposite sense. This law is more effective if a Yin organ is stimulated at a Yin time (midday to midnight) and if a Yang organ is stimulated at a Yang time (midnight to midday). e.g. If the kidney is tonified in the afternoon (Yin organ, Yin time) it will cause sedation of the large intestine. If the kidney (Yin) had been stimulated in the morning (Yang) the effect would not have been so great.

Although the law 'midday—midnight' stipulates that if the one organ is tonified then the other organ is automatically sedated, in actual practice the energetics are usually found to equalise each other so that both organs more nearly approach the normal. Hence, in the above example, if the kidney is tonified in the afternoon the large intestine will, as a result, be sedated. If, however, the large intestine were already in an under active state, it would be tonified by tonifying the kidney.

Physiological Relationships

There are relationships between the various organs which are not covered by the actual laws of acupuncture, but a physiological relationship between those in question is obvious at a glance. They are mentioned in Zhenjiu Dacheng (II, p. 18v):

Liver	to help its function, sedate the large intestine
Large intestine	If ill, tonify the liver
Spleen	If ill, disperse the small intestine
Small intestine	If ill, disperse the spleen

Relation of Meridian and Region of Body

A relationship between the meridians treated and a region of the body is part of ancient tradition. It is rarely used in practice today. Ling Tchou, Tsa tcheng loun stated in 250 B.C.:

'For diseases of the upper part of the body stimulate, above all, the meridian of the large intestine.
'For diseases of the central part of the body the meridian of the spleen.
'For diseases of the lower part of the body, the meridian of the liver.
'For diseases on the front of the chest, the meridian of the stomach.
'For the back, the meridian of the bladder.
'This is the most important part of the secret doctrine.'

VIII

THE MAIN CATEGORIES OF ACUPUNCTURE POINTS

The thousand or so acupuncture points may be divided into various categories, all points in each category having similar properties.

Points of Tonification

The point of tonification of a meridian is the 'mother' point of its own element, i.e. the liver belongs to the element wood. The 'mother' (preceding element) of wood is water. Therefore the point of tonification is the water point—liver 8 (see chapter VI).

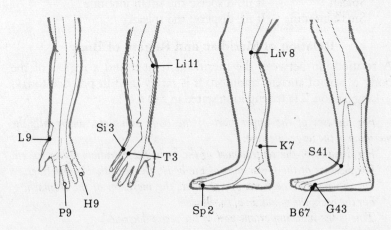

FIG. 8.1 Points of tonification

The first column in chapter VI, section 'treatment via law of five elements,' following this reasoning, gives the points of tonification of all meridians, which is printed below. The point of tonification is on the meridian whose function it controls (Fig. 8.1).

Meridian	Point
Lungs	point L9 (which is also the source)
Large intestine	point Li11
Stomach	point S41
Spleen	point Sp2
Heart	point H9
Small intestine	point Si3
Bladder	point B67
Kidney	point K7
Pericardium	point P9
Triple warmer	point T3
Gall bladder	point G43
Liver	point Liv8

When a point of tonification is stimulated various results take place, some direct and some indirect. The indirect effects are as a rule of secondary importance, so that sometimes they may be neglected; though it can happen that they are of such importance that they even overshadow the primary effect of the direct tonification of the meridian, there being no appreciable direct effect and an overwhelming indirect effect. It is for this reason that all the direct and indirect effects must be taken into account with each and every point stimulated, so that no unwished for results occur. The conditions revealed by the pulse diagnosis will decide which of the various actions and reactions will take place.

DIRECT RESULTS

(a) The meridian itself is tonified, e.g. if the point Heart 9 (H9) is tonified, the meridian of the heart is tonified. This is shown by a greater strength of the pulse of the heart.

This effect is by far the most important of all the effects produced by stimulating a point of tonification (e.g. H9).

INDIRECT RESULTS

(b) The meridian in rapport with the meridian tonified by the law 'husband-wife' is sedated if it is in excess, e.g. if the heart is tonified, the lung is sedated. This is because as a rule not much energy is created de novo; the deficiency in the heart is made up by passing a part of the excess of energy in the lung over to the deficiency in the heart; so that whereas before treatment the heart was deficient and the lung in excess, after the stimulation of point H9, both the lung and the heart meridians have an equal amount of energy.

This law only operates in cases where the 'wife' (the 'husband' H9, is stimulated) has an excess of energy. If the 'wife' (the lung in this case) has the same amount of energy as the 'husband' (heart), or even less energy than the heart, this indirect effect does not take place.

(c) The meridian in rapport with the meridian tonified by the law 'midday-midnight' is sedated, if it is in excess and if treatment is given at the correct time of the day.

The heart has its maximal energy at midday, the gall bladder has its maximal energy at midnight. All organs are connected with their opposite number, from which they are separated by twelve hours, by a secondary meridian through the medium of which the mechanism of the law 'midday-midnight' takes place. If the heart is tonified the gall bladder is therefore sedated.

This law only operates to any marked degree if:

1. The opposite element (gall bladder) has an excess of energy.

2. The meridian tonified (heart) is tonified at a period of the day which is in its own sign. In this case, the heart which is a 'solid' organ and therefore Yin, must be tonified at a Yin period of the day which is from midday to sunset.

Thus if the heart is tonified at H9 in the afternoon (time Yin), the gall bladder will, as a result, be sedated. This would not have happened at all and, if at all, to a lesser degree if H9 had been tonified in the morning or if the gall bladder had had the same amount or less energy than the heart.

Conversely, if the gall bladder were tonified at point G43 (its point of tonification) in the morning, the heart would be sedated (provided the heart were also in excess).

(d) Between certain meridians there are special connections via secondary meridians, that do not follow strict laws, and are not invariably operative.

In this case if the heart is tonified at H9, the vessel of conception is sedated.

(e) Relationship between meridians sometimes operate via the superficial circulation of energy.

If a meridian is tonified, the meridian which comes before it and after it in the order of the superficial circulation of energy is tonified. That is to say, if the heart is tonified at H9, the spleen and the small intestine meridians will be tonified. (According to Niboyet the tonification of the meridian before and after the one stimulated is preceded by a rapid sedation, as the energy from these two encircling meridians first rushes to the tonified meridian, before being tonified themselves by the excess).

(f) Tonification of a meridian entails tonification of the meridian before it and after it in the order of the circulation of the deep flow of energy in accordance with the plan of the pulse. In this case tonification of the heart would also cause tonification of the liver and pericardium meridians. But this effect is not as marked as that of the superficial circulation of energy. (Similarly to the previous example (e) there is a sedation before the tonification).

To sum up:

If the heart is stimulated at point H9 in the afternoon, the following results may be expected:

(a) The heart will be tonified, (if it was not in excess).
(b) The lung will be sedated, (if it was not deficient).
(c) The gall bladder will be sedated, (if it was in excess and the treatment was performed in the afternoon).
(d) The vessel of conception is sedated, (if in excess).
(e) The spleen and small intestine will be tonified, (if they were deficient).
(f) The liver and pericardium will be tonified, (if they were deficient)

These results are in conformity with the following acupuncture laws.

(a) Direct.
(b) The law of 'Husband-wife'.
(c) The law of 'Midday-midnight'.
(d) Special secondary meridian connections.
(e) Superficial circulation of energy.
(f) Deep circulation of energy (five elements).

Case History. A patient was seen who was suffering from heartburn and constipation. She had had typhoid fever forty years previously from which she nearly died. Since that time she has never felt well and lacked energy.

Pulse diagnosis revealed, amongst other things, a weakness of the pulses of the liver and large intestine. The liver and large intestine were tonified at their points of tonification—Liv8 and Li11. These points in

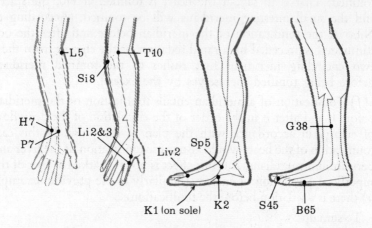

FIG. 8.2 Points of sedation

conjunction with other points, repeated over a considerable period, because of the chronicity of the disease, brought the patient back to a nearly normal state of health.

Points of Sedation

Each of the twelve main meridians has in contrast to its point of tonification, a specific point of sedation. This is invariably located on the meridian whose function it controls.

The point of sedation of a meridian is the 'son' point of its own element i.e. the small intestine belongs to the element fire. The 'son' (following element) of fire is earth. Therefore the point of sedation is the earth point—small intestine 8 (see chapter VI). The fifth column in chapter VI, section 'treatment via law of five elements', likewise gives the point of sedation of all meridians as also printed below (Fig. 8.2).

196

Meridian	Point
Lungs	point L5
Large intestine	point Li2 and Li3
Stomach	point S45
Spleen	point Sp5
Heart	point H7 (also source)
Small intestine	point Si8
Bladder	point B65
Kidney	point K1 and K2
Pericardium	point P7 (also source)
Triple warmer	point T10
Gall bladder	point G38
Liver	point Liv2

The effects are theoretically the reverse of the points of tonification, though this in practice will not always be found to operate, so that progress should be carefully followed by palpation of the pulse. It can sometimes happen that a point of tonification acts as if it were a point of sedation and vice versa.

Theoretically the effects expected should be:

(a) Direct stimulation—sedation.
(b) Stimulation in accordance with 'Husband-wife' law—tonification.
(c) Stimulation in accordance with the 'Midday-midnight' law (Yang organ in the morning, Yin organ in the evening)—tonification.
(d) Stimulation of special meridians—tonification.
(e) Stimulation in accordance with superficial circulation of energy —sedation.
(f) Stimulation in accordance with deep circulation of energy (five elements)—sedation.

Thus, if the liver were sedated at its point of sedation, point Liv2, the following would result:

(a) Sedation of liver, (if it were not already deficient).
(b) Tonification of spleen, (if it had been deficient before).
(c) Tonification of the small intestine (if Liv2 is sedated in the evening).
(d) Nil.

(e) Sedation of the gall bladder and lungs, (if these were in excess before treatment).

(f) Sedation of the kidney and heart, (if these were in excess before treatment).

Case History. The patient was lethargic in the morning, had frontal headaches, and palpitations with physical or even slight mental strain. Pulse diagnosis showed an over-activity of the gall bladder and an under-activity of the heart. The point of sedation of the gall bladder (G38) was stimulated in the morning which directly sedated the gall bladder; and at the same time indirectly tonified the heart via the law of midday-midnight (c). Her symptoms disappeared in ten minutes.

The Source

Each of the twelve main meridians has a third type of directive point called the source, which is located on the meridian that it controls. These are as follows (Fig. 8.3):

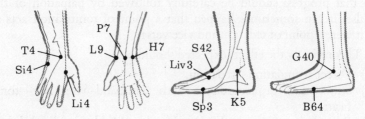

FIG. 8.3 Source points

Meridian	Point
Lungs	point L9 (also point of tonification)
Large intestine	point Li4
Stomach	point S42
Spleen	point Sp3
Heart	point H7 (also point of sedation)
Small intestine	point Si3
Bladder	point B64
Kidney	point K5
Pericardium	point P7 (also point of sedation)
Triple warmer	point T4
Gall bladder	point G40
Liver	point Liv3

The stimulation of the source point gives various results:

1. It may either cause direct tonification or direct sedation of the meridian on which it is placed. This type of amphoteric action distinguishes the source from a point of tonification or sedation which, as a rule, can only be tonified or sedated, as the name implies.

According to classical acupuncture the source is tonified if a gold needle is used, and is rotated clockwise, the needle being inserted in the direction of the current of energy along the meridian and the operation effected while the patient exhales. Similarly, the same point is sedated if a silver needle is used, if it is rotated anti-clockwise, and the needle is inserted against the direction of the current of energy along the meridian and the operation effected while the patient inhales.

In my experience the above factors are not of any great consequence. In fact in whatever way the source is stimulated it has the desired effect of re-establishing the balance of energy. If, for example, the kidney were underactive and the source of the kidney, point K5, were stimulated with either a silver or a gold needle, the kidney would be tonified. Once this direct effect of either tonification or sedation has taken place, the same interactions follow as for the points of tonification or sedation, following the same laws and conditions which governed their operations in the former instances, i.e. those of:

'Husband-wife'.
'Midday-midnight'.
Special secondary vessels.
Superficial circulation of energy.
Deep circulation of energy (five elements).

2. Stimulation of the source usually has a rapid effect.

3. If the point of tonification, or the point of sedation has been used and thereafter the source is utilised, the effect of the tonification or sedation is accentuated. e.g. If the kidney has been tonified by point K7, (its point of tonification) but the result is not sufficient, the source K5 if used, may reinforce the action.

Case History. A patient who had had polio as a child in one of his legs developed severe sciatica when an adult. Pulse diagnosis showed a weakness of the kidney pulse. This was tonified by putting a needle into the source of the kidney (point K5), which resulted in an immediate

relief of pain, but only to return when he started walking again. Various
other points were tried; the pain being relieved each time, only to reappear again. It was then found that one leg was an inch shorter than
the other. (The leg which had been affected by polio growing more
slowly). A raised shoe relieved the condition. This type of gross structural damage is not suitable for treatment by acupuncture.

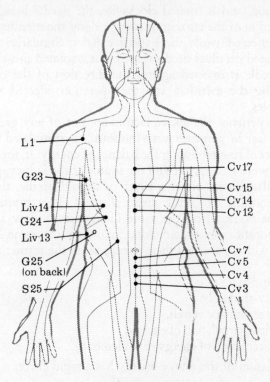

FIG. 8.4 Alarm points

Alarm Points

The points known as 'alarm points' are a series that occur on the
ventral surface of the abdomen or chest. They are (Fig. 8.4):

Meridian	Point
Lungs	point L1
Large intestine	point S25

Stomach	point Cv12
Spleen	point Liv13
Heart	point Cv14
Small intestine	point Cv4
Bladder	point Cv3
Kidney	point G25
Pericardium	point Cv15 (Discovered by Soulié de Morant)
Triple warmer (main)	point Cv5
Triple warmer (superior)	point Cv17
Triple warmer (middle)	point Cv12
Triple warmer (inferior)	point Cv7
Gall bladder (main)	point G24
Gall bladder (secondary)	point G23
Liver	point Liv14

All these points are located on the embryological anterior surface of the body. Only three points are on the meridian which they subserve, viz: Lung, gall bladder and liver, these three being organs which follow one another in the superficial circulation of energy, occupying the time from 11 p.m. to 5 a.m. Many of the points of alarm are located on a meridian the vessel of conception (Cv) which does not belong to the primary system of twelve meridians.

The alarm points have various functions:

1. The points are all situated on the ventral surface, and this being a Yin surface, they are typically associated with diseases of a Yin type. This is so marked that in old textbooks, only the five primary Yin organs (liver, heart, spleen, lung and kidney) are described as having an alarm point.

To quote Zhenjiu Yixue—'*The illnesses of the Yang act on the Yin. That is why the points of alarm are all in the Yin. The front of the abdomen and chest are Yin; that is why the points of alarm are there.*'

Yin diseases are those which are typically accompanied by cold, depression and weakness.

2. In the characteristic type of Yin disease the point of alarm becomes excessively tender. e.g. In many cardiac diseases the point of alarm of the heart (Cv14) (Fig. 8.4) which is about 1 inch below the xiphoid process of the sternum, is spontaneously tender.

I have mentioned earlier that an acupuncture point that needs treatment often becomes spontaneously tender. This tenderness is so exaggerated in the case of the points of alarm that it is used as a palpatory method of diagnosis in the following manner.

The patient is asked to lie flat and relaxed on a couch, with the chest and abdomen bare. The points of alarm are then palpated and if they are more tender than the surrounding tissues a functional disturbance of the organ which they represent may be deduced.

The area of tenderness and of superficial tissue changes as shown by palpation is considerably larger and more easily noticeable in the case of the alarm points than in that of the other types of acupuncture points when comparably activated. These two factors, taken together with the relatively greater increase in tenderness of this type of point, constitute useful diagnostic criteria.

The alarm point may become spontaneously painful, so that the patient is aware of it without it being pressed, more easily than in any other type of activated acupuncture point. Naturally this makes diagnosis easier.

3. Normally the point of alarm is considered a point of tonification, which, if stimulated, increases the energy in the meridian which it subserves.

The tonification of the meridian–organ concerned is followed to some extent by a tonification of the meridian which preceeds and follows it in the superficial circulation of energy and also the deep circulation of energy (five elements).

4. In my experience the point of alarm serves equally well as a point of sedation but care must be exercised in sedating an over-active alarm point as a hypertonification may unwittingly be the result, with an acute exacerbation of the condition being treated. This exacerbation can sometimes be avoided by stimulating the point of alarm for only a few seconds instead of the customary minutes.

5. Usually a qualitative increase in the Yang elements at the pulse will be noted. This is an uncertain response.

Illustration. In patients with diseases of the upper digestive organs, very frequently the point of alarm of the stomach, Cv12, (Fig. 8.4) becomes spontaneously tender. A needle put into this point may cause immediate relief of upper abdominal distension and nausea. The fundamental condition however will have to be treated by other points.

Associated Points

Qi Bo: *'If you press with your finger on these points, the pain of the corresponding organ is immediately relieved.'*

(Nei Jing, Ch. 51)

All meridians have an associated point on the back along the medial course of the bladder meridian on each side of the vertebral column. According to Qi Bo (Fig. 8.5):

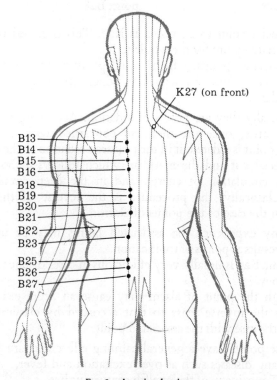

FIG. 8.5 Associated points

Meridian	Point
Lung	point B13
Pericardium	point B14
Heart	point B15
(Governing vessel	point B16)

Liver	point B18
Gall bladder	point B19
Spleen	point B20
Stomach	point B21
Triple warmer	point B22
Kidney	point B23
Large intestine	point B25
Small intestine	point B27
Bladder	point B28

One special point to be noted is K27. This is considered to act as the associated point for the whole series.

The associated points, which are all paravertebral on the dorsal surface, have certain characteristics which are in contrast to the points of alarm:

1. Classically they are points of sedation. According to the laws of acupuncture, once the meridian concerned with a particular associated point is sedated, it in turn causes a sedation of the meridian which precedes it and the meridian which follows it, both in the superficial circulation of energy and in the deep circulation of energy. Classically, the procedure is the reverse of that which operates in the case of the points of alarm.

2. In my experience the associated points may be used with excellent results as points of tonification.

e.g. Point B23 is usually very efficacious in cases of under-activity of the kidney.

Although the point of alarm may cause an acute exacerbation if used in the inverse sense to that accorded by classical theory, this is not the case with the associated point.

3. These points have a general calming effect and are therefore used in Yang diseases such as over excitation and fever.

Li Kao Tong-iuann of the twelfth century writes:

'To treat a disease caused by wind or cold, you must stimulate the associated point of a storage, hollow organ. In fact the illness entered by the Yang and then flowed through the meridians. If it started by a cold exterior it must finish by returning to the exterior by warmth.'

4. Chinese osteopathy uses these points to correct small displacements of vertebrae. The rationale is as follows:

In a disease of the descending colon, the associated point of the large intestine, B25 (Fig. 8.6), on the same side as the descending colon, i.e. the left, will together with other points become spontaneously tender. This causes a spasm of the muscles in the vicinity of point B25 on the left. These muscles which are adjacent to, and attached to, the fourth lumbar vertebra, cause it to be displaced towards the left.

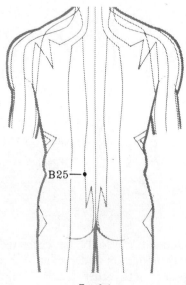

FIG. 8.6

Hence a disease of the descending colon may, under the correct conditions, cause as a secondary result a displacement of the fourth lumbar vertebra to the left, with, if the displacement is severe enough, resultant lumbago and possibly sciatica.

Only rarely does an internal disease cause a displaced vertebra for:

(a) Not all internal diseases cause tenderness of the associated point, and hence muscle spasm.

(b) The muscle spasm must be of a fairly severe degree.

(c) Before displacement occurs there must in general be associated factors which could operate to facilitate the displacement of a vertebra, such as a general metabolic disturbance causing osteo-porosis, or weakness of the paravertebral muscles, trauma, etc.

If the displacement of the fourth lumbar vertebra is only small it may be corrected by an acupuncture point (or medicine) that corrects the disease of the descending colon. It may also be corrected by stimulating point B25 on the left, though usually treatment of various secondarily effected points is also required.

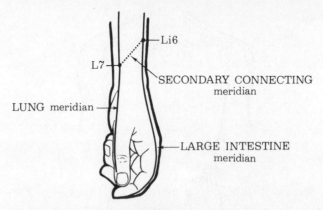

FIG. 8.7

A severe displacement can only be corrected by osteopathic manoeuvres or by manipulation under an anaesthetic. If the internal factor which, together with other factors, originally caused the displacement of the vertebra, are not treated at the same time as the displacement is corrected, there is a greater likelihood of a recurrence. This explains the too frequent recurrence of lumbago or sciatica if treated only by manipulation, osteopathy, corsets, etc. Conversely, under suitable conditions, the correction of the displaced vertebra may cure the primary internal disease.

This problem can, at times, present itself as the classical dilemma —which came first, the chicken or the egg? It is sometimes best to attack both ends of the problem at the same time.

Manipulative surgeons, osteopaths and masseurs, have often found that by manipulating vertebrae they can cure, or alleviate, internal diseases. This has been partially explained via neural reflexes connecting the diseased organ with the appropriate spinal segment. As all the important internal organs, (from the acupuncture point of view), have an associated point which is paravertebral, I think we can regard this fact as at least a partial explanation of the connection.

Illustration. Stage fright is sometimes due to an over-activity of the heart. The heart may be sedated in many ways; but as stage fright is an illness associated with nervousness the associated point is probably the best heart point to choose—point B15—between the shoulder blades.

'Connecting' Points

The so called 'connecting' points connect coupled meridians by a secondary meridian. e.g. There is a secondary meridian running from L7 to Li6, joining the lung meridian with the large intestine meridian (Fig. 8.7).

Coupled meridians are meridians which follow one another in the superficial circulation of energy and, at the same time, are of opposite sign, the one being Yin, the other Yang. It follows that the former lies on an embryological anterior surface, while the latter lies on an embryological posterior surface.

These coupled meridians thus constitute a unit of similarities and dissimilarities (Fig. 8.8).

Coupled meridians	Lungs	Yin	point L7
	Large intestine	Yang	point Li6
Coupled meridians	Stomach		point S40
	Spleen	Yin	point Sp4
Coupled meridians	Heart		point H5
	Small intestine	Yang	point Si7
Coupled meridians	Bladder		point B58
	Kidney	Yin	point K6
Coupled meridians	Pericardium		point P6
	Triple warmer	Yang	point T5
Coupled meridians	Gall bladder		point G37
	Liver	Yin	point Liv5

The vessel of conception, being the most Yin of any meridian and the governing vessel being the most Yang of any meridian, are also connected by their connecting points, these being Cv15 and Gv1 respectively.

There is also the so called Great Connecting Point of the spleen, Sp21.

Treatment of the connecting points can serve various purposes:

1. A disequilibrium between the two meridians of a couple may be corrected by only using one point. In this case either the connecting point of the deficient meridian is tonified or the connecting point of the over-active meridian is sedated.

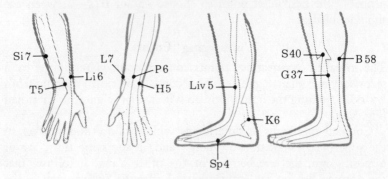

FIG. 8.8 Connecting points

If, for example, the liver is deficient, while the gall bladder is in excess, either the liver may be tonified at its first connecting point Liv5, or the gall bladder may be sedated at its connecting point G37. Thus two meridians are corrected by only using one acupuncture point.

It seems as if the connecting point on either meridian acts as a sort of short-circuit enabling the excess of energy to flow along the connecting vessel from one meridian to the other of a couple.

2. The connecting point controls the energy between the left and right halves of a meridian. e.g. If the left lung meridian has an excess of energy, while the right lung meridian is deficient in energy, these may be equilibriated by tonifying the connecting point of the lung meridian (L7) on the right side, or by sedating L7 on the left side—only one needle being used to produce the two effects desired.

3. The connecting point controls the flow of energy between organs related to one another by the law of 'midday-midnight'.

If the bladder meridian has an excess of energy while the lung is deficient, (bladder maximal activity 4 p.m., lung maximal activity

4 a.m.) the connecting point L7 of the lung may be tonified, and thus equilibrium between bladder and lung may be achieved.

When the connecting point is used in obedience to the law of 'midday-midnight', account need not be taken of Yin or Yang times of day, the reaction taking place equally well whatever time the point is stimulated.

If an exchange of energy is desired between the left lung and left functional part of the bladder, only the connecting point on the left side is utilised.

Case History. A patient had chronic bladder trouble over a period of twenty years, with frequency, nocturia, burning pain on urination, etc. The pulse diagnosis showed an irritable bladder with a wiry pulse. Treatment of the bladder meridian did not alter the condition for, as may be noticed frequently in acupuncture, the direct treatment of the diseased meridian, is often of no value. The bladder and kidney meridians are united via their connecting points—B58 and K6. Stimulation of the kidney connecting point, K6, regularised the pulse of the bladder. The treatment had to be repeated many times before a considerable improvement, though not complete cure, ensued.

GRAND PIQURE

By this method energy is drawn from one side of the body to the other via the connecting points.

If there is, for example, an excess of energy in the right stomach meridian, causing pain along part of its course, the connecting point on the opposite (left) side is stimulated—point stomach 40 (S40).

GRAND PIQURE COMBINED WITH TREATMENT ACCORDING TO THE LAW 'MIDDAY-MIDNIGHT'

The effect of the above example may be increased by stimulating the connecting point on the left side of the meridian connected to the stomach meridian by the law of 'midday-midnight'. This is the meridian of pericardium. Therefore its connecting point pericardium (P6) is stimulated only on the left.

Point of Entry and Exit

As mentioned previously, the energy Qi flows through the twelve meridians in a certain invariable sequence: lung, large intestine, stomach, spleen, etc.

This flow of Qi is always in the same direction starting at the point of entry of the lung meridian (Fig. 8.9), flowing along the lung meridian, and leaving again at the point of exit to enter the point of entry of the meridian of the large intestine; flowing along the meridian of the large intestine, to leave it again at the point of exit, to enter the meridian of the stomach at its point of entry etc., etc.

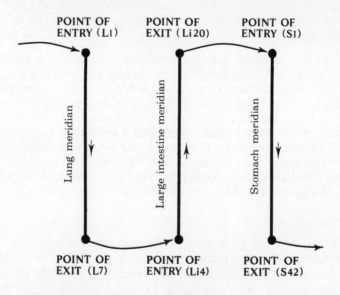

FIG. 8.9

The point of entry and the point of exit are usually the first and last points respectively of the meridian concerned, in which case, a secondary meridian unites the end of one meridian with the beginning of the next, along which the Qi flows. In some cases the point of entry or exit is not the end point of a meridian (though it is not far from it). In this case the main secondary meridian uniting the two meridians does not occur at the end point of the meridians. Nevertheless, the remaining distal portion of the meridian is not a cul-de-sac for the secondary meridian mentioned in the previous paragraph, uniting the end points of the meridians, is still operative, though it performs a function in this case secondary to the meridian connecting the points of exit and entry.

Tonification of a point of entry, tonifies the meridian concerned, provided the previous meridian has an excess of energy to pass on.

Sedation of a point of entry, under the reverse circumstances, is considered to sedate the meridian concerned. In my experience this effect is unreliable and unpredictable.

Sedation of a point of exit, sedates the meridian concerned, provided the following meridian is deficient in energy so that the excess energy of the sedated meridian may pass into it.

Tonification of the point of exit is considered to produce the same result as sedation.

The points of entry are more reliable in their effects than the points of exit (Fig. 8.10).

Points of Entry

Lung	point L1 (also point of alarm)
Large intestine	point Li4 (also source. *1st point is* Li1)
Stomach	point S1
Spleen	point Sp1
Heart	point H1
Small intestine	point Si1
Bladder	point B1
Kidney	point K1 (also point of sedation)
Pericardium	point P1
Triple warmer	point T1
Gall bladder	point G1
Liver	point Liv1

Points of Exit

Lung	point L7 (also 'Lo' point. *Last point is* L11)
Large intestine	point Li20
Stomach	point S42 (also point of tonification. *Last point is* S45)
Spleen	point Sp21
Heart	point H9 (also point of tonification)
Small intestine	point Si19
Bladder	point B67 (also point of tonification)
Kidney	point K22 (*Last point* K27)
Pericardium	point P8 (Alarm point of pericardium. *Last point* P9)

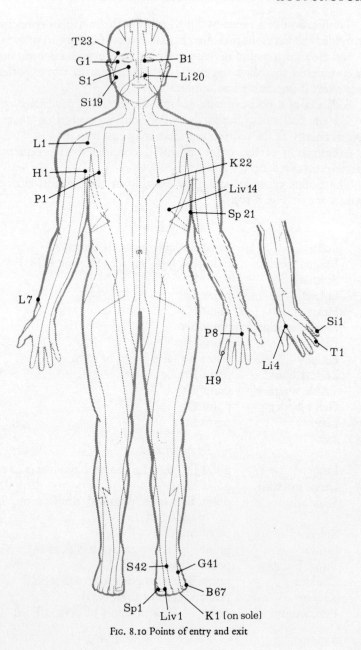

T 23
G 1
S 1
Si 19
B 1
Li 20
L 1
H 1
P 1
K 22
Liv 14
Sp 21
L 7
P 8
H 9
Si 1
T 1
Li 4
S 42
Sp 1
G 41
B 67
Liv 1
K 1 [on sole]

Fig. 8.10 Points of entry and exit

Triple warmer   point T23
Gall bladder   point G41 (*Last point* G44)
Liver   point Liv14 (Also point of alarm)

Example. Tonification of the point of entry of the small intestine (Si1) will tonify the small intestine, provided the meridian of the heart has an excess of energy to pass on.

Sedation of the point of exit of the triple warmer (T23) will sedate the triple warmer provided the gall bladder is deficient in energy.

Case History. In the skin disease, acne rosacea, the pulse of the large intestine is, amongst others, weakened. The point of entry of the large intestine, Li4, together with other points, were stimulated in a patient. Within a month the condition was about 90% cured, despite the fact that she had had this condition for many years.

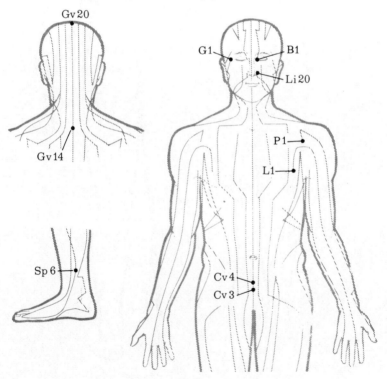

FIG. 8.11 Special meeting points

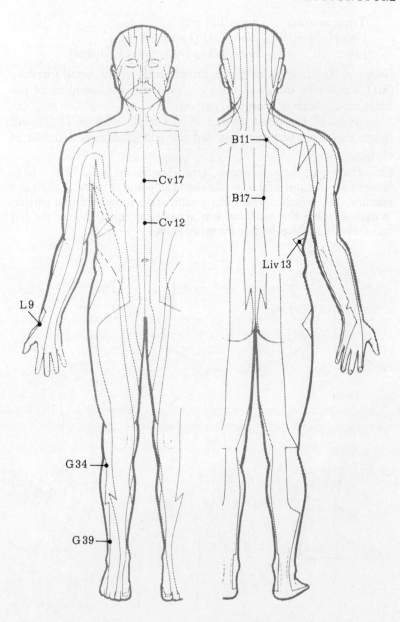

FIG. 8.12 Eight meeting points

Special Meeting Points

Stimulation of these points has an effect on a related group of meridians (Fig. 8.11):

Cv3 and Cv4	3 leg Yin and conception vessel
Gv20	3 leg Yang and governing vessel
Sp6	3 leg Yin
Gv14	7 Yang

The meeting point of the other related meridians is as follows:

Lung and Spleen	L1
Pericardium	P1
Small intestine and bladder	B1
Triple warmer and gall bladder	G1
Large intestine and stomach	Li20

Case History. A patient at hospital was suffering from a catarrhal nasal condition with hyperacidity. Pulse diagnosis showed a weak pulse of the large intestine and a bumpy wiry pulse of the stomach. The meeting point of the large intestine and stomach, point Li20, in combination with a more fundamental realignment of his fundamental energetics, cured the patient.

The Eight Meeting Points

The following eight points have a particular influence on the eight tissues mentioned; or, as the Chinese put it, 'the Qi of these eight tissues meet at the eight points.' They are (Fig. 8.12):

Solid organs (Zang)	Liv13
Hollow organs (Fu)	Cv12
Energy and/or breath (Qi)	Cv17
Blood	B17
Bones	B11
Marrow	G39
Muscles	G34
Vessels	L9

The Combining Points

The Nei Jing describes these points as:
'At the level of the combining points the energy of the six Yang

Fu penetrates into the interior of the body'. Again: 'The combining points rule the energies of the meridians.'

These points are (Fig. 8.13):

	Organ	Lower combining point	Upper combining point
3 Yang of foot	Stomach	S36	—
	Gall bladder	G34	—
	Bladder	B54	—
3 Yang of hand	Large intestine	S37	Li11
	Triple warmer	B53	T10
	Small intestine	S39	Si8

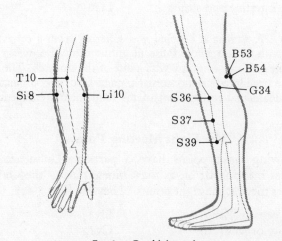

FIG. 8.13 Combining points

Frequently an organ-meridian may be disturbed in such a way that the disturbance is not seen at the extremities, but centrally in the abdomen and thorax. In these cases the combining points may be used.

Case History. A patient complained of intermittent swelling of the lower abdomen with no clear urinary symptoms. Pulse diagnosis revealed a wiry pulse of the bladder. The combining point of the bladder, point B54, in combination with subsidiary points, cured the condition.

The Points 'Window of the Sky'

The Nei Jing says:

'*All the energies Yang come from the Yin, for the Yin is earth. This Yang energy always climbs from the lower part of the body towards the head; but if it is interrupted in its course it cannot climb beyond the abdomen. In that case one must find which meridian is diseased. One must tonify the Yin (as it creates the Yang) and disperse the Yang so that the energy is attracted towards the top of the body and the circulation is re-established.*'

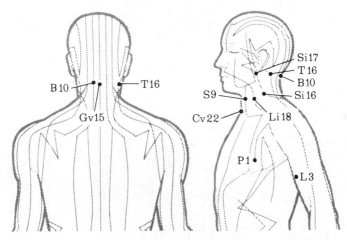

FIG. 8.14 Window of the sky points

The points used for this purpose are (Fig. 53):

S9	Li18
T16	B10
L3	Cv22
Gv15	Si16
Si17	P1

It will be noticed that all these points except for L3 and P1 are in the neck, which is the route whereby energy goes from the lower part of the body to the head.

The symptomatology according to the Nei Jing is as follows:

S9. Severe pain in the head, fullness of the chest, dyspnoea.

Li18. Loss of voice.

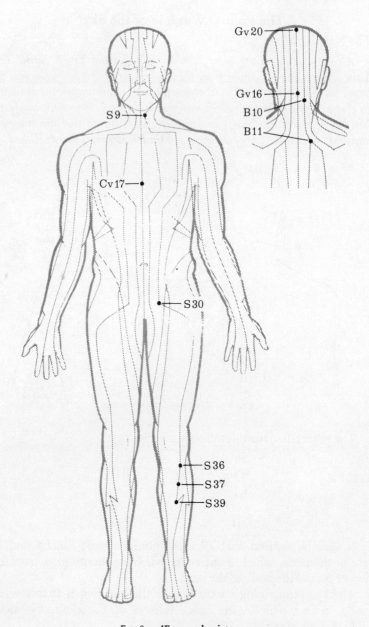

FIG. 8.15 'Four seas' points

T16. When the patient suddenly becomes deaf or cannot see clearly.

B10. Spasms, muscular contractions, fainting, when the patient's feet can no longer support the weight of the body.

L3. Great thirst (disharmony of liver and lung) nose bleeds or bleeding by the mouth.

Case History. A patient at hospital had lost his voice some months previously and felt light-headed. He felt as if his head and body were not properly connected. The point 'window of the sky' S9, repeated several times, in combination with subsidiary points, cured the patient. The first treatment only point S9 was used and caused a fluctuation between improvement and worsening of the condition. Thereafter (as the barrier had been opened) the appropriate Yin meridians (liver and kidney in this case) were tonified and the light-headedness disappeared.

The Points of the 'Four Seas'

The Nei Jing says:

'*Man possesses four seas and twelve meridians, which are like rivers that flow into the sea.*'

The four seas are:
1. The sea of nourishment.
2. The sea of blood.
3. The sea of energy.
4. The sea of the bone marrow.

1. 'The sea of nourishment is represented by the stomach. Its two principal points are S30 and S36 (Fig. 8.15).

If there is excess the patient has abdominal swelling. If there is emptiness he cannot eat.'

2. 'The sea of the blood is represented by the extra meridian, the 'penetrating vessel', which is the sea of the twelve meridians. Its points of liaison are B11 for the high part of the body and S37 and S39 for the low part of the body.

When there is an excess, the patient has the sensation that his body is greater in volume. When there is deficiency, the patient is affected, but cannot define what he feels.'

3. 'The sea of energy is represented by the region around the point Cv17. These points are in liaison with point B10 behind and S9 in front of the neck.

If there is excess, the patient feels pain in the chest, the face is red and there is breathlessness. If there is emptiness the patient cannot speak.'

4. 'The sea of bone marrow. Its point of liaison is localised on the summit of the head (probably governing vessel 20) and at the back of the head by point governing vessel 16.

If there is fullness, the patient feels as if he has an excess of energy.

If there is emptiness, the patient has dizzy bouts, noises in his ears, fainting, pain in the calf.'

It says further:

To sum up: 'One must be able to discern accurately if there is emptiness or fullness and puncture the points of the 'four seas' correctly, for thus one can regularise all the energies. But if one punctures incorrectly one can provoke grave trouble.'

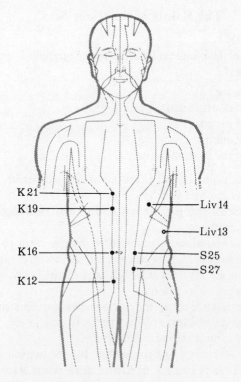

FIG. 8.16 Shokanten

Shokanten

The Japanese Shokanten, as described by Manaka*, are points on the abdomen that become tender if the greater, lesser or middle Yang or Yin become affected. As such, these points may be used both diagnostically and in the reverse, therapeutically (Fig 8.16).

Greater Yang	Small intestine/Bladder—K12.
Lesser Yang	Triple warmer/Gall bladder—S25.
Sunlight Yang	Large intestine/Stomach—S27.
Greater Yin	Lung/Spleen—Liv13.
Absolute Yin	Pericardium/Liver—Liv14.
Lesser Yin	Heart/Kidney—K16.

In addition, Manaka has described:

Lesser Yang	K21.
Absolute Yin	K19.

The Accumulating Points (Hung

The great gilded Buddhist temples in China are known as the 'Hung' and the name is also used for the accumulating points, for they are as important in the body as temples. They are described as 'gaps in the body where Qi and blood converge and collect' and are used in chronic disease (Fig. 8.17).

Meridian	Accumulating point
Lung	L6
Large intestine	Li7
Stomach	S34
Spleen	Sp8
Heart	H6
Small intestine	Si6
Bladder	B63
Kidney	K4
Pericardium	P4
Triple warmer	T7
Gall bladder	G36
Liver	Liv6

*IV Journees Internationales d'Acupuncture.

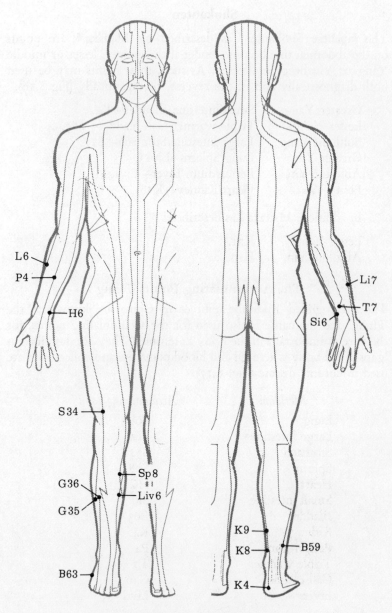

FIG. 8.17 Accumulating points

And for the extra meridians:—

Yin linking vessel	K9
Yang linking vessel	G35
Yin heel vessel	K8
Yang heel vessel	B59

The Five Categories

The Chinese give special names to five (or six) categories of points.

Category	Chinese name	Meaning
I	Well	Emerging
II	Gushing	Flowing
III	Transporting	Pouring
IV	Penetrating	Moving
V	Uniting	Entering

These names, and the meaning of them to the Chinese, image the

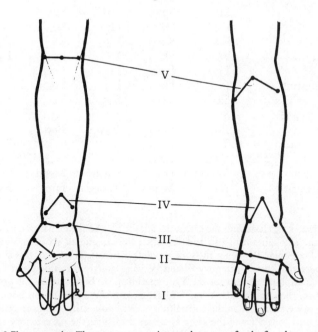

FIG. 8.18 Five categories. The acupuncture points are the same as for the five elements (Fig. 6.3)

flow of Qi along the meridian as the movement of water. The 'well' is the place whence the water emerges; the 'gushing' is its overflow; the 'transporting' point is where the water pours along; the 'penetrating' point where it moves. Finally, since water must find its way to union with the sea, the solid and hollow organs, we have the 'uniting point'.

The categories I, II, III, IV and V follow the points of the five elements: (for the Yin meridians) wood, fire, earth, metal, water; (for the Yang meridians) metal, water, wood, fire, earth, in that order from the tips of the fingers or toes to the elbow or knee (Fig. 8.18 and 8.19).

CATEGORY*

	I	II	III	IV	V
Lungs	L11	L10	L9	L8	L5
Spleen	Sp1	Sp2	Sp3	Sp5	Sp9
Heart	H9	H8	H7	H4	H3
Kidney	K1	K2	K5	K7	K10
Pericardium	P9	P8	P7	P5	P3
Liver	Liv1	Liv2	Liv3	Liv4	Liv8
Large intestine	Li1	Li2	Li3	Li5	Li11
Stomach	S45	S44	S43	S41	S36
Small intestine	Si1	Si2	Si3	Si5	Si8
Bladder	B67	B66	B65	B60	B54
Triple warmer	T1	T2	T3	T6	T10
Gall bladder	G44	G43	G41	G38	G34
Yin element	Wood	Fire	Earth	Metal	Water
Yang element	Metal	Water	Wood	Fire	Earth

*The system of classifying the categories adopted by Soulié de Morant and after him, in the first edition of this and my other books, utilised six categories; the additional category, IV, being the source points mentioned earlier in this chapter. Thus, under that system category III and IV were exactly the same point for the Yin meridians, but different for the Yang meridians. In both systems categories I, II and III are the same, whilst V and VI have become IV and V in this book. The five category system used in the 2nd edition of this book is the one more generally used in China today. I will therefore at a.later date, alter the six category system used in the present editions of my other books, to the five category system.

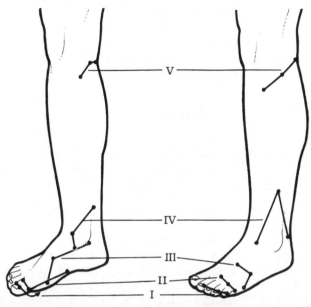

FIG. 8.19 Five categories. The acupuncture points are the same as for the five elements (Fig. 6.4)

Traditionally the following groups of diseases can best be treated by them:

I Region below heart full.
II Body hot.
III Body heavy, joints painful.
IV Dyspnoea, coughing, cold and hot.
V Rebellious Qi and diarrhoea.

Meeting Points

The meeting points have an effect on more than one meridian. For example bladder 1, as can be seen from the table, influences the small intestine and stomach in addition to the bladder itself.

It is difficult, if not impossible, to tell if a certain meeting point exerts its effect on several meridians directly, or indirectly via the normal laws of acupuncture. If the latter idea were correct, it should, of course apply to all points on the same meridian—in which case the conception of meeting points would be superfluous.

For the above reasons it is difficult to tell which are the various meridians effected by a meeting point, and opinions vary. Five traditional sources are given, which the reader may compare.

Likewise the meeting points given in my other books, are essentially but not quite the same, as in this volume.

Meeting Points

	1	2	3	4	5
L1	L	L, Sp	Sp	L, Sp	L, Sp
Li14	Li con	Li con	Li con	Si, B, Ya-l	Li con, Si, B, Ya-l
Li15	Li, Ya-h	Li, Ya-h	Li, Ya-h	Li, Ya-h	Si, Li, Ya-h, G
Li16	Li, Ya-h	Li, Ya-h	Li, Ya-h	Li, Ya-h	Li, Ya-h
Li20	Li, S	Li, S	Li, S	Li, S	Li, S
S1	Ya-h, Cv, S	Ya-h, Cv, S	Ya-h, Cv, S	Ya-h, Cv, S	Ya-h, Cv, S
S3	Ya-h, S	Ya-h, S	Ya-h, S	Li, S, Ya-h	Ya-h, S
S4	Ya-h, Li, S	Ya-h, Li, S	Ya-h, Li, S	Ya-h, Li, S	Ya-h, Li, S, Cv
S7	S, G		S, G	S, G	S, G
S8	G, Ya-l		G, S	G, S	G, S
S9				S, G	S, G
S30				Pen	Pen
Sp6	Sp, Liv, K	Sp, Liv, K	Sp, Liv, K	Sp, Liv, K	Sp, Liv, K
Sp12	Sp, Liv	Sp, Yi-l	Sp, Liv		Sp, Liv
Sp13	Sp, Liv, Yi-l	Sp, Yi-l	Sp, Liv, Yi-l	Sp, Liv, Yi-l	Sp, Liv, Yi-l
Sp15	Sp, Yi-l	Sp, Yi-l	Sp, Yi-l	Sp, Yi-l	Sp, Yi-l
Sp16	Sp, Yi-l	Sp, Yi-l	Sp, Yi-l	Sp, Yi-l	Sp, Yi-l

Ya-l = Yang linking vessel
Yi-l = Yin linking vessel
Ya-h = Yang heel vessel
Yi-h = Yin heel vessel
Pen = Penetrating vessel
Gir = Girdle vessel
con = connecting meridian

Taken from:
1. Jia yi ying
2. Wai tai mi yao
3. Tong ren yu xue tu jing
4. Zhen jiu da cheng
5. Lei jing tu yi
After Jingluoxue Tushuo by Hiu-jan and Zhu Ru-gong

	1	2	3	4	5
Si10	Si, Ya-l, Ya-h	Si, B, Ya-l Ya-h	Si, B, Ya-l, Ya-h	Si, Ya-l, Ya-h	Si, B, Ya-l, Ya-h
Si12	Si, Li, T, G	Si, Li, T, G	Si, Li, T, G	Si, Li, T, G	Si, Li, T, G
Si18	Si, T	Si, T	Si, T	Si, T	Si, T
Si19	Si, T, G	Si, T, G	Si, T. G	Si, T, G	Si, T, G
B1	Si, B, S	Si, B, S, Li	Si, B, T, G, S	Si, B, S, Ya-h, Yi-h	Si, B, S
B11	B, Si	B, T	B, G	B, Si, G, T	Gv con, B, Si
B12	Gv, B	Gv, B	Gv, B		Gv, B
B33		Liv		Liv, G	
B36	B	B, Si	B, Si	B, Si	B, Si
B59	Ya-h	Ya-h	Ya-h	Ya-h	Ya-h
B61		B, Ya-h		Ya-h	B, Ya-h
B62	Ya-h	Ya-h	Ya-h	Ya-h	Ya-h
B63	Ya-l	Ya-l	Ya-l	Ya-l	Ya-l
K3	Yi-h	Yi-h	Yi-h	Yi-h	Yi-h
K8	Yi-h	Yi-h	Yi-h	Yi-h	Yi-h
K9	Yi-l			Yi-l	Yi-l
K11	Pen, K	Pen, K	Pen, K	Pen, K	Pen, K
K12	Pen, K	Pen, K	Pen, K	Pen, K	Pen, K
K13	Pen, K	Pen, K	Pen, K	Pen, K	Pen, K
K14	Pen, K	Pen, K	Pen, K	Pen, K	Pen, K
K15	Pen, K	Pen, K	Pen, K	Pen, K	Pen, K
K16	Pen, K	Pen, K	Pen, K	Pen, K	Pen, K
K17	Pen, K	Pen, K	Pen, K	Pen, K	Pen, K
K18	Pen, K	Pen, K	Pen, K	Pen, K	Pen, K
K19	Pen, K	Pen, K	Pen, K	Pen, K	Pen, K
K20	Pen, K	Pen, K	Pen, K	Pen, K	Pen, K
K21	Pen, K	Pen, K	Pen, K	Pen, K	Pen, K
P1	P, G	P, G	P, G	P, Liv, T, G	P, G
T13		Li con	Li con	T, Ya-l	Li, T
T15	T, Ya-l	G, Ya-l	T, Ya-l	T, G, Ya-l	T, G, Ya-l
T17	T, G	T, G	T, G	T, G	T, G
T20	T, G, Li		T, G	T, G, Si	T, G, Si
T22	T, G, Si	T, G		T, G, Si	T, G, Si
G1	T, G, Si	T, G	T, G, Si	T, G, Si	T, G, Si
G3	T, G, S		G, S	T, G, S, Li	T, G, S

	1	2	3	4	5
G4	T, S	G, S	T, G, S, Li	T, G, S, Li	T, G, S, Li
G5				T, G, S, Li	
G6	T, G, S, Li	T, G, S, Li	T, G, S, Li	T, G, S, Li	T, G, S, Li
G7	G, B	G, B	G, B	G, B	G, B
G8	G, B		G, B	G, B	G, B
G9				G, B	G, B
G10	G, B		G, B	G, B	G, B
G11	G, B	T, G, B, Si	G, B	T, G, B	G, B
G12	G, B	G, B	G, B	G, B	G, B
G13	G, Ya-l	G, Ya-l	G, Ya-l	G, Ya-l	G, Ya-l
G14	G, Ya-l		G, Ya-l	T, G, Li, S, Ya-l	G, Ya-l
G15	G, B, Ya-l	G, B	G, B	G, B, Ya-l	G, B, Ya-l
G16	G, Ya-l	G, Ya-l	G, Ya-l	G, Ya-l	G, Ya-l
G17	G, Ya-l	G, Ya-l	G, Ya-l	G, Ya-l	G, Ya-l
G18	G, Ya-l	G, Ya-l	G, Ya-l	G, Ya-l	G, Ya-l
G19	G, Ya-l	G, Ya-l	G, Ya-l	G, Ya-l	G, Ya-l
G20	G, Ya-l	G, Ya-l	G, Ya-l	G, Ya-l, T	G, Ya-l
G21	T, Ya-l	T, G, Ya-l	T, G, Ya-l	T, G, S, Ya-l, T	T, G, S, Ya-l
G24	G, Sp		G, Sp, Ya-l	G, Sp, Ya-l	G, Sp, Ya-l
G26	G, Gir			G, Gir	G, Gir
G27	G, Gir			G, Gir	G, Gir
G28	G, Gir	G, Gir	G, Gir	G, Gir	G, Gir
G29	G, Ya-h	G, Ya-h	G, Ya-h	G, Ya-h	G, Ya-h
G30	G, S			G, S	G, S
G36	Ya-l	Ya-l	Ya-l	Ya-l	Ya-l
Liv13	Liv, G	Liv, G	Liv, G	Liv, G	Liv, G
Liv14	Liv, Sp, Yi-l	Liv, Sp, Yi-l	Liv, Sp, Yi-l	Liv, Sp, Yi-l	Liv, Sp, Yi-l
Cv1	Cv, Gv, Pen	Cv, Gv, Pen	Cv, Gv, Pen	Cv, Gv, Pen	Cv, Gv, Pen
Cv2	Cv, Liv	Cv, Liv	Cv, Liv	Cv, Liv	Cv, Liv
Cv3	Cv, Liv, Sp, K	Cv, Liv, Sp, K	Cv, Liv, Sp, K	Cv, Liv, Sp, K	Cv, Liv, Sp, K
Cv4	Cv, Liv, Sp, K	Cv, Liv, Sp, K	Cv, Liv, Sp, K	Cv, Liv, Sp, K	Cv, Liv, Sp, K, S
Cv7	Cv, Pen	Cv, Pen, K		Cv, Pen, K	Cv, Pen, K
Cv10	Cv, Sp	Cv, Sp	Cv, Sp	Cv, Sp	Cv, Sp

	1	2	3	4	5
Cv12	Cv, Si, T, S	Cv, Si, T, S	Cv, Si, T, S	Cv, Si, T, S	Cv, Si, T, S
Cv13	Cv, S, Si	Cv, S, Si	Cv, S, Si	Cv, S, Si	Cv, S, Si
Cv17				Cv, B, K, Si, T	
Cv23	Cv, Yi-l	Cv, Yi-l	Cv, Yi-l	Cv, Yi-l	Cv, Yi-l
Cv24	Cv, S	Cv, S	Cv, S	Cv, Gv, S, Li	Cv, S
Gv1			K, G	K, G	K
Gv13	Gv, B	Gv, B	Gv, B	Gv, B	Gv, B
Gv14	6 Yang, Gv	6 Yang, Gv	6 Yang, Gv	6 Yang, Gv	6 Yang, Gv
Gv15	Gv, Ya-l	Gv, Ya-l	Gv, Ya-l	Gv, Ya-l	Gv, Ya-l
Gv16	Gv, Ya-l	Gv, Ya-l	Gv, Ya-l	Gv, Ya-l, B	Gv, Ya-l
Gv17	Gv, B	Gv, B	Gv, B	Gv, B	Gv, B
Gv20	Gv, B	Gv, B	Gv, B	Gv, 6 Yang	Gv, B, T, G, Liv
Gv26	Gv, Li, S	Gv, Li	Gv, Li,	Gv, Li, S	Gv, Li, S
Gv28				Gv, Cv, S	Gv, Cv

Origin and End Points

Ma Chen-tai's school of thought during the Ming dynasty, compares the meridians to a river. The origin point is the source of the river; the end point is the lake into which the waters of the river accumulate at the end of its course. These points are only given for the three lower Yin and Yang; the origin in each case being at the ends of the toes, the end points of the trunk or the face. (Fig. 8.18).

Meridian (river)	Origin	End
Bladder	B67	B1
Stomach	S45	S8
Gall bladder	G44	Si19
Spleen	Sp1	Cv12
Kidney	K1	Cv23
Liver	Liv1	Cv18

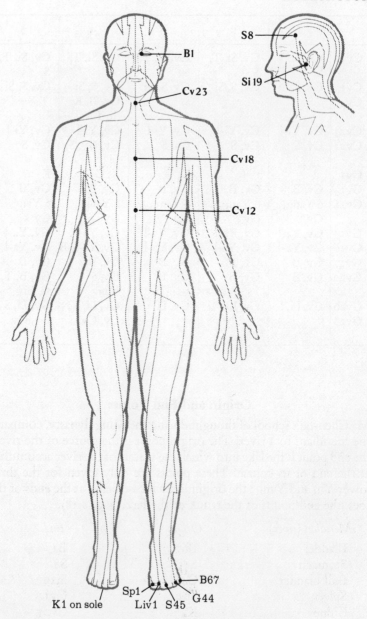

S8

Si 19

B1

Cv23

Cv18

Cv12

B67

Sp1

K1 on sole

Liv1   S45   G44

FIG. 8.20 Origin (light print) end and (heavy print) points

Root and Side Effect Points

Ma Chen-tai also discussed the root of a disease or meridian and its side effect or fruit. This is envisaged not as the main effect but as the possible side effect of a disease, or as the manifestation of a disease affecting the meridian. The root points are on the limbs, the side effect points on the trunk or head (Fig. 8.21).

Meridian	Root	Side Effect
Bladder	B59	B1
Gall bladder	G44 and G43	Si19
Stomach	S45	S9 and S4
Spleen	?Sp6	B20 and Cv23
Kidney	K8	B23
Liver	?Liv4	B18
Small intestine	Si6	B2
Triple warmer	T3	T23
Large intestine	Li11 and Li14	Li20
Lung	L9	L1
Heart	H7	B15
Pericardium	P6	P1

Selection of Acupuncture Points

Acupuncture points that are near the site of symptoms often have a greater local effect especially in painful conditions.

Points that are far away, especially the important points below the knee and elbow, often have a greater systemic effect.

Often the associated and alarm points stimulated together have a greater effect than each alone.

Some like to combine the source and connecting points.

The accumulation point and the appropriate one of the eight meeting points may be combined advantageously. For example S34 the accumulating point of the stomach may be used with Cv12 the meeting point of the Yang hollow organs (Fu) in epigastric pain with heartburn.

SUMMARY OF SOME OF THE MORE IMPORTANT TYPES OF ACUPUNCTURE POINT

	WOOD / METAL	FIRE / WATER	EARTH / WOOD	METAL / FIRE	WATER / EARTH	TONIFICATION	SEDATION	SOURCE	ASSOCIATED	ALARM	CONNECTING	ACCUMULATING	ENTRY	EXIT	LOWER MEETING PT.	UPPER MEETING PT.
Lung	L11	L10	L9	L8	L5	L9	L5	L9	B13	L1	L7	L6	L1	L7		
Spleen	Sp1	Sp2	Sp3	Sp5	Sp9	Sp2	Sp5	Sp3	B20	Liv13	Sp4	Sp8	Sp1	Sp21		
Heart	H9	H8	H7	H4	H3	H9	H7	H7	B15	Cv14	H5	H6	H1	H9		
Kidney	K1	K2	K6	K7	K10	K7	K1	K6	B23	G25	K5	K4	K1	K22		
Pericardium	P9	P8	P7	P5	P3	P9	P7	P7	B14	Cv17	P6	P4	P1	P8		
Liver	Liv1	Liv2	Liv3	Liv4	Liv8	Liv8	Liv2	Liv3	B18	Liv14	Liv5	Liv6	Liv1	Liv14		
Large intestine	Li1	Li2	Li3	Li5	Li11	Li11	Li2	Li4	B25	S25	Li6	Li7	Li4	Li20	S37	Li11
Stomach	S45	S44	S43	S41	S36	S41	S45	S42	B21	Cv12	S40	S34	S1	S42	S36	
Small intestine	Si1	Si2	Si3	Si5	Si8	Si3	Si8	Si4	B27	Cv4	Si7	Si6	Si1	Si19	S39	Si8
Bladder	B67	B66	B65	B60	B54	B67	B65	B64	B28	Cv3	B58	B63	B1	B67	B54	
Triple warmer	T1	T2	T3	T6	T10	T3	T10	T4	B22	Cv5	T5	T7	T1	T23	B53	T10
Gall bladder	G44	G43	G41	G38	G34	G43	G38	G40	B19	G24	G37	G36	G1	G41	G34	

EIGHT EXTRAORDINARY VESSELS

	MASTER	COUPLED	ACCUMULATING	CONNECTING
Conception vessel	L7	K3		Cv15
Governing "	Si3	B62		Gv1
Penetrating "	Sp4	P6		
Girdle "	G41	T5		
Yin heel "	K3	B62	K8	
Yang heel "	B62	K3	B59	
Yin linking "	P6	Sp4	K9	
Yang linking "	T5	G41	G35	

THE FOUR SEAS

	COUPLED	ACCUMULATING
Sea of nourishment	S30	S36
Sea of blood	B11	S37
Sea of energy	Cv17	B10
Sea of marrow	Gv20	Gv16

MEETING POINTS

3 Lower Yang & Du mo	Gv20
3 Lower Yin	Sp6
7 Yang	Gv14
3 Lower Yin and Ren mo	Cv3 Cv4
Lung and spleen	L1
Pericardium and liver	P1
Small intestine and bladder	B1
Triple warmer and gall bladder	G1
Large intestine and stomach	Li20

EIGHT MEETING POINTS

Zang	Liv13
Fu	Cv12
Qi	Cv17
Blood	B17
Bones	B11
Marrow	G39
Muscles	G34
Vessels	L9

WINDOW OF THE SKY

S9 Li18 T16 B10 L3 Gv16 Cv22 Si16 Si17 P1

233

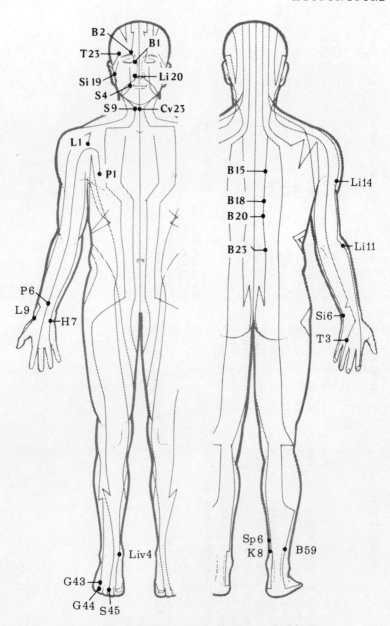

FIG. 8.21 Root (light print) and side effect (heavy print) points

IX

PULSE DIAGNOSIS

The pulse diagnosis is the key-stone of Chinese traditional diagnosis. It is described in detail in the ancient treatises (Fig. 9.1).*

'One should feel whether the pulse is in motion or whether it is still.'

'When the upper pulse is abundant, then the rebellious Qi rises. When the lower part is abundant, then the Qi causes a swelling in the abdomen. If the pulse appears to stop then the Qi has decayed.'

(Su Wen, Ch. 17.)

'The "feon" pulse is like a weak wind that puffs up the feathers on the back of a bird, flustering and humming; like the wind that blows over autumn leaves; like water that moves the same swimming piece of wood up and down. . .

'If the pulse (at position III, left, deep) of the kidney is slightly hard. . . resistant. . . it is normal. If it is very hard, as hard as a stone, there will be death. . .'

(Hübbotter, P. 179)

A doctor skilled in its practice would—without ever speaking to or seeing the face or body of his patient and with no more contact than a hand thrust through a hole in a curtain to give access to the radial artery of the wrist—be able to arrive at a reliable diagnosis in a matter of minutes.

It can be used to confirm a diagnosis already arrived at by clinical

*Chinese pulse diagnosis, Sung dynasty. After Ilse Veith. The Yellow Emperor's Classic of Internal Medicine, 1949. Williams and Wilkins, Baltimore.

圖之診仰診覆

脉人他診

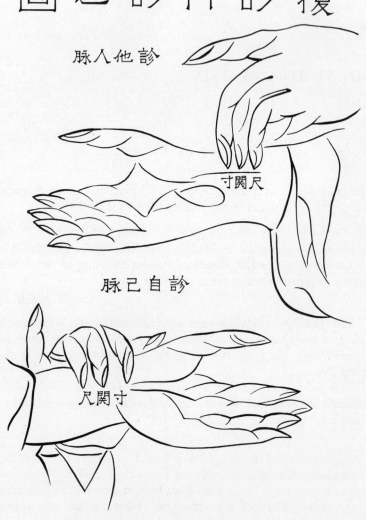

寸關尺

脉己自診

尺關寸

Fig. 9.1

and laboratory methods. It can be of very great benefit in a case where, although the patient is obviously ill, it has not been possible to arrive at a conclusive diagnosis in spite of thorough clinical and laboratory investigations.

It is so sensitive a method of diagnosis that not infrequently it will register past illnesses so accurately that a doctor is in a position to recount the past history of his patient's health (even though it involve illness he suffered fifty years previously) and to warn him of illness to be expected in the future, whether it be in several months' or in several years' time.

But such results as these can only be obtained under the correct conditions and within specific limitations, which must be strictly adhered to, so that not too much, nor too little, is expected of this method.

To those who do not understand its working, it can seem like magic. A patient who has been told by his doctor that at some time in the future he will develop a disease, though there is at the time no obvious indication to suggest it, may well conclude, when the 'prophecy' comes true, that his medical advisor has access to the secret mysteries of Nature.

To African Pygmies, utterly ignorant of the laws of aeronautics, an aeroplane taking flight like a giant bird above their heads, can

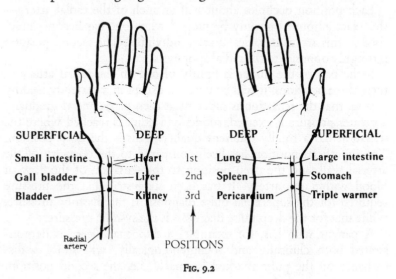

FIG. 9.2

237

only be explained in terms of magic. So we Europeans in our turn, observing some of the things the Pygmies can do and being ignorant of the processes which make them possible, either dismiss them casually from our minds or apply to them that same word of 'magic'. In reality, both conclusions are no more than misconceptions and both are due to insufficient knowledge.

The pulse diagnosis is both a science and an art. The scheme in Fig. 9.2 describes how pulse diagnosis works, though in actual practice it can only be satisfactorily learnt by demonstration and continuous correction from a doctor who has mastered the technique.

The pulse at the radial artery of the wrist is divided into three zones, each of which has a superficial and a deep position.

Left hand			Right hand	
Superficial	*Deep*		*Deep*	*Superficial*
		Positions		
Small intestine	Heart	1st	Lung	Large intestine
Gall bladder	Liver	2nd	Spleen	Stomach
Bladder	Kidney	3rd	Pericardium	Triple warmer

Each position occupies about half an inch of the radial artery—the exact amount can only be judged when one has become practised in this art, as it varies in each individual. The second position is roughly opposite to the radial apophysis.

If the ball of the finger is lightly placed on the radial artery in these three positions, it will be noticed, except in a perfectly healthy person, that the sensation is different at each place, and if gradually a greater pressure is exerted, suddenly a point is reached where the sensation has a totally different quality. This is the deep position. The superficial position has been compared to the elasticity of the arterial wall, and the deep position to the sensation of the flow of blood within the artery. It has been suggested that the pressure required for the superficial pulse diagnosis is the diastolic pressure, while that for the deep pulse diagnosis is the systolic pressure.

A patient who has, for example, a duodenal ulcer, as demonstrated both clinically and roentgenologically, will show a disturbance on the pulse marked 'stomach', i.e. the second position,

The standardised interpretation of the pulse given overleaf, is not shared by all authors, as the accompanying table shows. Taken from:

		1	2	3	4	5	6	7	8
Left radial artery	1st Deep	H	H	H	H	H	H	H	Sternum (Cv17)
	1st Superficial	Si	Si	Si	Sternum (Cv17)	H	Sternum (Cv17)	Pericardium connection	H
	2nd Deep	Liv	Liv	Liv	Liv	Liv	Liv	Liv	Liv
	2nd Superficial	G	G	G	G	G	Diaphragm	G	G
	3rd Deep	K	K	K	K	K	K	K	Si B
	3rd Superficial	B	B	B	Si	B Li	Si B	B Li	K
Right radial artery	1st Deep	L	L	L	L	L	L	L	Middle of chest
	1st Superficial	Li	Li	Li	Middle of chest		Middle of stomach	Middle of chest	L
	2nd Deep	Sp	Sp	Sp	S	Sp	Sp	Sp	S
	2nd Superficial	S	S	S	Sp	S	S	S	Sp
	3rd Deep	Gv4	Gv4	T	K	K	K	Gv4 T	Li
	3rd Superficial	B	T	Pericardium connection	Li	T Si	Li	Si	K

1. Wang shu-he 2. Li dong-yuan 3. Hua bo-ren 4. Li shi-zhen 5. Yu jia-yan 6. Li shi-cai
7. Zhang jing-yae 8. Yi zong jin jian.   Taken from Zhongyixue Gailun.

superficial, right. Similarly, as discussed later, other diseases show on other pulses, though not always with an obvious correlation.

There is some doubt as to the existence of both a superficial and a deep position in pulse diagnosis. As the superficial and deep position belong to coupled organs, the theory can in either case be easily adapted.

Case History. A girl with asthma missed so many of her lessons that discussions were in progress about sending her to a special school for the handicapped. From the point of view of acupuncture asthma may be due to a dysfunction of the lung or spleen or heart or kidney or liver or a non-specific type. Each one of the above six varieties has to be treated differently, and the pulse diagnosis is one of the best methods of differentiation. In this case the spleen was at fault, which when treated cured her asthma.

The Various Qualities

1. The pulse is different in every individual. There is no absolute norm, and something that may be normal for one individual, is pathological for another. Thus, the basic fundamental norm for each individual must be judged from experience, otherwise an attempt could be made to correct something which is normal so that disease would result.

It is, for example, perfectly normal for certain people to be vivacious and quick, and this is reflected in the quality of the radial pulse. For others, it is more normal to be of a phlegmatic temperament, and this is again reflected at the radial pulse. If an attempt be made to apply an artificial standard norm, to 'correct' these different (but in each case normal) pulses by 'appropriate' sedating or tonifying acupuncture points, disease will result. It is, after all, normal for an African to be black and a European to be white—an Albino African is ill.

2. All the pulses in ensemble may be plethoric, in which all the twelve basic pulses beat too strongly and feel over-full. This is known as 'total plethora of Yin and Yang'.

All the superficial pulses in ensemble may be plethoric. This is called 'total plethora of Yang'.

All the deep pulses in ensemble may be plethoric. This is 'total plethora of Yin'.

3. All the pulses in ensemble may be much too weak. This may be called 'total' weakness of Yin and Yang'.
Similarly we have:
'total weakness of Yang', and
'total weakness of Yin'.

4. If the pulses in position I are more powerful than the pulses in position III, Yang is more powerful than Yin. Similarly, if position III is stronger than position I, Yin is in excess of Yang.

5. If the pulses on the right radial artery are stronger than those on the left radial artery, there is excess of Yang. Conversely, if those on the left are stronger than those on the right, there is an excess of Yin.

Specific Qualities

Classically there are twenty-eight different qualities, though less than this is sufficient for ordinary practice.

'When the pulse of the spleen is soft and even, well separated, as the footsteps of a chicken touching the ground; it is called regular. When the pulse is full, the frequency increases, like a chicken lifting its feet; then one speaks of disease.'

(Jia Yi Jing, Vol. IV, Ch. 1a)

What might be called an artistic sense is a prerequisite for some of the finer points in pulse diagnosis, as frequently pulse conditions are felt which have not been felt before, or are not described in books (Fig. 9.3).

Essentially the pulse acquires the same quality (in an artistic sense) as the organ which it represents. For example, I once felt the pulse of a doctor who did not tell me his symptoms or the result of investigations. The pulse of his stomach was like thickened, wet, soggy, blotting paper. I was unable to think of the diagnosis (it obviously being not a stomach ulcer, carcinoma or hyperacidity). The doctor then told me that he had, as diagnosed gastroscopically, hypertrophic gastritis. The similarity (artistically speaking) between a hypertrophic gastric mucosa and thickened, wet, soggy, blotting paper are obvious. If my imagination had been a little livelier at the time, I am sure that I could have made the full diagnosis without the doctor concerned saying anything.

1. A particular quality developed on only one flank of the same radial artery in the same position, e.g. a plethoric heart pulse which

is more marked on the left side (lateral), suggests (to those who think they are differentiates) that the left side of the heart is more strained than the right as is usual in hypertension.

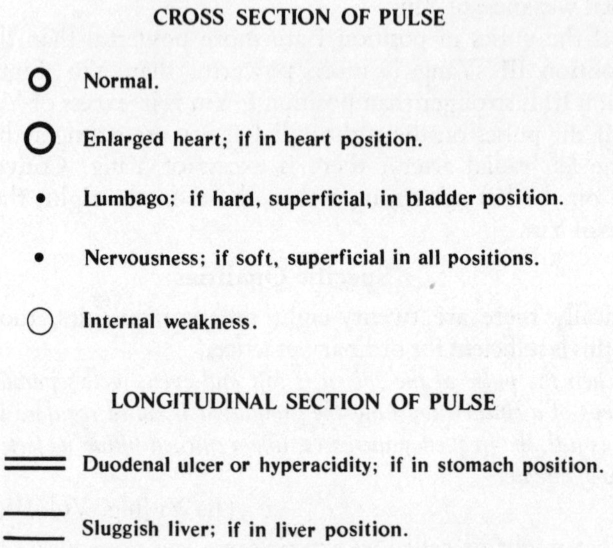

CROSS SECTION OF PULSE

O   Normal.

O   Enlarged heart; if in heart position.

•   Lumbago; if hard, superficial, in bladder position.

•   Nervousness; if soft, superficial in all positions.

○   Internal weakness.

LONGITUDINAL SECTION OF PULSE

≡   Duodenal ulcer or hyperacidity; if in stomach position.

—   Sluggish liver; if in liver position.

Fig. 9.3

2. The disturbance in the proximal or distal part of the pulse is more marked. For example, in the case of the pulse of the large intestine, a disturbance in the distal part of the pulse is suggestive of disease of the anus, rectum or descending colon; of the middle part, of the transverse colon; and the proximal part of the pulse for the ascending colon. These qualities are difficult to appreciate.

3. A healthy person is one in whom the pulse flows smoothly, without turbulences or kinks, which has a certain tension but is yet

Normal pulse   Ropy pulse

Fig. 9.4

compressible and elastic, and which has the same characteristics throughout its depth (Fig. 9.4 left).

A person who has a pulse like that described above is, physiologically speaking, perfectly healthy: if he has had diseases in the past, they have become fully healed, nor has he any latent diseases which are due to become active and develop obvious symptoms, giving objective findings. This type of person is not likely to have any serious illness and will probably live a long time. If he becomes ill there will be a disturbance in only one or two places on the pulse; this disturbed pulse position, whatever other qualities it may have, retains its elasticity, signifying that the disease can relatively easily be cured. If a diseased pulse position has a certain hard and brittle quality, the disease is harder to cure.

It is taught that on occasions in the course of a serious disease and shortly before death, the pulses become normal.

Only on rare occasions have I myself felt a perfectly normal pulse in someone who was ill. This illustrates that although the pulse is accurate to an astonishingly high degree it is not, any more than anything else, a hundred per cent foolproof. For this reason, and as a double check, it is usually advisable to take a history, make a physical examination, laboratory investigations, etc. as suggested by the individual case.

A history, physical examination and laboratory investigations are useful in directing one's attention to what one might expect to find on pulse diagnosis. So much may be found on the pulse that it is useful to have some other means to act as a pointer in discriminating between their relative importance. It should not be forgotten that the pulse divides diseases into twelve basic categories—and no more.

4. Diseases whether they be physical, physiological or mental show themselves on the pulse, provided the disease has a physiological effect.

If, for example, someone has had tuberculosis of the lungs, which has been fully healed so that the physiological function of the lungs is perfectly normal, the pulse of the lungs will be normal, despite the fact that a chest X-ray may show a few healed scars in the parenchyma of the lungs. The pulse is normal because the scars (unless extensive) do not influence the physiological function (and hence health and disease) of the lungs; just as the physiological function of the skin is not influenced (to any appreciable degree) by the healed scars of a few minor skin abrasions. If the tuberculosis were still active, or the healed scars so extensive as to influence pulmonary function, it would show on the pulse.

A diabetic will, if untreated, have an abnormal pulse. If his pulse is felt at such an interval after taking insulin that his blood sugar-insulin balance is perfect, the pulse will be so near to normal, that an abnormality will be missed unless one is specifically looking for it. If the pulse is felt a few hours before or after this ideal insulin balance, the abnormality of the pulse will be detected more easily, though of course not as easily as in the uncontrolled diabetic.

A substantial proportion of mental diseases, contrary to certain opinion, is really physiological, and hence can be treated by acupuncture. It is, for example, well known that anyone who is livery is liable to be depressed, in which case the depression can be cured by treating the liver. (The liver symptoms may not be present, but show themselves on the pulse of the liver.) A depression which has a purely circumstantial cause (e.g. bankruptcy) does not show itself on the pulse. Mental diseases are discussed in detail elsewhere.

5. A pulse which is ropy in outline (Fig. 9.4 right) and consistency is a sign of general, chronic, physiological unbalance. People with this type of pulse are very difficult to cure.

If a person who has enjoyed good health for most of his life becomes ill, the pulse of the diseased organ becomes abnormal, while the pulses as a whole, remain normal and smooth.

The person with a ropy pulse may not even have a specific disease that can be localised, though as a rule it occurs in people who, for many years, have taken drugs in excessive amounts, or whose habit of living has included anything else that might undermine their general health. Sometimes a ropy pulse occurs in elderly people who have had many illnesses affecting several bodily systems, all of which have been only partly cured.

6. The hollow pulse. Certain pulses are hollow, the examining finger feeling a normal resistance on light application, but immediately greater pressure is applied the finger, as it were, falls through into a hollow. This pulse signifies, in general, a deficiency state.

7. The wire pulse. Sometimes all the pulses, or only the superficial or deep, or even an isolated pulse become taut, hard and thin, like the E string of a violin.

This pulse signifies spasm and pain. In a patient who has pain or spasm, it is natural to tighten up, which also occurs in the pulse which becomes hard and tight like a wire.

The wire pulse is typically seen on the bladder pulse in lumbago or sciatica. Nervous people may have all their superficial pulses wiry.

8. A hard, round, incompressible pulse, usually signifies a stone, whether it be biliary or renal. Occasionally the size of a stone can be judged in this way, and if it is judged small enough to be able to pass along the biliary ducts, the gall bladder may be stimulated to expel it.

9. A blown up pulse may occur in the stomach due to aero-gastria; similarly the cardiac pulse may be blown up in cardiac strain or hypertrophy.

10. A coarse and rough pulse may be the result of cold weather. This condition disappears after the patient has been in a warm room for about half an hour.

11. The pulses become deeper in winter and in diseases associated with hardening and cold.

12. The pulses are more superficial in the summer and in febrile diseases.

13. Sometimes the pulse may be split longitudinally in two, which is more often noticed with the pulse of the gall bladder than with any other. I do not know the significance of this characteristic apart from the fact that it is associated with weakness. Possibly it indicates a non-synchronisation of the functions of the left and right biliary systems.

The Method of Utilising Physiological and Other Relationships

The more one feels the twelve basic pulses, the more does one have the impression that what is felt is not the specific organ concerned, such as the heart or the liver, but rather the basic 'conception' behind it, rather like Goethe's idea of the 'Urpflanze'.

Though obviously more than twelve organs or parts of the body can be effected by disease, with extremely few exceptions, they all show on the twelve basic pulses.

I think this can best be understood if the human being is considered as being in essence the result of the interplay of twelve basic forces which, in the course of embryonic development (and phylogenetic evolution), arrange the different individual cells and groups of cells to form twelve basic physiological and anatomical entities. The way that cells or groups of cells move during embryonic development along the most complicated paths is suggestive of some underlying force directing their movements.

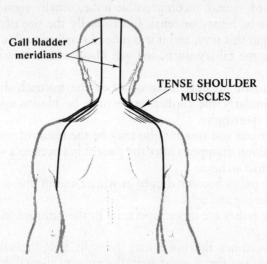

Gall bladder
meridians

TENSE SHOULDER
MUSCLES

FIG. 9.5 Due to mental tension the shoulder muscles may tighten. The gall bladder meridian runs over these muscles; and hence the gall bladder or its coupled organ the liver, should be treated to relax the muscles

Embryologists explain this by the concepts of chemotaxis or polarity but these are probably only a very partial answer. Perhaps this can best be made clear by an example:

A disturbance in the liver pulse may be caused by:

(a) Disease of the liver itself—congestion, cirrhosis, carcinoma, etc.

(b) Haemorrhoids—the portal circulation, of which the haemorrhoidal veins are a part, passes through the liver. Hepatic congestion should always be treated first and only later the safety valve—the haemorrhoids.

(c) People who bruise easily. Presumably the clotting factors, such as prothrombim, are not sufficiently produced by a weak liver.

(d) Biliousness, nausea and vomiting.

(e) Migraine. Migraine (the usual type) is generally basically due

246

to liver (and gall bladder) disturbance with the associated nausea. Most people with migrainous types of headache are first bilious and then some years later develop migraine.

(*f*) Weak eyesight, pain in or behind or around the eyes, black spots in front of the eyes, zig-zags, etc. This may be explained via the traditional relationship between the eye and the liver (see chapter on five elements).

(*g*) Excessive muscular tension, especially around the shoulders and neck (Fig. 9.5) (see chapter on five elements).

(*h*) Inability to wake up fresh in the morning, however early one has gone to bed.

(*i*) Certain types of asthma, hay fever, skin rashes and other allergic or 'stress' symptoms. Probably due to the manufacture of antibodies and other factors in the liver and spleen (Fig. 9.6).

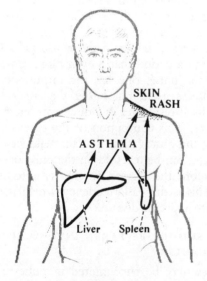

FIG. 9.6

The above-mentioned diseases may cause the disturbance of other pulses in addition to that of the liver. In addition most diseases have various causes, some of which will not affect the liver and therefore will not register on the liver pulse.

There are, of course, many more diseases which register as a disturbance on the pulse of the liver, but for the purposes of this discussion no more need be mentioned.

It will be noticed that most of the diseases or symptoms mentioned above (*a*) to (*i*) are related, (whether it be physiologically, anatomically, or by various laws of acupuncture) to the liver. The liver is the one factor that unites all these diseases, even though some of them may superficially not seem to have any relation to one another.

Similarly, if all the diseases of mankind are considered (excluding those few that have no physiological effect), it will be found that they all cause the alteration of one or several of the twelve basic pulses, and are hence related to the twelve basic organs. Anyone who is able to carry out the pulse diagnosis accurately, may prove the above statement to himself.

This fundamental conception that the human being is divisible into twelve basic physiological systems, to which other factors are subservient, is a gift for which we are indebted to the ancient Chinese of prehistoric times, for it is described in such detail in one of the oldest medical books in the world (The Nei Jing), that its origin must lie in a period that is even more remote.

When feeling the pulse, one has the impression, that what is felt is not the disease itself, but rather the entelechy behind the disease, showing itself only later as a disease in one or other branch of the basic twelve. This conception of the entelechy of disease is also suggested by the observation that the tendency to one of the basic twelve diseases can be foretold on the pulse diagnosis, months or even years before the disease or any symptoms or objective findings occur. This is the basic tendency which is only at a later date specialised into a specific disease.

FACTORS THAT SHOULD BE TAKEN INTO ACCOUNT WHEN PALPATING THE PULSE

Certain difficulties may be encountered in pulse diagnosis which may, in certain circumstances, necessitate relegating the pulse diagnosis to a secondary position.

Naturally the easiest pulse to palpate is that of the healthy middle-aged person, where the pulse is fairly elastic. In little children care must be taken because of the smallness of the pulse. In the aged plaques of atheroma in the radial artery may confuse the picture. It seems, as a rule, that if an atheromatous plaque is located specifically at a certain pulse position, then the organ system represented is diseased.

In certain people a dilation of the radial artery may occur at a particular pulse position. It might be considered that this dilation is merely secondary to a localised weakening of the radial artery and therefore dismissed. Experience usually shows, however, that the organ represented by the dilated segment is rather severely diseased and is fairly resistant to treatment.

In marked hypo or hypertension the pulse is either so uniformly weak or strong, that individual characteristics are difficult to palpate, unless the hypo or hypertension are first treated.

External influences must always be considered: Drugs, excessive food or drink, running, emotion, etc.

MODERN THOUGHTS

The above chapter describes the Chinese pulse diagnosis in the traditional manner, which as much else does not correspond to my own experience.

I do not distinguish between the superficial and deep positions. Hence the liver and gall bladder, the bladder and kidney, and the stomach and spleen are each regarded as one, not a pair. The lung and large intestine pulse I regard as only the lung pulse for reasons given in Chapter 1, of Scientific Aspects of Acupuncture. Likewise, the heart and small intestine pulse I regard as only the heart. The pericardian and triple warmer positions I disregard.

Although I still find Chinese pulse diagnosis important, its importance is not as great as suggested in this chapter.

THE 28 MOST COMMONLY USED PULSE QUALITIES*

1. Floating — The pulse gives a sensation of floating on the surface of the skin; it responds to the finger when pressed lightly.

A Floating pulse is associated with Yang pulses, generally being found with the Exterior symptoms of Wind Evil lodging outside. If Floating but without strength, then it is a pointer to Empty symptoms.

2. Sunken (Deep) — The pulse gives the impression of being sunken between the muscle and bone; is only felt if pressed heavily.

A Deep pulse belongs to the category of Yin pulses, and is generally found with Interior symptoms of Evil Qi dormant internally. However, this pulse may also occur with Qi obstructed, Empty symptoms, etc.

3. Slow — The pulse is slow, only 3 beats to each breath.

The Slow pulse is also in the grouping of Yin pulses, generally to be found with inner organs Yin Cold symptoms. If a Floating pulse is associated with slow characteristics, then Yang is Empty outside; if a Deep pulse is associated with the Slow type, then Fire is decayed in the inside.

4. Rapid — The pulse is quick and feels urgent; 6 beats to each breath.

The Rapid pulse type is one of the Yang pulses; it is generally found with Fu Heat symptoms. If the pulse has little strength and

*The name in brackets e.g. (Deep) is an alternative translation as used in 'The Treatment of Diseases by Acupuncture'. In this book and whenever possible elsewhere I will not in future use the name in brackets, but only the main translation e.g. Sunken.

characteristics of the Floating and the Rapid type occur together, a disease of Yin Empty type is indicated; if on the other hand it is strong with at the same time the qualities found in Deep and Rapid types of pulse, then an over-abundance of Fire and Heat internally is denoted.

5. Slippery The pulse is felt to come and go, with a flowing, round and slippery movement.
(a) If the blood is over-abundant, a Slippery pulse will be found. But pregnant women also have this type of pulse and in these cases it is not an indication of disease.
(b) The Slippery type of pulse can also be found in instances where the patient has Phlegm symptoms and where undigested food is left in the body tracts. It may also occur with Evil Qi extreme.
Whether this type of pulse does or does not indicate disease, can be established from other accompanying symptoms. Diseases associated with this pulse usually respond easily to treatment.

6. Choppy (Rough) The movement of the pulse is felt as choppy and rough.
This type of pulse is found in cases where the Blood is deficient and the Jing injured. It may also occur in company with Qi obstructed or Cold and Damp symptoms.

7. Empty The pulse comes with a floating and soft movement. It disappears on pressure.
This pulse is associated with Blood Empty symptoms. It may also be found in illnesses due to Summer-heat.

8. Full The pulse feels full and forceful, long, big and hard.
This is a type found in cases of Evil abundant symptoms, and it may also occur with the

Fire symptoms of Evil abundant or Evil Full, obstructed and congealed.

9. Long

The pulse is felt as extraordinarily long, straight up and down, exceeding the extent of the original position.

This pulse is a sign of overflowing, and is present in symptoms denoting over-abundance, together with Qi rebellious Fire. If long, yet clear and round, as though feeling along a thin cane to the tip, it is a sign of health and not disease.

10. Short

The pulse feels short, choppy and little, seeming to have no head or tail, the middle arising suddenly and seeming unable to fill its natural place.

This is a sign of deficiency. It is also seen in cases where Original Qi is Empty and impoverished.

11. Overflowing

The pulse give the impression of being overflowing and large, filling the area below the doctor's finger; though abundant and large when coming, the movement loses its fullness and force as it passes.

The pulse is present in cases where symptoms suggest conditions of Evil Abundant and Fire Vigorous. If overflowing but without strength it suggests the cause of disease is Empty Overflowing and is a sign of Fire floating and Water dried up.

12. Minute

The pulse feels blurred, very fine and soft, almost imperceptible, as though about to be cut off, though it is not.

A pulse of this type when associated with Lost Yang symptoms, and where Qi and Blood are much decimated, cannot be reversed unless dealt with without delay.

13. Tight

The pulse is felt as taut and strong.

This pulse is found in conjunction with Cold

Evil symptoms. It may also be associated with pain symptoms.

14. Slowed-down The movement of the pulse is broad, slow and even, with no great change in pace.
This pulse denotes the presence of stomach Qi, and in general is not a disease pulse. It may also occur in Damp Evil diseases.

15. Hollow The pulse gives the sensation of being shaped like an onion stem; either floating or deep with a hollow area in the middle.
This pulse is present in cases where there has been great loss of blood such as haematemesis, epistaxis, menorrhagia, etc.

16. Bow-string (Wiry) The sensation given by this type of pulse is that of pressing on the string of a fiddle, felt bouncing directly beneath the finger.
This type of pulse is found together with liver Wind symptoms. It can also be present with pain symptoms in Phlegm-fluid diseases.

17. Leather This type of pulse is felt as large with a bow-string quality, yet hasty. It is obtained superficially but not when pressed hard. The sensation is that of pressing on the skin of a drum, the outside stiff and the inside hollow. Such a pulse denotes diseases due to an extreme excess of Exterior Cold. It is also found where there is loss of sperm or blood in men and miscarriage in women.

18. Firm (Hard) This pulse is large, with a bow-string and hard quality. It can only be obtained deeply. This type of pulse is an indication of Qi-accumulation diseases.

19. Weak-floating A pulse which feels very fine and soft, yet floating, only obtained when pressed lightly. Such a pulse is found with Yin Empty symptoms. It can also indicate the cause of disease as Kidney Empty, Marrow exhausted, where the Jing is impaired.

20. Weak This pulse is felt as fine and small, yet deep. It can only be located when pressed heavily. When pressed lightly it is no longer felt.

This type of pulse occurs in association with Yang decayed symptoms. Where it occurs in the course of a protracted disease it should not be construed as a sign of danger.

21. Scattered This pulse gives an effect of being floating, disordered and scattered; if the middle depth is selected, it gradually becomes hollow, and if pressed heavily, it ceases to be discernible.

This pulse is found in cases where the kidney Qi has been undermined and destroyed. There is always great danger in disease which shows a scattered pulse.

22. Fine The pulse is felt like a thread, fine and soft, but more evident than a Minute pulse.

A pulse associated with decayed Qi. It may also occur where there are symptoms due to Damp. If found in conjunction with disease due to debility and absence of vitality, the disease is severe.

23. Hidden (Buried) The pulse appears to be hidden. If you push the muscle and feel the bone then you begin to get its shape.

Such a pulse occurs in cases where the cause of disease has penetrated deeply into the organs. If the cause can be traced to a type of Yin Evil having been checked on the exterior and to the Yang Qi being isolated in the interior, then the pulse will become normal once sweating has taken place.

24. Moving This pulse can be detected in the 2nd position, shaped like a bean. Its movement is slippery and rapid.

	This pulse is associated with pain symptoms and is also present in disease due to fright.
25. Hasty	The movement of the pulse is sudden and hasty, halting at times. This pulse is present in conjunction with Fire symptoms. It is also seen with disease due to an obstruction of Qi.
26. Knotted	The pulse moves slowly and gradually, sometimes halting. This is a type of pulse which occurs in cases where the natural flow of the bodily process has been interfered with, causing an accumulation, congealing and obstruction.
27. Intermittent	The pulse is felt only intermittently. At times it almost stops, unable to regulate itself, and moves again only after a long time. Such a pulse denotes that the Zang Qi has been impoverished and destroyed. Its presence is indication that the disease has already become dangerous.
28. Fast (Hurried)	The pulse gives the effect of being hurried and anxious, 7 or 8 beats to each breath. It feels extremely agitated and urgent. This pulse indicates a serious over-abundance of Yang Qi, and Yin Qi diminished to the point of exhaustion. It is a warning of the danger of sudden death.

Nowadays the 28 pulse qualities described above are often classified under 6 groups, as it is often nearly impossible to make some of the finer distinctions. There are also other methods of grouping the pulse qualities. The 6 are:

Floating (1)*	Slow (3)	Slippery (5)
Sunken (2)	Rapid (4)	Choppy (6)

*The numbers are the same as for the 28 pulse qualities overleaf.

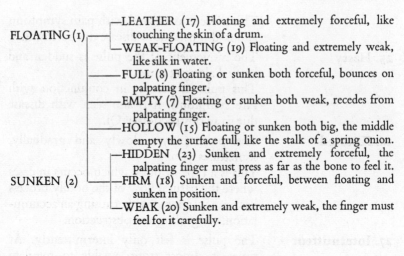

FLOATING (1) —
—LEATHER (17) Floating and extremely forceful, like touching the skin of a drum.
—WEAK-FLOATING (19) Floating and extremely weak, like silk in water.
——FULL (8) Floating or sunken both forceful, bounces on palpating finger.
——EMPTY (7) Floating or sunken both weak, recedes from palpating finger.
——HOLLOW (15) Floating or sunken both big, the middle empty the surface full, like the stalk of a spring onion.
—HIDDEN (23) Sunken and extremely forceful, the palpating finger must press as far as the bone to feel it.

SUNKEN (2)
—FIRM (18) Sunken and forceful, between floating and sunken in position.
—WEAK (20) Sunken and extremely weak, the finger must feel for it carefully.

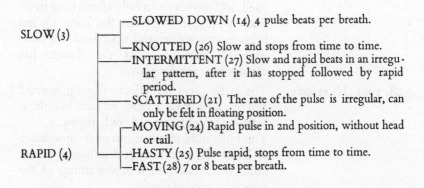

SLOW (3)
—SLOWED DOWN (14) 4 pulse beats per breath.

—KNOTTED (26) Slow and stops from time to time.
——INTERMITTENT (27) Slow and rapid beats in an irregular pattern, after it has stopped followed by rapid period.
——SCATTERED (21) The rate of the pulse is irregular, can only be felt in floating position.
—MOVING (24) Rapid pulse in 2nd position, without head or tail.

RAPID (4)
—HASTY (25) Pulse rapid, stops from time to time.
—FAST (28) 7 or 8 beats per breath.

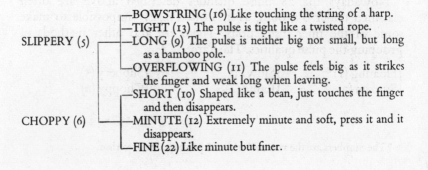

SLIPPERY (5)
—BOWSTRING (16) Like touching the string of a harp.
—TIGHT (13) The pulse is tight like a twisted rope.
—LONG (9) The pulse is neither big nor small, but long as a bamboo pole.
—OVERFLOWING (11) The pulse feels big as it strikes the finger and weak long when leaving.
—SHORT (10) Shaped like a bean, just touches the finger and then disappears.

CHOPPY (6)
—MINUTE (12) Extremely minute and soft, press it and it disappears.
—FINE (22) Like minute but finer.

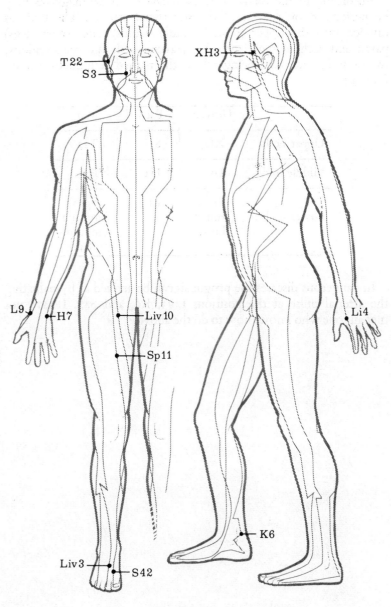

FIG. 9.7

According to the *Su Wen, sanbu jiuhou lun* pulse diagnosis may be performed on several of the superficial arteries. The body is divided into the upper (head), middle (hands), and lower (legs) parts; and each of these into the heaven, earth and man regions; the pulse in each case being felt at the named acupuncture point (Fig. 9.7).

	Heaven	Earth	Man
Upper body	XH3	S3	T22
Middle body	L9	Li4	H7
Lower body	Liv10 (women Liv3)	K6	Sp11 (stomach symptoms S42)

In dangerous diseases the prognosis can be arrived at by palpating the arterial pulse at the positions Liv3, K6, and S42. I have not met anyone who knows how to do the above.

X

THE CAUSE OF DISEASE

Since the 17th century, the general tendency in Western medicine has been to search for a purely physical cause in every human ailment. We attribute infections to bacteria or viruses. We consider that certain diseases (e.g. beri-beri, and some anaemias) result from deficiency states in the body and others from injuries to internal organs (as diabetes supervenes on an injured pancreas.) Even mental disease is either traced to a wholly physical cause, such as the secretion of an abnormal chemical within the body, or thought to be a condition of the mind produced by, and confined to, the mind alone.

In the Middle Ages, on the other hand, the cause of disease was more often seen as cosmological than physical, as directly due to forces outside rather than inside man. Sickness was the punishment meted out by Heaven to the evil-doer; the mentally deranged were possessed by the powers of darkness or suffering under a magic spell. The conjunction of stars and planets at a man's birth conditioned the physical weaknesses and the diseases likely to accompany them, which he would bear with him to the grave. The world in which man lived was malignant as well as benign; certain places were centres of healing but others were centres of disease; aches and agues emanated from subterranean streams and among the fruits of the earth grew also its poisonous plants.

In a sense, Chinese medicine combines these two attitudes. Among their many systems for the classification of disease, the most important is that which divides its causes into outer and inner 'influences', the former being meteorological conditions in the widest sense, the latter the emotions. Those relatively few diseases which fitted neither category were entered under miscellaneous headings.

The Meteorological Cause of Disease

When I was a doctor practising orthodox medicine, I used to think that changes in the weather had very little to do with disease; but, since becoming acquainted with Chinese theories on the subject, I have noticed how often, in a scarcely perceptible way, the weather actually does influence disease. It is, of course, a well-known fact that women with cystitis or an irritable bladder are more troubled in a cold season and that a particular type of migraine always occurs at mid-day in tropical countries. But the body seems to react to something more than simple changes in the climate. A patient suffering from that type of lumbago which becomes more acute in cold weather will notice that, though the temperature in his room may remain constant, his pain increases as the temperature outside falls. It would seem that a fall of temperature is not the only cause of his discomfort and that the body is influenced to just as great a degree by some subtle simultaneous change in the environment.

The Chinese divided the different meteorological conditions into what they called the 'six excesses', thus:—

WIND

Wind, since it belongs to the element 'wood', is the ruling element of spring (see chapter on five elements), and it is for this reason that wind diseases occur most often at this time of year. 'Evil wind' as the Chinese call it, is able to enter the body more easily when unaccustomed temperatures have dilated the pores of the skin.

The symptoms of 'wind injury' are coughing, headache, blocked or running nose, sneezing, etc. What is known as greater Yang Penetrating Wind brings dislike of cold, sweating, headache and a floating and slowed down pulse.

Wind may be associated with, or caused by, other 'evil' conditions. It may result from cold producing 'wind-cold' or originate from heat becoming 'wind-heat' and in both cases the consequent symptoms will be a mixture of the component elements. Such mixtures occur more often in wind conditions than in the other meteorological states. What is called 'inner wind' may also occur, producing 'phlegm-fire hot and abundant' or 'blood-empty wind-moving' symptoms of fainting, nervous spasms, vertigo, numbness, distortion of mouth and eyes with stiffness of the spine. Here the wind, since it is created within the body, does not belong to the wind of meteorology.

COLD

Cold, associated with the element 'water', is therefore the dominant of the six excesses during the winter, though it may also appear at other times of the year. It is a Yin evil and most likely to injure the Yang Qi of a patient.

When cold evil affects the exterior of the body, it may give rise to the symptoms of fever with a dislike of cold, breathlessness without sweating, headache, pains in the body and a tight and floating pulse. When the cold evil enters the meridians, it produces cramps and pain in the bones and muscles, and when it invades the solid and hollow organs, diarrhoea, vomiting, intestinal noises and abdominal pain.

But there is a type of 'inner cold' which, being created within the body, does not belong to the six excesses. This is known as 'Inner Zang Yang Qi empty and weak' and the symptoms (vomiting, diarrhoea, coldness of the limbs, rapid pulse and grey complexion) are caused by empty Yang creating inner cold.

'*If the evil is in the stomach and spleen... the Yang Qi is deficient, Yin Qi excessive; the intestines therefore murmur and the abdomen is painful*'.

(Ling Shu, wuxie pian)

SUMMER HEAT

Summer heat, belonging to the element 'fire', is naturally predominant at the full height of summer.

'*In heaven there is heat, in earth there is fire... their nature is summer heat.*'

(Su Wen, wuyunxiang dalun)

'*On the extreme days of early summer there are warm diseases, on the extreme days of late summer, summer heat diseases.*'

(Su Wen relun)

The chief symptoms of these summer heat diseases are headache, excessive body-heat, parched mouth, palpitations and consequent awareness of the heart action, spontaneous sweating and a rapid and overflowing pulse.

There are various types of this disease. A man who faints, after working hard or taking a long walk on a hot day, will be suffering from the type called 'penetrating summer heat', which comes under the category of 'Yang summer heat.' If, on the other hand, in the full heat of summer he has too cold a drink, the Yang Qi will be exhausted by the Yin cold and he will suffer from the 'penetrating cold of summer heat', in the 'Yin summer heat' category. This may give him an unpleasant sensation of chilliness, a dull ache in the head, abdominal pain with vomiting, and he may perspire freely. Summer heat may also combine with dampness to produce a red or white vaginal discharge, or dysentery, vomiting, abdominal pain and muscle spasm.

DAMP

Damp, belonging to the element 'earth', is the controlling meteorological condition of late summer. The various ailments which derive from it are classified as upper, lower, exterior or interior dampness, all characteristically heavy, muddy, greasy and blocking in their nature. They are often contracted after exposure to fog, after wading or working in water or being drenched with rain or from living in a damp place.

In 'upper damp' disease the head feels heavy, the nose is blocked, the face yellow and there is dyspnoea. In 'lower damp' there is oedema of the ankles and a thick vaginal discharge. 'Exterior damp' brings a sensation of alternating coldness and heat, spontaneous sweating, general weariness and lethargy; the joints ache and the limbs and body are swollen and puffy. 'Interior damp' is accompanied by a full, melancholic sensation in the chest, the vomiting of foul smelling food, swelling of the abdomen, jaundice and diarrhoea.

There is another type of dampness which is created internally, and hence not among the six excesses. It is caused by the consumption of wine, tea, cold melons or sweet greasy foods, all of which impede the function of the spleen.

DRYNESS

Dryness, belonging to the element 'metal', is the dominant meteorological state of autumn. A distinction is drawn between 'cool dryness' and 'warm dryness.'

'In mid-autumn it begins to grow cool, the west wind blows in an easterly direction and there is much wind dryness disease. . . If the weather is fair for a long time and there is no rain, the autumn Yang is sunny. Those who are affected by it will often have warm dryness disease.'

(Tongsu Shanghan lun)

The symptoms of cool dryness disease are a slight headache, a dislike of cold, coughing, absence of sweat and a blocked nose. In warm dryness disease the body feels hot, the mouth is parched, there is sweating, coughing, a pain in the throat and chest, blood in the sputum and sneezing with a dry nose.

In addition there is internal dryness, which is not among the six excesses. This is due to excessive loss of fluid from sweating, vomiting or diarrhoea, a condition in which the skin is dry, wrinkled and withered, the mouth and lips dry and cracked and the stomach fluid also dried up. What the Chinese call 'diabetes' ('wasting and thirsty disease' and others with similar symptoms), with hiccoughing, dry and hard stools, severe paralysis of the legs, convulsions and haemoptysis also occurs.

FIRE

The five meteorological conditions mentioned above can all, in extreme circumstances, be transformed so as to come under the element 'fire'. In most instances this will mean a more acute form of the disease. In, for instance, 'wind heat' disease the symptoms of a fixed look in the eyes, spasm of the limbs, curvature of the spine etc. are all due to the simultaneous increase in intensity of both wind and fire. The palpitations, facial flush, sweating, body heat and incessant thirst of 'penetrating summer heat' are really due to the transformation of summer heat to 'fire'. The exhaustion and depression which may accompany warmth and heat diseases will (if the change to 'fire' takes place) produce symptoms of burning lips and dry tongue, incoherent speech and mental confusion. If dryness changes to the element of fire, it will burn the lungs and cause coughing and blood-spitting. The deep red tongue and the awareness of heart-action, noticed in some fever patients, is caused by the cold evil changing to 'fire'.

In addition to, but distinct from, the above is 'internal fire', which has nothing to do with the six excesses. If 'wind' is very violent, liver fire is said to 'rise'. Many people in a fit of rage will go red in the face and feel a sensation of heat rising from the upper abdomen. Excessive eating and drinking will cause stomach fire to collect inside; excessive sexual activity causes the 'minister fire' to move wildly; deep feelings of grief or compassion will cause fire to arise in the lungs.

DORMANT QI

'If one is injured by cold in winter, then in spring one will have a warm disease. If one is injured by wind in spring, then in summer one will have diarrhoea. If one is injured by heat in summer, then in autumn one will have intermittent fevers. If one is injured by damp in autumn, then in winter one will have coughs.'

(Su Wen, yingyang yingxiang dalun)

The above quotation illustrates the Chinese belief that a disease' entering the body at one season, may remain dormant and not produce symptoms till a later season. Strictly then, a patient injured in spring (a wood season) by dormant wind (the excess pertaining to wood) will show symptoms of wind (wood) in the following summer.

A 'dormant evil' is able to enter the body because of a general weakness or lack of resistance in the patient; 'an empty place', as the Chinese put it, 'is that which contains evil'. For example, heavy manual work in winter will dilate the pores and cause sweating, so that 'cold evil' can easily enter through the skin. Similarly, a patient with weak kidneys is a ready prey to dormant 'cold evil' since the kidneys belong to the element water and are particularly susceptible to cold. The Chinese say that the dormant Qi is roused to activity by the body's response to seasonal changes: the Yang Qi begins to move outward in spring, the Yin Qi to move internally in autumn. Sometimes the dormant evil wakens of its own accord.

GENERAL CONSIDERATIONS

It goes without saying that everybody is not affected alike by the five meteorological conditions (the six excesses); indeed, some exceptionally healthy people are not affected by any of them.

Moreover, of two patients, the first may be attacked by one particular 'evil' while the second, immune from that 'evil', will succumb to another, just as one man will be afflicted by influenza, another by a duodenal ulcer, a third by cancer and a fourth remains perfectly healthy. As a rule the six excesses, like the dormant Qi, can only affect an already weakened part of the body. One of the aims of preventive acupuncture (see ch. XII) is to keep the body as fit as possible so that these weaknesses are strengthened sufficiently early.

'*Wind, rain, cold and heat, unless they find the body weak, cannot by themselves do injury to man.*'

(Ling Shu, baibing shisheng pian)

Abnormal weather conditions are, from the meteorological point of view, the commonest cause of disease: sudden cold in summer, for instance, or warmth in winter. All doctors will have noticed that many patients are liable to fall ill when there is such a change in the weather, if it is particularly unusual for the time of year. If the low temperature is fairly consistent throughout the winter, flu or colds will be comparatively rare but a sudden fall of temperature at midsummer may well produce an epidemic of them.

'*Though wind Qi can create the myriad things, it can also harm them, as water can float a vessel but can also sink it.*'

(Yinkui yaolue)

Nor should the climate of the place in which one lives be overlooked. The cold and dryness of central Canada, the humidity of Singapore, the intermediate temperatures of England, where draughts and dampness are sometimes emphasised by inefficient heating, are all factors in the diseases from which different patients suffer.

The six excesses are able to invade the body only if the Protecting Qi is weakened. For the function of the Protecting Qi is to '*warm the flesh, moisten the skin, nourish the space between the skin and the flesh and control the opening and closing of the pores. It performs the function of protecting the exterior*'. The Nourishing Qi, which flows along the meridians, nerves and blood-vessels, is auxiliary to the Protecting Qi; if it is weakened it will in turn weaken the Protecting Qi, and here again disease is more likely to result.

The pulse, in pulse diagnosis, reflects the season and therefore also those adverse influences which might be expected at that time.

'On a spring day the pulse is floating, like a fish swimming on the waves; on a summer day it is superficial (in the skin), drifting like a surplus of the myriad things; on an autumn day it is below the skin, like an insect creeping into its winter shelter; on a winter day it is in the bone (deep), hidden like an insect hibernating.'

The Seven Emotions

In the previous section the outer (or meteorological) causes of disease were discussed. We now turn to the inner (emotional) causes.

Modern medicine might use the word 'psychosomatic' to describe the diseases considered in this section, as they are physical results of uncontrolled emotion; those in the previous section might be given the label 'somatopsychic', being mental diseases resulting from outer or physical causes.

As already mentioned, there is considerable interplay between the physical and the mental. An illness with a purely physical cause may produce both physical and mental symptoms; an illness of the mind may also produce disease in the body. Rheumatoid arthritis for, example, may have its insidious onset within the system, just like any other physical disease, or it may be precipitated by an emotional shock such as a broken engagement.

If the emotions are kept within the normal limits no disease results. If they are so powerful as to be uncontrollable, giving a man the feeling of being 'possessed' and of having his life governed by them, they will injure the body. A passing emotion, even a violent one, is harmless enough; if it is allowed to dominate the mind for any length of time it may well give rise to some physical disease. If a person, normally healthy in mind and body, is depressed by some distressing circumstance, he will recover from his depression as soon as the situation which caused it alters for the better. If, however, the situation persists for some time and the sufferer has some weakness which lowers his resistance, he will continue to feel depression even when its cause is removed. Because it has lasted for so long, the depression has either caused a weakness or aggravated some mild inherent one. Once this physical deterioration has begun it cannot be cured by purely mental means, such as will-power, except by a remarkably strong-minded person, and an easier course to adopt is first to correct the physical weakness. Then, provided the patient is capable of making some effort to help himself, the mental condition will right itself of its own accord.

The effect of the various emotions on Qi, the energy of life, are thus described:—

'If there is anger, then Qi rises; if there is joy, then Qi slows down; if there is grief, then Qi dissolves; if there is fear, then Qi descends; if there is fright, then Qi is in disorder; if there is over-concentration, then Qi congeals.'

(Su Wen, fengtong lun)

'Joy injures the heart, anger injures the liver, over-concentration injures the spleen, anxiety injures the lungs, fear injures the kidneys.'

(Su Wen, yinyang yingxiang dalun)

These quotations not only show the effect of the emotions on Qi but specify the particular organ injured by them, a point of practical importance. For, if anger injures the liver, then the patient who is always losing his temper over trifles can be cured by the correct treatment of his liver.

The heart is the central organ, as far as the seven emotions are concerned, and is often implicated by an emotional disturbance which primarily affects a different organ.

'If there is grief and anxiety, the heart is affected; if the heart is affected, the five Zang and the six Fu tremble.'

(Ling Shu, kouwen pian)

EXCESSIVE JOY INJURES THE HEART

'When one is excessively joyful, the spirit scatters and is no longer stored.'

(Ling Shu, benshen pian)

Most readers will, I am sure, have observed the fact that being deliriously happy or laughing uncontrollably does indeed give one the feeling described in the quotation as a 'scattering' of the spirit; one cannot, as it were, hold oneself together. On Chinese pulse diagnosis, people who laugh excessively will often (though not always) be found to have an overactive heart. In certain circumstances excessive joy can also affect the lungs.

'If the lungs are joyful and happy without limit, then this will injure the animal soul.'

(Ling Shu, benshen pian)

EXCESSIVE ANGER INJURES THE LIVER

If a naturally irritable person is faced with a problem he cannot solve or finds that his affairs have not gone according to plan, he may fly into a violent rage. Then *'Qi rebels and rushes upwards and anger and fire suddenly erupt'*.

'Qi and blood rebel upwards, causing man to feel joy and anger.'

(Su Wen, sishiji nicong lun)

The flushed, 'full-blooded' person, such as the conventional image of the butcher or the beer-swiller, is in fact more quickly roused to anger than the average man.

'If blood has a surplus then there is anger.'

(Su Wen, tiaojing lun)

Not only does anger come more easily to such a man than to the average but *'great anger can injure blood fluid and, if Yin blood is deficient, then water does not submerge wood, so that liver fire is even more vigorous.'* In these circumstances his body, which is deficient in Yin but full of 'fire', will react with fury to the most trivial provocation.

Although dysfunction of the liver is the typical predisposition, there are (as with everything else) often other causes of this abnormal anger:—

'Anger belongs basically to the liver. There are some though who say that anger originates in the gall bladder. This is correct if one considers that the liver and gall bladder are coupled organs, and although the liver is the stronger of the two, the decisions which are taken by the liver are essentially made in the gall bladder.' (See 'The Meridians of Acupuncture', ch. XII)

'Some say that blood unites above, Qi unites below, and that one whose heart is troubled and alarmed is prone to anger. They consider that Yin is conquered by Yang, so that disease reaches the heart.'

'There are some who say that, if the kidneys are abundant and angry for a long time, this will injure one's will-power. There are others who say that, if evil Qi invades the kidney meridian, the person in question is angry without reason, for anger starts in the Yin and then affects the kidneys. Hence anger may be produced by dysfunction of the liver, gall bladder, kidneys or heart.'

(Zangshi leijing)

EXCESSIVE ANXIETY INJURES THE LUNGS

If one observes oneself carefully, one will notice that a certain type of emotion, best described by the word 'anxiety', causes one to hold one's breath, to breathe shallowly, irregularly, or only in the upper part of the chest. This same type of anxiety can also affect the large intestine, since the large intestine and the lungs are coupled organs, and so produce ulcerative colitis, a condition to which over-anxious people are notoriously prone.

'In one who has anxiety the Qi (meaning both energy and air) is blocked and does not move.'

(Ling Shu, benshen pian)

Anxiety can also sometimes affect the spleen, for the lung and the spleen are respectively the arm and leg greater Yin organs and easily influence one another.

EXCESSIVE CONCENTRATION INJURES THE SPLEEN

The type of over-concentration referred to in this context is an obsessive concern with a particular problem. The sufferer from it cannot stop thinking about this problem; it occupies his mind from dawn till dusk and is still nagging at him as he falls asleep. He is almost literally buried as he broods on it behind locked doors, oblivious to the world around him.

A careful distinction must be made, however, between a man who is thus isolated by excessive concentration and one who is driven to this state by an inner fear.

EXCESSIVE GRIEF OR SORROW

Grief or sorrow may be caused by distress, vexation and suffering.

'If the heart Qi is empty, then there is sadness.'

(Su Wen, benshen pian)

'If Jing and Qi unite in the lungs, then there is sadness.'

(Su Wen, xuanming wuqi lun)

'If the liver sadness moves into the middle, then it injures the spiritual soul.'

(Ling Shu, benshen pian)

'If sadness is too extreme, then the pericardium is cut off from the rest of

the body. If this happens, then Qi moves inside, and once this begins the heart collapses.'

(Su Wen, nue lun)

'*If there is sadness, then the pericardium is in distress; the lungs spread and its lobes move; the upper warmer (lung and heart) does not penetrate; nourishing and protecting Qi do not scatter; hot Qi is in the middle, so Qi dissolves.'*

(Su Wen, futong lun)

These quotations show that the division of the seven emotions into the five elements is not mathematically exact.

EXCESSIVE FEAR INJURES THE KIDNEYS

Fear can be aroused by a tension in one's emotional balance. Chinese medicine held that one is particularly vulnerable to fear, if there is some deficiency of kidney Qi or of Qi and blood or if the will-power is weak and the spirit frightened. The kidneys are the storehouse of the will-power, as is the heart of the spirit. If the blood is deficient, then the will-power wanes; if the will is weak, one is prone to fear; if one fears, then the spirit is frightened.

'*If the spirit is injured, then fear is to blame.'*

'*If the Qi of the kidney meridian is deficient, then one is prone to fear.'*

'*If blood is deficient, then there is fear.'*

EXCESSIVE FRIGHT

Fright is produced by a sudden encounter with the alarming and unexpected, like the noise of a near explosion or the sight of an appalling accident. This marks the distinction between 'fright' and 'fear', for fear does not happen suddenly; it is born from what one already knows or expects.

'*If there is fright, then the heart has nothing on which it can rely, the spirit has nothing to which it can turn, thoughts have nothing on which they can settle. Hence Qi is in disorder.'*

(Su Wen, jutong lun)

Again, fright as one of the seven emotions does not fit into the classification of the five elements. The above quotation shows that it chiefly affects the heart; but, if the fright persists for any length of time, it ceases to be either sudden or unexpected. It has become a fear, and will therefore affect the kidneys.

Miscellaneous Causes of Disease

EXCESS OF FOOD AND DRINK

The Chinese consider food to be the main source of energy in post-natal life. They believe that the stomach extracts the essence from ingested food and water and that this essence is then distributed to the rest of the body by the spleen, the coupled organ of the stomach.

Over-eating will affect the digestion and give a sense of fullness in the epigastrium, heartburn, a bad taste in the mouth, putrid breath, loss of appetite and irregular defecation. If food with too strong a taste is eaten, it may produce damp heat and phlegm, with the symptoms of belching, intestinal noises, excessive phlegm with a sensation of heaviness in the chest, and ulcers.

If one eats decaying food, one may get dysentery. If food is too cold, the Yang Qi of the stomach and intestines will be injured and the patient may suffer from stomach-ache, vomiting, swelling of the abdomen and a sense of suffocation and fullness in the epigastrium. Over-indulgence in hot and pungent foods may cause the stomach and intestines to accumulate heat and the stools to be dry and congealed. It may even result in bleeding haemorrhoids.

An excessive addiction to any one of the five flavours will suppress the function of the organ which it subjugates (see ch. VI). Too much sour (wood) food can injure the spleen (earth); too much bitter (fire) food can injure the lungs (metal); too much sweet (earth) food can injure the kidneys (water); too much hot (metal) food can injure the liver (wood); too much salty (water) food can injure the heart (fire) (Fig. 10.1).

The above system should be compared with that mentioned near the end of chapter VI where an excess injures its own element, i.e. 'sour injures the muscles (liver, wood). . .' As with most things in Chinese medicine, sometimes one set of laws are followed and sometimes another. The experienced physician is the one who knows what will be the outcome with the particular patient he is treating.

Prolonged over-indulgence in alcohol can produce acute alcoholism or delirium tremens, and also a certain kind of general debility which renders the patient liable to many types of acute disease. Hunger and thirst sufficiently prolonged are also among the causes of disease.

PHYSICAL LABOUR

Man's body is so constructed that too little physical exercise will impair its health. In Chinese terms, the blood and energy flowing through the meridians and blood-vessels grows sluggish. On the

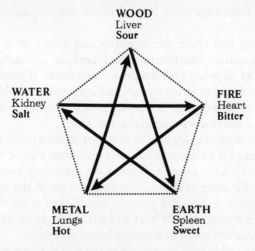

FIG. 10.1

other hand, excessive physical labour also has its dangers. It injures the spleen and can produce muscular exhaustion, lethargy in speech, breathlessness after exertion, slight fever, spontaneous sweating and abnormal awareness of the heart-beat.

'*If there is exhaustion, then Qi wastes away.*'

(Su Wen, jutong lun)

'*Looking for a long time injures blood; standing for a long time injures bones; walking for a long time injures muscles.*'

(Su Wen, benbing lun)

UNREGULATED SEXUAL ACTIVITY

Chinese philosophy, especially Taoism, which is so closely interwoven with Chinese traditional medicine, is largely based on the idea of the balance and harmony of life. Too much or too little in any direction will interfere with this balance. Thus too much or too little food, too much or too little exercise, and likewise too much or too little sexual activity, all these will endanger the harmony which is health.

'If sexual intercourse passes the norm... then it will injure the kidneys.'
(Ling Shu, xieqi zangfu bingxiang pian)

The 'essence' of life is stored in the kidneys. Excessive sexual activity weakens the essence of life and lowers the body's resistance to infection.

'The kidney Yin and kidney Yang are deficient, or the Yin is empty and fire vigorous, or destiny fire is small and weak, or Yin and Yang are both injured.' Such excess can produce the symptoms of coughing up blood, aching bones, hot flushes, night sweats, palpitations, lumbago, weak knees, coldness in the extremities, nocturnal emissions, impotence, irregular periods, menorrhagia or vaginal discharge. All the above symptoms have, of course, in many cases quite other causes; nor need any patient feel uneasy lest his doctor should take them as evidence of a life abandoned to lecherous orgies!

EPIDEMICS

The Chinese recognised the existence of epidemics and divided them into two main groups. The first group includes all those epidemics caused by abnormal climatic conditions: unseasonable cold or heat, excessive wind or rain, drought, floods or mountain mists at the wrong time of year. The second group consists of those epidemics due to poor hygiene: lack of cleanliness, dirt and refuse, putrefying bodies left too long unburied.

The evil energy (Qi) held responsible for these epidemics went under various names: Heterodox Qi, Perverse Qi, Confused Qi, Poison Qi, Demon Qi etc. These were thought of as invading the body from the outside, an idea which modern theories of bacteria or viruses as the causes of infectious disease do not contradict.

WOUNDS AND INSECT BITES

Under this heading come those diseases caused by accidents, snakebite, insect stings and bites, rabies etc.

WORM INFESTATION

Chinese books usually give a fairly full description of diseases caused by worms. Such diseases were common in China, owing to the use of fresh, uncomposted night-soil. In my opinion Western medicine is superior to traditional Chinese medicine in its classification and description of helminthic diseases, so it is unnecessary to elaborate further on the topic here. One of the greatest benefits Western knowledge has given to China has been the prevention of helminthic diseases by adequate sanitation, drainage systems and general cleanliness.

PENETRATING POISONS

Included in this group are all diseases due to the consumption of poisonous berries, wood alcohol, bad or poisonous fish, bad meat etc. In addition to the above are poisonous medicines, inaccurate prescriptions, or overdoses of normally beneficial medicines.

HEREDITY

This class describes the ordinary hereditary diseases which are dealt with in any Western book on medicine. It also includes shocks suffered by the mother during pregnancy:—

'If the man's mother had a severe fright while she was pregnant and the Qi ascended but did not descend. . . then this would cause the child to have epilepsy.'

(Su Wen, qibing lun)

XI

DISEASES THAT MAY BE TREATED
BY ACUPUNCTURE — STATISTICS

Theoretically it is possible to help or cure by acupuncture any disease that can be affected by a physiological process. Duodenal ulcer, acne vulgaris, migraine, for example, are all the result of physiological process, and as such may be cured: the duodenal ulcer, by reducing the amount of acid produced by the stomach; the acne, by increasing the function of the lungs and hormonal regulation; the migraine, by increasing the function of the liver.

A trouble that is purely anatomical and uninfluenceable by a physiological process, such as a kidney stone, advanced osteo-arthritis, a fully formed cataract, cannot be treated by this means. Human physiology is such that it is hardly ever possible for des-tructive changes in bones to be repaired—though it is obviously possible to affect the circulation, swelling and muscle spasm around an arthritic joint, without though altering the bone very much. In a cataract the protein of the lens of the eye has become denatured, a chemical change that cannot be reversed under the normal con-ditions of life.

The capacity for the regeneration of the new tissue in the human being must be taken into account when judging the possibility of a cure. It must be remembered that the human has less power of regeneration than any animal, and vastly less than the lower animals. A flat worm will completely regenerate itself if it is cut in half longitudinally or transversely (so that two flat worms are made out of one); if the tail of a rain worm is cut off, it will partially regrow; the fin of a lung fish will grow again if it has been broken off; similarly the limbs of an amphibia (if cut under experimental conditions.) The human organism has not this same regenerative power. His creative energy has been transferred to the power of thought.

From the point of view of Chinese medicine, there is often no essential difference between a physical and a mental disease:

1. A physical dysfunction can cause a mental disease.
2. A mental dysfunction can cause a physical disease.
3. A physical dysfunction can cause a physical disease.
4. A mental dysfunction can cause a mental disease.

To give an example:

A If someone lives in depressing circumstances for a *short* time, then the depressing circumstances affect this mode of thinking, and he becomes depressed. If then after a short while the depressing circumstances disappear, then the patient can usually readjust himself mentally and the depression disappears.

B If, on the other hand, the depressing circumstances continue for a *long* time, then the depressed mind of the patient will eventually affect the liver (see relation between the liver and depression in the chapter on the five elements). Once the liver is affected, even if the original depressing circumstances are removed, the depression will remain. This depression can only be cured if the liver is treated—provided the depressing external circumstances have also been removed.

C If someone harms his liver, by, for example, eating a poison that destroys part of the liver, then the patient may (1) have predominantly physical symptoms such as jaundice, ascites, pruritis, or he may (2) have predominantly mental symptoms such as depression or an uncontrollable anger. In this instance whether the patient has physical or mental symptoms the liver would have to be treated physically.

To take another example of a mental disease which is really a physical disease and can therefore be treated by acupuncture: Most people who have various disturbances which include 'fear' have an underactivity of the kidney (many frightened children are bed wetters—kidney; after a fright most people wish to pass urine—

kidney). Actors with stage fright, teachers with lack of confidence, others before interviews, examinations, driving tests, people who are afraid to leave their house to meet strangers—all these are often kidney weaknesses which may be cured by treating the kidney. The law of the five elements, described earlier, indicates which organ is the culprit for the five main categories of mental diseases.

Case History. A regular colonel left the army at 45 and had to start civilian life. This involved interviews with many prospective employers. A certain degree of nervousness would be normal under the circumstances, but he was excessively nervous, so that he became unbearable at home. Pulse diagnosis showed an underactive kidney, which when treated reduced the excessive nervous tension, to one of normal proportions.

Case History. During the course of a takeover bid a patient's nerves were so shattered that he started shaking to such an extent that he could not pour out a cup of tea. The whole takeover bid was from his point of view jeopardised by his excessive nervous reaction, shaking hands, sleeplessness, fits of suicidal depression, etc. In his instance there was a dysfunction of the lung and heart which was quickly cured, and I am glad to say the patient's part of the firm prospered. He thanked me afterwards especially as he had been dragged to see me against his will by his wife.

One of the great contributions of Chinese medicine is its ability to link physical and mental diseases, whereby it is often found that a physical disease has a mental cause, and a mental disease a physical cause. In either case they may be treated by acupuncture.

In acupuncture psychologists would have a powerful weapon with which to treat their patients in a rational manner instead of rolling tranquillisers down their throats, passing electric currents through their brains, or discussing those parts of their sex life which they would rather forget. The role of the psychologist will still remain though in what has been classified above as 2 a mental dysfunction causing a physical disease, and 4 a mental dysfunction causing a mental disease. Quite apart from the above considerations, a good clinician should know which method (tranquillisers, E.C.T., psycho-analysis, acupuncture etc.) to apply in a given case.

The list of illnesses given below may be found in most books on acupuncture; some authors mention more, some less. Among the diseases listed some may be cured in nearly every case treated, while others may only yield to treatment in a small proportion of the patients treated. The duration of the disease, the amount of damage done, the general constitution of the individual patient must be taken into account. In some diseases, which have progressed too far for it to be possible to effect a cure, it may be possible to arrest the disease so that it does not progress any further; or a disease which is severely incapacitating may, at least, be partially cured or relieved, so that the man or woman may continue living a reasonably normal life.

Vague feelings of malaise, not feeling 100% fit but not really ill, not having enough energy or drive, etc., etc., are really all preclinical symptoms of disease, which, if they persist long enough, will quite likely result in actual disease. These vague preclinical symptoms can usually be precisely recognised by the pulse diagnosis (as discussed in the chapter on Preventive Medicine), and immediately treated. The increased sense of both physical and mental well-being that may thus be achieved, is a major contribution of acupuncture.

It is often said that 'the patient's psyche does not matter'. This is not true. It is not true for ordinary medicine nor for acupuncture, though some people (I think quite erroneously) consider that an objective diagnosis cannot be made unless the thoughts and feelings of both patient and doctor are disregarded, and a medical consultation is conducted like a test-tube experiment. It is well known to anaesthetists that the dose of anaesthetic required, especially for light anaesthesia, may have to be either doubled or halved according to the mental attitude of the patient—whether he wishes to become unconscious or whether he resists. The speed of recovery after an operation or the chances of life or death for a person who is very seriously ill are, as most doctors will agree from their own experience, partly a matter of the will power of the patient.

It is sometimes assumed that the mind is subjective, irresponsible and unreal, a negligible factor in medicine, since it cannot be measured; while the body is objective, measurable and real. To the acupuncturist they are but two facets of the same problem. Under certain circumstances one facet is more important, while at other times the other.

Some who have not experienced or seen the results of acupuncture get the impression that this is little more than hypnotism. This is by no means the case for:

(a) Acupuncture will work if the patient is completely uncon-scious under a general anaesthetic.

(b) There are certain sensitive people who notice the effect of a needle within a few seconds. As an acupuncture point is small it is occasionally possible to miss the exact spot, whereupon the sensitive patient, if he has already had experience of the treatment, will remark that it is not working. The acupuncturist can verify this by the pulse diagnosis. This should, in any case, be repeated as a routine after all the acupuncture needles are in place, for the pulse should alter within seconds of the needle being put in. If the needle is then readjusted by $\frac{1}{10}$th inch the sensitive patient will at once feel the difference, which may be verified by the pulse diagnosis.

(c) Occasional cases of spontaneous cures may be attributed to accidental injuries to acupuncture points. This is rarely the case as at any one time only a few acupuncture points are active—and they are small. An injury over a large area which may include one or several acupuncture points seems to have no specific effect. The stimulus must be localised to have an effect.

Tropical diseases, of which most European acupuncturists have no practical experience, are not mentioned in the index.

Various acute surgical emergencies such as appendicitis, peri-ιonitis, etc. and various other potentially lethal diseases are not mentioned in the index, for although the acupuncturist may well be able to treat them (as is done in China today), most European acupuncturists will, as a matter of principle, not treat these diseases, as acupuncture is new to Europe. In addition, many of these acute emergencies can be well treated by orthodox medicine.

Some people say one cannot cure a chronic disease. This though is quite wrong. An expert acupuncturist may cure it as easily as: taking out a thorn, or wiping away snow flakes, or untying a knot, or pulling out a cork. Even if a disease is of long duration it can be cured; those who say it is incurable do not know acupuncture properly.

(Jia Yi Jing, Vol. II, Ch. 1a)

Duration of Treatment

The number of treatments required to effect a cure varies con-siderably. The average patient when seen by the acupuncturist for the first time does not, as a rule, have merely one disease, but in addition a variety of mild chronic complaints which do not in-capacitate him, but simply make life less pleasant. It is a flare-up of these mildly chronic ailments that actually brings the sufferer to the doctor. The patient may have, for example, dyspepsia, a bitter taste in the mouth, frequent headaches, insomnia, brittle nails, and an irritable mood that he cannot control. One or more of these symptoms will have become acute; for instance, the dyspepsia may have developed into a duodenal ulcer.

All these symptoms (in one individual patient) including the duodenal ulcer, will take an average of about seven treatments to cure (or if a cure is not possible, to ameliorate).

Once a patient has been completely cured of his various ailments and the pulse is normal, provided he is seen by the doctor for a check-up every six months (as described in the chapter on pre-ventive medicine), his basic health will then, as a rule, remain satis-factory. If he should then (with a basically sound health) develop an illness it can usually be cured in relatively few treatments—even a single one sometimes being sufficient.

Certain difficult diseases, especially if they have been in existence over a substantial portion of the patient's life, have a hereditary tendency or have resulted in anatomical changes, may easily take more than seven treatments to cure or ameliorate.

A disease of short duration, provided the causes, which may not be apparent, are also of short duration, will probably take less than seven treatments.

A very small proportion of patients who do not improve while they are being treated, may notice an amelioration or even a cure some months later—seemingly the healing process may be very slow.

Response to Treatment

The speed of response varies considerably from patient to patient, and with each disease.

Certain patients feel a response within a few seconds of the first needles being in place the first time they come for treatment. Others may have to be treated four or possibly even more times, for the first response to be felt.

The effect of a single treatment may be noticed during the treat-ment or several days later.

After a treatment nothing tangible may be noticed. At other times there may be an increase in energy, a lightness and buoyancy due to the stimulating effect of the treatment. In some people there is a great feeling of relaxation which may be followed by a pleasant drowsiness due to the sudden release of tension.

Occasionally, and in certain people, there is a reaction before the improvement starts. This may seem, if it is not understood, to be a worsening of the condition. A reaction may be compared to what happens in the case of an infection deep in the hand which first becomes an acute boil (seemingly a worsening of the condition—the reaction) before it discharges its accumulated pus to the exterior. The infection in the hand could also have been cured by the absorption of the infection into the blood stream. In the latter case the improvement would have progressed smoothly without a reaction. With or without a reaction the end result is the same, though the acupuncturist naturally always tries to effect a cure the smooth way. Certain chronic conditions however have, of necessity, to be brought to an acute stage (the reaction) for it to be possible to cure them. On rare occasions a reaction may be experienced after every treatment. The following letter illustrates an extreme example.

Dear Dr. Mann,   26.3.70
The effects of your last treatment were so extraordinary I think you'd like to know about them!

For 48 hours I suffered a great deal of severe pain—Codis twice in the night and once or twice next day failed to ease it and my spine and neck and back got worse and worse.

At one moment on the second day I thought I was going to seize up as I've done before and I thought 'I *must* get to Dr. Mann' for a needling, only to be brought up short by remembering it was the needling that had brought it on.

Then it passed and steadily I improved till every one of the symptoms—waves of nausea, livery-ishness, *pains went and even, for the first time in years, I found myself able to drink an ordinary amount of wine (strongly disapproved of for me by my medicos who prefer that I take 'purple hearts') without any subsequent heaviness or other liver symptoms.

*She was unable to walk far.

'Cheers!' Well done and thank you very much!
With all good wishes from a grateful and rejuvenated old lady.
Yours sincerely.

The improvement that is noticed during a course of acupuncture does not follow a steady course. As a rule the degree of improvement and its duration increases with each treatment till the stage is reached where the improvement persists and becomes a cure that lasts. The improvement from the first treatment may last minutes, hours or days, the effect lasting longer with each repetition. Some patients improve rapidly at the beginning of treatment but may take a long time to achieve that extra little bit that makes the cure; others improve slowly at the beginning and then take a sudden turn and are cured in no time. The majority follow an intermediate course. Most often there are various ups and downs during treatment and there is rarely an absolutely steady improvement—nature does not know straight lines. Not infrequently there is a setback at some stage of the treatment, which is then overcome by altering the acupuncture points used.

The final result rests with the individual doctor, his knowledge and ability of the subject.

Below is a list of some of the commoner conditions treated. The easier ones have a higher degree of success than the more difficult; but at times the seemingly impossible can be cured, while the easy may prove intractable.

HEAD

Neuralgia, headaches, migraine, fainting, trigeminal neuralgia (sometimes), tics, spasms.

LIMBS AND MUSCULATURE

Fibrositis, muscular rheumatism, sciatica, lumbago, swelling, discoloration, cramps, intermittent claudication, cold hands and feet (sometimes), oedema, writers' cramp, weakness, some types of trembling, neuralgia of shoulders and arms, tennis elbow, early rheumatoid or osteoarthritis, weakness or feeling of excessive heaviness of limbs, frozen shoulder.

DISEASES THAT MAY BE TREATED BY ACUPUNCTURE

DIGESTION

Duodenal and stomach ulcer, hyperacidity, gastritis, dyspepsia, inability to eat ordinary food, non digestion of food, no appetite, undigested stools, pale stools, eructations, wind, abdominal distension, bad breath, dry mouth, bad taste in mouth, heartburn, pyloric spasm, nausea, vomiting, rectal prolapse, constipation, diarrhoea, various types of colic, atony, perianal pain or itch, haematemesis, underfunction of liver, tender liver, hepatitis, chronic cholecystitis, colitis, ulcerative colitis, pancreatitis, nausea and vomiting of pregnancy, vomiting of children and infants, abdomen feels cold.

RESPIRATORY SYSTEM

Asthma, bronchitis, tracheitis, shortness of breath, pulmonary congestion, recurrent colds, coughs and mild pulmonary infections.

CARDIO VASCULAR SYSTEM

Angina pectoris, pseudo angina pectoris, pain or heaviness over cardiac area, fainting, palpitations, certain valvular defects, arterial spasm, phlebitis, lymphangeitis, adenitis, pallor, pins and needles, poor circulation, fainting, feels easily cold.

GENITO URINARY SYSTEM

Renal insufficiency, pyelitis, cystitis, some types of renal colic, lumbago, bladder irritation and spasm, bed wetting, lack of control of bladder, early prostatic hypertrophy.

SEXUAL SYSTEM

Pelvic pain, painful periods, irregular periods, flooding, vaginal pain, itching, menopausal trouble, hot flushes, ovarian pain, impotence, frigidity, sterility, lack of sexual desire, nymphomania, pollution, mastitis, menopausal loss of hair (sometimes).

EYES

Weak eyesight, tired after reading a book a short time, not optical defects, black spots and zig-zags in front of eyes, pain behind or around eye, conjunctivitis, blepharitis, iritis (sometimes).

EAR, NOSE AND THROAT

Hay fever, rhinitis, nose bleeding, sneezing, loss of smell (some types), sinusitis, catarrh, tonsillitis, laryngitis, loss of voice, pharyngitis.

SKIN

Acne, itching, eczema, urticaria, abscesses, herpes, neurodermatitis, etc., may also help psoriasis.

NERVOUS SYSTEM AND PSYCHIATRIC FACTORS

Nervousness, depression, anxiety, fears, obsessions, timidity, stage fright, neurasthenia, wish to die, agitation, outbursts of temper, yawning, excessive loquacity, sleeplessness, nocturnal terror, many neuralgias, facial palsy, neuralgia after shingles (sometimes), petit mal (sometimes), trembling, trigeminal neuralgia (sometimes).

GENERAL STATE

Anaemia, general fatigue, lassitude, excessive perspiration, excessive sleep, excessive yawning, sensitive to changes in temperature, travel sickness, post operative weakness, weakness after severe diseases, insomnia.

CHILDREN

Most of the more common diseases of children, excepting the infectious diseases. Children respond quickly. An important aim of acupuncture is to achieve and maintain healthy childhood, as much ill health of later years can then be avoided. Bed-wetting, fear of the dark, bad tempered or frightened states, inability to learn properly at school, underdevelopment, stunted growth (sometimes), cyclic vomiting and acidosis in infants.

GENERAL HEALTH

Most patients who have been treated by acupuncture notice a considerable improvement in their general health. This is because acupuncture can correct those minor disturbances in health which are undetected by other methods of diagnosis, and which if they remained untreated could in later years easily turn into a serious overt and easily recognised disease. The sensitivity of Chinese pulse diagnosis (see section on Preventive Medicine) makes it possible to detect minor disturbances, enabling immediate treatment to be given at an early stage.

Reactions

A few patients experience a reaction after treatment and feel temporarily worse before they are better. This is more likely to happen after the first treatment than subsequent ones.

The reaction may manifest itself as an aggravation of the patients usual symptoms, or sometimes as merely fatigue. This passes off in a few hours or days, though on very rare occasions it might last weeks. After the reaction there is sometimes a return to the patients initial state of health, though more often it is followed by an improvement or even a remarkable improvement.

In acupuncture one often tries to strengthen the diseased part of the body, one tries to make the lazy parts work again. This might be compared to someone digging a garden or riding a horse after a long period of inactivity. The lazy muscles ache after such exercise, just as the lazy organs of the body might revolt at strong acupuncture treatment.

Reactions are rare, but they can be nearly totally avoided by giving a weaker acupuncture treatment, which might require though two, three or four times as many treatments. There are some illnesses which are so severe or ingrained that a patient cannot respond, without at any rate one reaction, to initiate the process of healing.

If there is no response to treatment, a doctor may try to induce a reaction to stimulate the curative process. Once there has been a reaction the physician will usually reduce the strength of treatment so that there are no subsequent reactions.

It should be remembered that reactions are rare, the symptoms may be mild or severe, but there is no damage and it is all temporary.

STATISTICS

On the whole, the following statistics, are in my opinion somewhat optimistic; though they may if diluted be used as a rough guide. I know of no statistics, in China or the West, which correspond with my present-day experience of acupuncture. I have little doubt, now that a greater number of doctors are practising acupuncture in the West, that more accurate statistics will in the ensuing years be published. These will be incorporated in later printings of this book.

It should not be forgotten that acupuncture is mainly suitable for diseases which are physiologically reversible, i.e. it may cure asthma; it may help (but not cure) the early stages of chronic bronchitis; whilst the later stages of chronic bronchitis, bronchietasis or emphysema are not helped except in so far as they have an element of spasm.

A The following statistics of Mauries* (Marseille) may act as a guide. It consists of all (625) the patients he treated in a specified period who had been previously diagnosed and treated by doctors other than acupuncturists, with little or no success. It does not include patients who visited Dr Mauries before they had seen another doctor; so that the possible statistical error of a spontaneous cure despite treatment is at least partly negated. Patients whom he has not been able to contact, or who have left his district, have not been included. Despite the fact that the diagnosis has been made by at least two doctors in each case, it will be obvious to the reader that some of the criteria used in diagnosis and the meaning attached to a particular diagnosis are a little different from those usually employed in England, for which due allowance should be made.

*(Actes des Ill eme Journées International d'Acupuncture).

286

Rheumatic and allied diseases	No. treated	Cured	Improved	Failure
Lumbago	29	19	6	4
Sciatica	25	15	4	6
Facial neuralgia	11	6	4	1
Rheumatism of several joints	36	19	11	6
P.C.E.	5	3	1	1
Cervical arthritis	9	5	3	1
Pain in heel of foot	2	2	—	—
Interscapular neuralgia	1	—	—	1
Gout of big toe	2	2	—	—
Tennis elbow	1	—	—	1
Arthrosis deformans	1	—	1	—
Generalised vertebral arthritis	3	2	1	—
Coccydynia	2	—	—	2
Arthritis of knee	14	9	1	4
Mandibular arthritis	2	1	—	1
Frozen shoulder	4	2	1	1
Rheumatism of knee and ankle	1	1	—	—
Coxarthritis	1	—	—	1
Intercostal neuralgia	3	2	—	1
Hernia of lumbar disc	1	—	—	1
Traumatic lumbar pain	1	—	—	1
Arthritis of shoulder	5	3	2	—
Cervico-brachial neuralgia	5	4	1	—
Post-menopausal rheumatism	1	1	—	—
Rheumatism of ankle	2	2	—	—
	167	98	36	33

i.e. 80% cured or improved

Pulmonary diseases	No. treated	Cured	Improved	Failure
Hay fever	9	6	—	3
Emphysema	10	3	4	3
Chronic bronchitis	3	1	2	—
Asthma	38	24	8	6
Cough due to hypertension	1	1	—	—
	61	35	14	12

i.e. 80% cured or improved

Urology	No. treated	Cured	Improved	Failure
Cystitis	2	2	—	—
Incontinence	8	2	3	3
Renal colic	1	1	—	—
	11	5	3	3

i.e. 72% cured or improved

E.N.T.	No. treated	Cured	Improved	Failure
Streptomycin tinnitis	1	—	—	1
Chronic sinusitis	1	1	—	—
Chronic tracheitis	2	1	—	1
Chronic laryngitis	1	1	—	—
Chronic otorrhea	1	1	—	—
Catarrhal deafness	1	1	—	—
Allergic oedema of larynx	1	1	—	—
Post menopausal deafness	1	—	—	1
	9	6	0	3

i.e. 66% cured or improved

Gynaecology	No. treated	Cured	Improved	Failure
Dysmenorrhea	5	5	—	—
Hypermenorrhea	1	1	—	—
Menstrual trouble	1	1	—	—
	7	7	0	0

i.e. 100% cured or improved

Diseases of arteries and veins	No. treated	Cured	Improved	Failure
Arteritis of leg	3	—	2	1
Circulatory disturbance in a man	1	1	—	—
Circulatory disturbance in a woman	2	1	—	1
	6	2	2	2

i.e. 66% cured or improved

288

Cardiology	No. treated	Cured	Improved	Failure
Cardiac asthma	2	—	—	2
Paroxysmal tachycardia	1	1	—	—
	3	1	0	2

i.e. 33% cured

Digestive tract	No. treated	Cured	Improved	Failure
Gastralgia	3	3	—	—
Diarrhoea with food	1	1	—	—
Vomiting due to megaoesophagus	1	—	—	1
Peptic ulcer	1	1	—	—
Vomiting of infants	3	3	—	—
Chronic diarrhoea	2	2	—	—
Constipation	8	5	—	3
Biliary atony	6	5	1	—
Gastric ulcer	4	2	1	1
Habitual vomiting	1	1	—	—
Cholecystitis in a colonial	1	1	—	—
Gastralgia in a syphylitic	1	1	—	—
	32	25	2	5

i.e. 84% cured or improved

Neurology	No. treated	Cured	Improved	Failure
Littles disease	1	—	1	—
Results of hemiplegia	6	—	5	1
Myelitis	1	—	—	1
Para-facial spasm of Meige	1	—	1	—
Epilepsy	1	—	1	—
Tabetic pains	1	1	—	—
Parkinson's disease	3	—	—	3
Atrophy due to polio	1	—	1	—
Spasmodic quadriplegia due to cervical disease	1	—	1	—
Disseminated sclerosis	3	—	—	3
	19	1	9	9

i.e. 52% of improvements including one cure.

Endocrinal diseases	No. treated	Cured	Improved	Failure
Diabetes mellitus	3	—	—	3
Diabetes insipidus	1	—	1	—
Hyperthyroidism	1	—	1	—
Too short in stature	1	—	1	—
Adrenal insufficience	1	1	—	—
Pagets disease	1	—	1	—
	8	1	4	3

i.e. 62% cured or improved.

Neuro-vegetative disequilibrium (syncope, tachycardia, globus hysteria, spasms, lassitude, etc., etc.)

	No. treated	Cured	Improved	Failure
General neuro-vegetative disequilibrium	208	151	23	34
Post operative functional disturbances	3	3	—	—
Nervous hypertension	12	11	1	—
Neurasthenia	5	2	2	1
Vomiting of pregnancy	1	1	—	—
Angina pectoris	2	2	—	—
Neuritis of pregnancy	1	—	—	1
Pruritis ani	1	—	—	1
Eczema	1	1	—	—
'Floaters'	1	—	—	1
Demencia praecox	1	1	—	—
Plexalgia	1	1	—	—
Yawning	2	2	—	—
Excessive sleepiness	1	1	—	—
	240	176	26	38

i.e. 84% cured or improved.

Diverse diseases	No. treated	Cured	Improved	Failure
Quinche's oedema	3	3	—	—
Taenia	1	1	—	—
Excessive loss of weight	2	2	—	—
Amyotrophia	1	—	1	—
Furunculosis	2	2	—	—
Hiccups	1	—	1	—
Idiopathic headaches	6	3	2	1

Aphthous stomatitis	1	—	—	1
Non cardiac oedema of ankles	1	—	—	1
Seborrhea	1	—	—	1
Asthenia and anaemia	2	2	—	—
Bad at mathematics	4	4	—	—
Vertigo	1	1	—	—
Psoriasis	1	—	—	1
Obesity in a woman	1	1	—	—
Ophthalmic herpes zosta	1	1	—	—
Insomnia	3	2	1	—
	32	22	5	5

i.e. 84% cured or improved.

B The following statistics are taken from the Department of Surgery, Chung Shan Medical College, Canton, China.* They are concerned with the treatment of thirty-six cases of acute appendicitis, ten of appendicular abscess and three of perforated appendix with general peritonitis. They were treated mainly by acupuncture; though ten of them were treated by traditional Chinese herbs or a combination of both methods.

I. DURATION AFTER ONSET OF ILLNESS

Duration	Acute appendicitis	Appendicular abscess	Perforated appendix
2-6 hours	5		
6-12 hours	5		
12-24 hours	9	1	
24-48 hours	5		2
48-72 hours	4	2	1
4 days	2	1	
6 days	1		
7 days		2	
8 days		1	
10 days		1	
15 days		2	
Records unavailable	5		
	36	10	3

*Chinese Medical Journal 79: 72–76, July, 1959.

2. TEMPERATURE ON ADMISSION

Temperature	Acute appendicitis	Appendicular abscess	Perforated appendix
Normal	11		
High	24	9	3
37.1-38°C	17	3	
38.1-39°C	5	6	3
39.1-40°C	2		
Records unavailable	1	1	
	—	—	—
	36	10	3

3. W.B.C. ON ADMISSION

W.B.C.	Acute appendicitis	Appendicular abscess	Perforated appendix
7,000 or less	4	—	—
7,000-10,000	8	1	—
10,000-20,000	19	6	2
20,000-30,000	1	2	1
30,000-40,000	1	—	—
Records unavailable	3	1	—
	—	—	—
	36	10	3

4. SYMPTOMS AND SIGNS OF ACUTE APPENDICITIS
CASES BEFORE TREATMENT

	No. of cases	%
Rigidity of abdominal muscles in right lower abdomen	24	66.6
Tenderness on pressure of right lower abdomen	36	100
Rebounding pain in right lower abdomen	36	100

5. CONDITION OF ACUTE APPENDICITIS CASES AFTER
TREATMENT (Only those with complete record included)

Duration	Disappearance of abdominal pain	Normal blood picture	Normal temp.
< 24 hours	9	7	12
< 2 days	6	4	2
< 3 days	5	4	3
< 4 days	2	2	2
5-7 days	5	1	—
8 days	1	—	—

6. DURATION OF HOSPITALISATION IN ACUTE APPENDICITIS CASES

Hospital days	No. of cases
Emergency cases not hospitalised	3
2 days	4
3 days	3
4 days	6
5 days	8
6 days	5
8 days	1
11 days	1
12 days	1
13 days	1
22 days	1
	36

41.7%

78.7%

Conclusion: Good results obtained in all cases. No untoward complications were observed.

C L. J. Milman, E. D. Tikochinskaia and N. P. Bobrova (Acupuncture Laboratory of the Bechterev Psychoneurological Institute and the Polyclinic No. 5 in Leningrad)* treated thirty-five cases of physical sexual malfunction, which had proved resistant to ordinary treatment. Twenty-six of these were cured or improved.

*Russian Acupuncture Conference, Gorki, June 1960.

Of these twenty-six, twenty-four came for a re-check one-and-a-half years later; and of these twenty-four, twenty-one had remained cured or improved.

D Professor U. G. Vogralik (Gorki Medical Institute) states the following statistics:*

Disease	No. of Patients	Greatly improved or completely cured	Improved	No change	Treatment continues
Peptic ulceration	48	37	3	2	6
Spastic colitis	5	2	1	1	1
Bronchial asthma	54	3	31	14	6
Thyrotoxicosis (mild & severe)	12	3	6	1	2
Cardiac neurosis	16	0	5	8	3
Angina pectoris	18	7	7	4	—
Angina pectoris (sclerotic)	24	5	11	8	—
Rheumatic coronaritis	2	1	0	1	—
Erythraemia	23	6	11	4	2
Trigeminal neuralgia	13	4	4	1	4
Glaucoma	35	20	4	3	5
	250	88	83	47	29

E At one time, when I practised acupuncture in hospital, we analysed and published the following results:†

The statistics given below refer to 40 consecutive patients seen at the Ear, Nose and Throat Department. In each case the main symptom was headache. We chose headache, as this symptom, with some exceptions, is difficult to cure by Western medical methods,

*Russian Acupuncture Conference, Gorki, 1959.
†Felix Mann and Anthony Halfhide. Medical World, April 1963.

while a reasonably permanent cure or considerable alleviation can be achieved by acupuncture in about 80 per cent of the patients treated.

Patients were referred to the Department by their general practitioners or from other departments of the Hospital. They were first seen by one of us (A.H.), and a thorough ENT investigation was made: this included almost invariably an x-ray examination of the sinuses. Where the headache was found to be due to ENT disease, such as sinusitis, and amenable to orthodox ENT methods, patients were treated by A.H. without using acupuncture. Such cases are not included in the figures. Other cases excluded were those in which the headache was of minor importance and cases of chronic suppurative otitis media, cranial tumour and so on.

All the patients had been treated for headache without much success by at least two doctors—their GP and a member of the ENT Department. Many of them had been to one or several other departments of the Hospital as well. Only those cases were treated by acupuncture (by F.M.) in which orthodox medicine had failed or achieved only a slight improvement.

We have not tried to classify the headaches into various types, as the usual definitions are too arbitrary and do not fit in with what we consider to be the important symptoms. Some doctors might have classified about half the patients as having migraine, other doctors, tension headaches, others neuralgia. Two of the headaches were specific—trigeminal neuralgia and supraorbital neuralgia.

The results, as recorded in the table, were as follows: 3 patients ($7\frac{1}{2}$ per cent) showed no improvement or aggravation; 5 ($12\frac{1}{2}$ per cent) showed moderate improvement; and 32 (80 per cent) were cured or showed considerable improvement. We have adopted this classification as many of the patients have had headache for a large part of their lives and the cause usually goes back several years further. Those very severe cases—those patients who before treatment had spoken of suicide, had stopped work, or were living in a semi-conscious state under constant analgesia usually still have an occasional mild headache, and so could be described perhaps as 70 to 99 per cent cured. A few with moderately severe headache still have a very occasional mild one—much as a patient cured of pleurisy may have an occasional pleuritic pain in cold or damp weather.

TABLE Analysis of cases treated by acupuncture for various types of headache and other symptoms or diseases

Various types of headache					Other symptoms or diseases in the same patient			
Patient	Sex	Duration of headache (years)	Number of treatments	Result	Symptom or Disease	Duration (years)	Number of treatments	Result
J.D.	F	1	1	+ +	Vertigo	1⁴/₁₂	1	+
M.E.	F	7	1	+ +				
N.G.	M	5	2	+ +				
M.H.	M	10	12	+	Asthma	14	15	+
R.L.	M	15	7	+ +	Lumbago	?	?	+ +
D.L.	F	2	14	+ +	Biliousness	2	14	+ +
L.O.	F	2	6	+ +	Heartburn	2	6	+ +
B.P.	F	1½	5	+ +	Tinnitus	8/52	3	+ +
M.Q.	F	½	2	+ +	Asthenia	2	9	+ +
H.S.	M	8	4	+ +				
E.S.	F	8	4	+ +				
E.T.	F	20	8	+ +	Allergic rhinitis	20	8	+
P.T.	M	4	9	—				
H.T.*	F	3	1					
A.W.	F	20	4	+ +	Anosmia	2	4	+
H.N.	M	1	14+	+	General debility	1	14+	+
J.T.	M	10	7	+ +	Allergic rhinitis	10	7	+
D.H.	M	20	4	+ +	Biliousness	?	7	+ +
D.B.	M	2	10	+ +	Asthenia	?	10	+
P.C.*	M	1	1					
R.D.	M	15	3	+ +				
M.G.	F	1	8	+ +				
F.E.	M	10	8	+ +	Hypochondria			
G.C.	F	?1	12	+ +	This was a case of trigeminal neuralgia			
A.H.	F	9/12	3	+ +	This was a case of supraorbital neuralgia			
G.H.	F	6	3	+ +				
R.H.	F	3	6	+ +	Hysterical aphonia	30	6	+ +
M.K.	F	3	15	+	Allergic rhinitis	3	15	+
T.L.	M	9/12	4	+ +	Asthenia			
K.M.	M	5	2	+ +				
J.M.	M	4	4	+	Allergic rhinitis	?	4	+
A.N.	F	12	8	+ +	Biliousness	12	8	+ +
E.S.	F	3	7	—				
M.S.	F	20	12	+ +	Allergic rhinitis	20	12	+
A.W.	F	5	3	+ +	Biliousness	5	3	+ +
L.P.	F	5	2	—				
E.A.	M	17	6	+ +	Biliousness	?	6	+ +
C.L.	F	8	9	+ +	Anosmia	?	8	+
D.M.	F	1	4	+ +	Very sleepy	1	4	+ +
A.M.	M	15	17	+				
V.H.	F	5	11	+ +				
R.W.	M	10	8	+ +				

+ + cured or considerable improvement — no improvement or aggravation
+ moderate improvement * did not continue treatment

Some patients, particularly those with severe symptoms of long duration, will probably have a mild recurrence of their headaches after several months or several years of freedom. These can usually be cured in one to three treatments. In the most difficult case there may be several recurrences, each being milder and separated by a longer interval until, in the end, the condition is completely cured, or at least nearly so.

In certain patients with headache due to diseases which cannot be cured by either Western medicine or acupuncture (there are none in this statistical series), it is sometimes possible to alleviate the headache. As the basic condition cannot be cured, constant 'pep up' treatments will be required *ad infinitum*—helpful perhaps but unsatisfactory.

As can be seen from the table, many of the patients had other symptoms or diseases which were treated at the same time as the headache. (Only the main additional symptom is noted in the statistics.) Mostly the treatment of the other symptoms took the same number of treatments as the headache—thus patient L.O. (7th down) needed a total of 6 treatments to cure both the headache and the heartburn. Sometimes the other symptoms took longer or shorter to cure or alleviate than the headache. Where there was little difference in the number of treatments required to treat both symptoms, the greater number of treatments has been put down under both headings. Where there is a question mark the relevant fact had not been noted in the case history.

F Ten of us* analysed the results of treatment of 1000 consecutive patients. The more rarely treated conditions were not included, so as to obviate spurious conclusions from a small review. Sometimes it was difficult to know under which heading to put a single patient for several had a multiplicity of diseases and symptoms. As a rule the disease for which the patient primarily went to the doctor has been included in these statistics.

*Felix Mann, Raymond Whitaker, Bernard Perlow, Robert Graham, James Rentoul, Gerald King, Rankin Martin, Henry Kobner, Lawrence Hyman, David Blake.

ANALYSIS OF 1,000 CONSECUTIVE PATIENTS TREATED BY
ACUPUNCTURE COMPILED BY 10 DOCTORS

	Total number of patients	Cure or considerable improvement.	Moderate improvement.	No result or slight improvement.
Headache, migraine	119	71	22	26
Neuralgia, trigeminal neuralgia	12	2	8	2
Lumbago, sciatica 'slipped disc'	67	31	16	20
Organic neurological diseases	30	6	5	19
Gastritis, peptic ulcer	41	15	18	8
Constipation	9	4	2	3
Colitis	11	6	2	3
Haemorrhoids	9	6	2	1
Osteo-arthritis, rheumatoid arthritis, ankylosing spondylitis	196	52	89	55
Muscular rheumatism, brachial neuralgia, cervical spondylosis	95	33	4	8
Gout	ᴄ 9	5	3	1
Metatarsalgia, tennis elbow	8	7	0	1
Asthma	57	25	17	15
Chronic bronchitis, pulmonary dyspnoea	11	6	3	2
Hay fever, vasomotor rhinitis	51	20	20	11
Tonsillitis	10	5	3	2
Angina pectoris	8	2	3	3
Intermittent claudication	5	0	3	2
Cramp in calves	7	5	0	2
Hypertension	10	0	5	5
Varicose veins	5	0	3	2

	Total number of patients	Cure or considerable improve-ment.	Moderate improve-ment.	No result or slight improve-ment.
Other organic vascular disorders	6	0	1	5
Cystitis, irritable bladder	8	5	1	2
Prostatism	9	3	3	3
Dysmennorrhoea	26	14	4	8
Vaginal discharge	11	7	1	3
Hot flushes	9	5	2	2
Nausea and vomiting of pregnancy	7	5	2	0
Impotence	27	7	7	13
General psychiatric	30	9	11	10
Claustrophobia	6	4	1	1
Unfounded fears	9	5	2	2
Endogenous depression	13	6	4	3
Excessive tension	16	8	4	4
Mental apathy	11	5	3	3
Insomnia	11	4	3	4
Premature senility (early stage)	15	10	1	4
Liver dysfunction	11	6	3	2
Food allergy	8	4	2	2
Car sickness	9	7	0	2
Acne	10	5	3	2
Blepharitis	6	4	3	0
Urticaria	5	4	1	0
Tinnitus	7	1	1	5
	1000	439	290	271

G   The following 1518 cases were treated by Dr Johannes Bischko, in the E.N.T. department of the Vienna Allgemeine Poliklinik which is under the direction of Prof E. H. Majer. The period of observation was from 22.12.58 to 21.4.71. Of the 1518 patients treated, 1037 had a single disease whilst 481 had two diseases. All patients were treated in the out-patients department. Those patients who did not continue treatment have been added to the no result column.

Diagnosis	No. of cases	No. of treatments	Good result	+ –	No result
Tinnitus	309	16 to 25	105	124	80
Symptoms after middle ear operations	74	10 to 15	21	7	46
Lesions of inner ear	36	10 to 20	4	9	23
Presbycusis	72	8 to 16	27	32	13
Vertigo	96	8 to 15	66	19	11
Menière's disease	36	10 to 15	18	12	6
Facial paralysis	57	10 to 25	23	23	11
Anosmia	8	10 to 20	6	1	1
Hayfever	25	6 to 15	17	5	3
Sinusitis	259	4 to 11	200	36	23
Symptoms after sinus operation	84	5 to 10	33	19	32
Trigeminal neuralgia	118	2 to 20	73	31	14
Vasomotor headaches	189	4 to 10	129	43	17
Migraine - cervical	117	4 to 13	81	19	17
Migraine – ophthalmic	13	4 to 15	7	4	2
Migraine – vascular	88	4 to 20	63	15	10
Spastic torticollis	17	10 to 30	14	3	—
Stutter	71	4 to 15	48	13	10
Spastic dysphonia	102	4 to 15	66	32	4
Bronchial asthma	38	6 to 15	25	7	6
Ozaena	9	4 to 12	4	3	2

XII

PREVENTIVE MEDICINE

In ancient China a first class physician was one who could not only cure disease but could also prevent disease. Only a second class physician had to wait until his patients became ill so that he could then treat them when there were obvious symptoms and signs.

It is for this reason that the doctor was paid by the patient when he was healthy and the payment was stopped when he was ill. This was so much so that the doctor had to give the patient free of cost the medicines required, medicines which he, the doctor, had paid for out of his own pocket.

'*To administer medicines to diseases which have already developed and to suppress revolts which have already developed is comparable to the behaviour of those persons who begin to dig a well after they have become thirsty, and of those who begin to make their weapons after they have already engaged in battle. Would these actions not be too late?*'

(Su Wen, Ch. 2)

This type of preventive medicine is based in acupuncture on the pulse diagnosis, which, as already mentioned, presents in its early stages, rather the entelechy of disease than the disease itself.

It is well known that the person who will at a later date develop, for instance, hypertension, exhibits certain mental symptoms (a certain stiff walk and fixedness of ideas), many years before the hypertension as such shows itself and similarly with other diseases. This type of preclinical symptomatology is so vague and uncertain that, on the whole, little use can be made of it.

The pulse diagnosis, on the other hand, is a certain indication of preclinical disease. A little consideration will show that before a disease develops with physical signs and objective findings, there will be, possibly for months or years beforehand, some physiological disturbance that is too slight to cause overt symptoms. But, even at this stage, the pulse registers a definite abnormality.

The acupuncturist will at this preclinical stage treat the patient, using acupuncture points dictated to him solely by the pulse diagnosis.

For preventive medicine of this type to be effective, the patient must, of course, see the doctor at regular intervals. In my experience a healthy person with a reasonable constitution need only have his pulse felt every six months; which is the same interval at which one should visit a dentist. Once a year is enough for the exceptionally healthy.

One additional advantage of this preventive routine is that the whole general level of health is maintained at a higher level. It can give not only the absence of disease, but a positive feeling of well-being with an abundance of physical and mental energy.

Very often people are not actually ill, but feel a little below what they sense should be ideal health. This is, in reality, the preclinical stage of disease which may take very many years till it is seen as an overt disease. If this person is correctly treated, not only is the slight fatigue, etc. cured, but in addition he is spared the consequences of later developing an obvious disease.

The length of life may be increased with less cerebral sclerosis and its attendant evils:

The Yellow Emperor once addressed T'ien Shih, the divinely inspired teacher: '*I have heard that in ancient times the people lived to be over a hundred years, and yet they remained active and did not become decrepit in their activities. But nowadays people only reach half of that age and yet become decrepit and failing. Is it that mankind is degenerating through the ages and loses his original vigour?*'

Qi Bo, the chief physician, answered: '*In ancient times those people who understood the ways of nature, patterned themselves upon the Yin and the Yang. . .*'

(Su Wen, Ch. 1)

When treating patients with early signs of ageing and cerebral sclerosis (such as apathy, inability to follow an argument and feeling generally decrepit), the response (if the process is not too advanced) is often remarkable, with a return of mental agility and youthfulness which is noticed by friends who do not even know that the patient has seen a doctor. Nevertheless, earlier diagnosis and treatment, as in preventive medicine, would probably have given even better results.

Parents who are healthy normally beget children who are also healthy. This is one of the most important aspects of preventive medicine for children who are born robust and healthy, have, as a rule, less disease later in life and on the whole a healthier mental outlook. If adults become ill, who were robust as children, they are easier to cure. The diseases which are hardest, and sometimes well nigh impossible to cure completely, are in those who were born weaklings and who were ill during the first few years of life.

For preventive acupuncture to be effective, the initial treatment must have been successful, so that the pulse has become normal. It may not be possible to completely cure someone who has been ill for many years; though the patient may say he is cured as he has no symptoms. In this case the pulse will still show a slight abnormality which cannot be corrected. In this type preventive acupuncture is only partially effective. If the patient had been seen earlier, preventive acupuncture would have been fully effective.

We have to face the fact that, in our modern civilization, with its many influences which are detrimental to health, by no means all diseases can be prevented though most acupuncturists find that not only is the general level of health heightened, the basic germ plasma of the next generation improved, and expectation of life increased, but also a substantial proportion of disease prevented. This type of preventive medicine applies particularly to the chronic and degenerative diseases and not to such an extent to the infective diseases or those caused by external agents, except insofar as the general resistance has been increased.

Various additional factors should not be forgotten: Exercise, naturally grown food that is not poisoned or devitalised, good air, enough relaxation and enough thought:

Modern man drinks wine like water, leads an irregular life, engaging in sexual intercourse while he is drunk, thus exhausting his vital forces:

they do not know how to preserve their vital forces, wasting their energy excessively, seeking only physical pleasure, all of which is against the rules of nature. For these reasons they reach only one half of the hundred years and then they degenerate.

(Su Wen, Ch. 1)

My more recent experience suggests that the yearly or half-yearly visits are unnecessary and that in most instances it is just as effective if one only returns for treatment when the symptoms reappear. If one returns early before the symptoms are advanced, one treatment is often enough. The early symptoms often manifest themselves merely as fatigue and lethargy, rather than the more obvious symptoms of a disease.

Most of the diseases that occur in a particular individual are different symptoms of the same basic illness. So, if a patient who was originally treated for one illness develops another, his symptoms may often be relatively quickly alleviated.

SECTION 3

The Meridians of Acupuncture

CONTENTS

The above twelve groups are each sub-divided into:

PHYSIOLOGY

Traditional Chinese and Western Scientific Conceptions
This section includes translations from Chinese texts, correlations with Western medicine and case histories

SYMPTOMS AND SIGNS

Symptomatology; *Main Meridian Symptoms*; Symptoms of Excess; Symptoms of Insufficiency; *Cold, Hot, Empty, Full Symptoms*; *Connecting Meridian (Luo) Symptoms*; Symptoms of Excess; Symptoms of Insufficiency; *Muscle Meridian Symptoms*

COURSE OF MERIDIANS

Course of Meridians; *Main Meridian*; *Principal Course*; *Special Details*; *Connecting Meridian (Luo)*; *Muscle Meridian*;*Divergent Meridian, Yang and Yin*
This section listed as coupled meridians under the Yang meridian

IMPORTANT POINTS

CHAPTER I

THE GENERAL FEATURES
OF THE MERIDIANS

Recognition of what are called the 'meridians' of the human body is one of the fundamentals of the theory and practice of acupuncture, the form of medical treatment originally developed in ancient China, but now gradually finding a respected place in Western medicine. The meridians need to be conceived as the paths of circulation and influence of certain forms of essential energy (called in Chinese Qi) in the body. This flow of essential energy, Qi, along the meridians, might in reality be a wave of electrical depolarisation travelling along a fibre of the autonomic nervous system: the Qi being the electrical phenomenon, the meridian the fibre of the autonomic nervous system. In this book I will adhere to the traditional Chinese description as without it the Chinese conception of disease cannot be understood.

For the purposes of general exposition, the meridians can be best regarded as a communications system, a system consisting basically of meridian complexes, each being associated with a particular physiological unit of the body, the units being the twelve basic organs distinguished as such in Chinese medicine, i.e., the lungs, the large intestine, the stomach, the spleen, the heart, the small intestine, the bladder, the kidneys, the pericardium, the triple warmer, the gall bladder and the liver.

The Chinese normally speak of the meridians in pairs and they distinguish the members of each pair by reference to the arm or leg, thus indicating the main location of the particular meridian instead of the particular organ to which it is related:

Sunlight Yang $\begin{cases} \text{arm—large intestine} \\ \text{leg—stomach} \end{cases}$

Lesser Yang $\begin{cases} \text{arm—triple warmer} \\ \text{leg—gall bladder} \end{cases}$

Greater Yang $\begin{cases} \text{arm—small intestine} \\ \text{leg—bladder} \end{cases}$

Greater Yin $\begin{cases} \text{arm—lung} \\ \text{leg—spleen} \end{cases}$

Absolute Yin $\begin{cases} \text{arm—pericardium (circulation-sex)} \\ \text{leg—liver} \end{cases}$

Lesser Yin $\begin{cases} \text{arm—heart} \\ \text{leg—kidney} \end{cases}$

Thus the small intestine meridian is referred to by the Chinese as the Arm Greater Yang, and the bladder meridian as the Leg Greater Yang. Used on its own the term Greater Yang would refer to the two meridians jointly.

The twelve main meridians are traditionally arranged in a certain order, following the sequence in which Qi flows from one meridian to another, and also following the sequence of the times of maximum and minimum activity of the meridians and organs.* Thus arranged the two ways of naming meridians become more obvious to the reader.

The Greater Yang (small intestine and bladder) is not coupled with the Greater Yin (lung and spleen) as might be expected but with the Lesser Yin (heart and kidney). The small intestine and heart on the one hand, and the bladder and the kidney on the other hand, are coupled meridians (Sovereign Fire and Water).

The Chinese system of identification moreover indicates that there are functional relationships between the meridians in each pair, and clinical experience shows that these organs or meridians are in fact related to one another. For instance, the kidney (foot Lesser Yin meridian) and heart (arm Lesser Yin meridian) sometimes have a reciprocal effect: in cardiac failure there is often oliguria; in renal failure there is not infrequently secondary cardiac failure.

The relationships between one organ and another should not however be taken as fixed and invariable features of the system. The laws and relationships of the meridians merely illustrate the possibilities that one organ or meridian has of exerting an effect on its fellows. There are, as it were, only certain routes whereby one

*For details see: *Acupunture: The Ancient Chinese Art of Healing*.

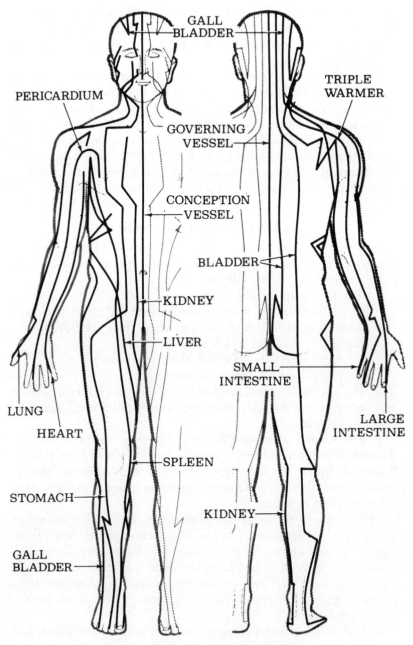

THE 12 OR 14 IMPORTANT MERIDIANS

organ can affect another, these routes being formulated into laws. Some of these routes are more direct than others, so that whereas there are many possibilities, only certain of them occur at all frequently in practice.

The implication is merely that, if a patient has say a cardiac disease, one should keep one's eyes open for any renal complications. There are of course other possibilities, for if the patient has primarily a cardiac disease it may have an effect on the gall bladder via the law of mid-day and midnight, or on the small intestine for the heart and small intestine are coupled organs, or on the spleen via the superficial circulation of energy, and the spleen may likewise be affected in a primary disease cardiac disease via the law of the five elements.

Classification of Meridians

The twelve meridian complexes described broadly in the foregoing paragraphs comprise complexes of different types of meridians and these are classified traditionally as follows:

Main meridians (of which there are twelve)
Branch meridians (of varying number with each main meridian)
Connecting meridians—Luo—(of which there are fifteen)
Muscle meridians (of which there are twelve)
Divergent meridians (of which there are twelve)
Extra meridians (of which there are eight)

The whole series of meridian complexes permeates both the surface and the interior of the body and forms what is called in Chinese 'the meridian network'.

In practice and when used by itself, the term 'meridian' usually denotes either the meridians in general, or simply the main meridians. These are by far the most important, and their influence can be regarded as in the nature of a common denominator of the associated other types of meridians.

The courses of the main meridians are located on the surface of the body by reference to a series of acupuncture points. Apart from two meridians known as the Conception Vessel and Governing Vessel, which are described later, the main meridians are the only ones which have their own acupuncture points; the other-categories of meridians are influenced indirectly through the points on the main meridians.

In both Chinese and European charts of acupuncture points and meridians, each meridian normally is represented as a line joining consecutive numbers of the same meridian. For example, one section of the meridian of the spleen joins points Spleen 13 to Spleen 14. According to the Chinese, however, the spleen meridian makes a deviation at this point and goes from Spleen 13 to Conception Vessel 2, then on to Conception Vessel 3, and only then finally on to Spleen 14. In my 'Anatomical Charts of Acupuncture Points, Meridians and Extra Meridians',* only the direct course of the main meridians is shown. In this present book, the deviations of the main meridian from the direct meridian are shown both in the text and in the drawings. In the text of this book the differences between the direct route and the devious route connecting with points on other meridians can be discerned, as the direct course consists of only the consecutive numbers on the same meridian. In the drawings at the back of this book the deviations to other meridians have been shown by both *lettering and numbering* the points on the other meridians, while the meridian under discussion has only a *number* (in heavy type) at a few of its representative points.

In addition, the main meridians have branches (which, as the deviations, are also not shown on my acupuncture charts) but are shown in the drawings at the back of this book as a dotted line. Most but not all of these branches go to acupuncture points on other meridians and these points, like those of the deviations, are lettered in addition to being numbered.

Before going on to describe the functions of each of the twelve meridian complexes in the succeeding chapters, it is appropriate to outline the chief characteristics of each of the particular types of meridians of which the complexes are composed, and to mention a number of features relevant to practical application. The remaining sections of this chapter are devoted to this purpose and, at this point, I should mention the following. This is that, in describing both the functions and the positions of the meridians in this book, I have more or less adhered to the classical tradition. In practice, however, I have not infrequently noticed that the sphere of influence of the meridians is not entirely consistent with the traditional view. The anatomical differences also imply that there are many more branch meridians than those described, some of them being of con-

---

*Also published by William Heinemann Medical Books Ltd. Republished now as Atlas of Acupuncture.

siderable clinical importance. When I have been able to systematise them, the physiological and anatomical differences will be described in later editions of this book.

THE MERIDIAN COMPLEX

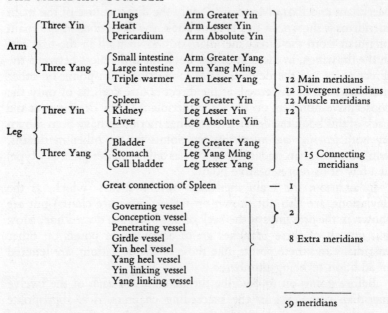

The Main Meridians

The main meridians permeate the body by the following two methods:

a. The Yang meridians control the exterior of the body, the Yin meridians the interior. The exterior and interior meridians are paired with one another as coupled meridians. For example, the large intestine (Yang meridian) with the lung (Yin meridian).

The Fu (Yang organ) and the Zang (Yin organ) are supposed to have a direct connection. The meridians also are connected with one another, this taking place at the tips of the fingers and toes. For example, the lung and large intestine meridians are connected between the thumb and index finger; likewise the stomach and spleen meridians are connected between the second toe and the big toe.

b. There is a connection between arm meridians and leg meridians. This occurs in two places: one is on the head, where the arm Yang meet the leg Yang, and the other on the front of the chest, where the arm Yin meet the leg Yin meridians.

The main meridians run both up and down the limbs, and the Qi flows from one meridian into the next in succession, until the whole circuit is completed, thereafter flowing into the first one again. In half of the main meridians (*i.e.*, the three upper Yang and three lower Yin meridians) the flow is centripetal; in the others it is centrifugal.

The Connecting Meridians (or Luo)

Each of the twelve main meridians has a Luo point and an associated Luo meridian. The functions of the latter are to connect with coupled meridians.

One part of the Luo meridian is connected to the coupled meridian, running from the Luo point of the one meridian to the Luo point of the coupled meridian. For example, Lung 7 is connected to Large Intestine 6. This part of the Luo meridian is always below the elbow or knee.

The other part, which most have, roughly follows the course of the main meridian for a short distance, and controls the part of the body that it traverses.

The Luo meridian of the Governing Vessel connects with the Vessel of Conception and the kidney meridian. The Luo meridian of the Vessel of Conception connects with the Chong mo. The spleen has the so-called Great Luo, which connects with all the other 14 Yin and Yang Luo.

The connecting (Luo) meridians are supposed to run a superficial course through the body. Some authorities have said that it is possible to see whether the Luo are full or empty, but this idea may have arisen amongst the early acupuncturists through confusing the Luo with veins, for veins can easily be seen when they are full of blood and disappear when there is little blood in them.

As these meridians run on the whole superficially, and have a relatively short course with few inter-connections, their symptomatology relates mainly to the surface of the body and not so much with the severer and more complicated diseases of the internal abdominal organs.

The Muscle Meridians

The muscle meridians, as their name implies, run superficially along the surface of the muscles; they pass from joint to joint. The diseases which they influence are mainly those affecting the surface of the body, such as muscular rheumatism and the neuralgias.

The muscle meridians do not have any connections with the internal organs and thus do not influence internal diseases. There is moreover no reciprocal interior and exterior relationship amongst the muscle meridians.

The muscle meridians start at the extremities of the limbs, thence running centripetally with a meeting point at most major joints en route, and terminating on the abdomen, thorax or head. The leg 3 Yang muscle meridians unite on the cheek; the leg 3 Yin muscle meridians unite at the genitalia; the arm 3 Yang muscle meridians unite at the side of the head; the arm 3 Yin muscle meridians unite on the chest.

This purely centripetal course is different from that of the main meridians.

The Divergent Meridians

The divergent meridians usually leave their parent meridian above the knee or elbow, thereafter traversing the interior of the body and connecting with the coupled interior organ. For instance, the bladder divergent meridian is connected to the kidney. Most of the divergent meridians then emerge at the neck. The Yang divergent meridians join their parent main meridian and then continue their course as the main meridian. The Yin divergent meridians likewise link up with the coupled Yang meridian. For example, the divergent meridians of the bladder and kidney meridian both join the bladder main meridian at the back of the neck, their subsequent course being continued only by the main bladder meridian.

From this it may be seen that the divergent meridians connect the internal Zang and Fu and also that coupled divergent meridians are closely inter-twined. The flow of Qi along all divergent meridians is cephalad, as opposed to that of the main meridians.

The divergent meridians enable the Yin main meridians to have an effect on the head, for all of the arm or leg main Yin meridians stop short on the chest, and none reaches the head directly. For example, although it does not reach the head the kidney divergent meridian has an effect on the head because it joins the bladder main meridian at the nape of the neck, thus enabling the bladder main meridian to transmit any effect of stimulating the kidney meridian.

The Extra Meridians

Six of the eight extra meridians, or 'strange meridians' as they are called in Chinese, have no acupuncture points of their own. They use the acupuncture points of the twelve main meridians. They do not have a circulation of energy. The exceptions are the Governing Vessel and Conception Vessel, which not only have their own acupuncture points but also have their own circulation of energy.

The eight extra meridians have no reciprocal connections between the solid and hollow organs, or the interior and surface of the body. Their function is supposed to be like that of a lake, regulating the excess or deficiency of water in the rivers—the main meridians.

Practical Application

The Meridian Complex

Traditionally the various types of meridians are described as being separate entities: the muscle meridians having a certain function, the connecting meridians (Luo) another function, etc., etc. For practical purposes, however, I do not think there is much difference between the various types.

If, for example, a patient has a symptom which is at least partially localised over the cheek, this might suggest a dysfunction of the bladder muscle meridian, which unites there. If pulse diagnosis and other symptoms or signs also indicate a dysfunction of the bladder, the diagnosis is confirmed, and the disease may be treated via acupuncture points on the bladder main meridian (or points on other meridians which have an indirect effect on the bladder).

The above example shows that the specialised types of meridians extend the range of activity of the main meridians. In my view it is best to regard the specialised types as an extension of the main meridian bearing the name of the same organ. For example, the use of an acupuncture point on the gall bladder main meridian has its field of activity extended to the connecting, muscle, divergent and branch meridians of the gall bladder. In reverse, a symptom along or near any of the above specialised meridians indicates a disturbance of the gall bladder—in the Chinese sense.

Many parts of the body are not near any particular one of twelve main meridians, but if these are taken together with all the other meridians (a total of 59), practically every part of the body is covered.

The Vessel of Conception and Governing Vessel could be counted as a special addition, for they have their own acupuncture points, thus making a total of fourteen important meridians. The other six extra meridians do not seem to fit in with the above classification. It is possible that they channel the influences of particular points, such as K3, which have a large sphere of activity. Alternatively they may act as communications between various meridians, and would therefore be classified under the meridian to which they have the greatest affinity, e.g., the Dai mo as part of the gall bladder complex.

In many parts of the body, several meridians each belonging to a different member of the main twelve run over the same region of the body. Where this occurs, detection of the offending meridian entails not only noting the pulse diagnosis, the symptoms and signs, but also a knowledge of the principles of physiology and pathology. In every such instance all the above factors must be considered, the relation of the meridians to the diseased area being but one of the many factors. These often contradict one another and need to be weighed in the light of clinical experience.

The Organ Affects the Meridian and the Meridian Affects the Organ

The meridians are, as it were, the threads that link the various phenomena observable in acunpuncture, both in diagnosis and in treatment.

A patient may have a disease of the heart, and amongst other things this is usually accompanied by pain down the inside of the arm roughly following the course of the meridian of the heart. There may also be pain going up the throat to the eye, or over the chest to the middle of the abdomen, these pains following the course of the branches of the main heart meridian or of the muscle or connecting or divergent heart meridian. If an acupuncture point on the heart meridian is stimulated in this type of case, the disease of the heart (provided it is the type of cardiac disease that may be treated by acupuncture) will be cured, or at least ameliorated.

A reverse order of events may occur in a patient who has, say, a Colles fracture at the wrist, which has happened in such a way that there is a particularly tender place over the meridian of the heart. In such a case the patient, who previously had no cardiac symptoms, may suddenly develop palpitations or have a feeling of constriction in the chest, or dyspnoea on exertion. (This will not happen in the majority of Colles fractures; it will only happen in those with the point of maximum tenderness over the heart meridian.) This patient too may be cured by stimulating an acupuncture point on the meridian of the heart, using the meridian either on both sides, or on the same side as the injury, or preferably only the opposite side.

Thus a disease or dysfunction of the heart may cause symptoms along one or other of the meridians belonging to the heart complex; and in reverse, something that irritates a certain point on the heart meridian may give rise to cardiac symptoms or even disease. In either type of case, whether the disease originated in the heart or by irritation of the heart meridian, the dysfunction may be corrected by stimulating acupuncture points on the meridian of the heart.

This is one of the special advantages of acupuncture, for it enables diagnosis and treatment to be so closely allied that they are practically one and the same thing, i.e., if you have made a diagnosis, you more or less automatically know the treatment. Similarly, and in reverse, if you are not sure of the diagnosis, and try a certain treatment which then works, you automatically know the diagnosis.

The Meridians and Cellular Pathology

Western medicine is based on the ideas of cellular pathology as first expounded by Virchow. In this one distinguishes as minutely as possible the type of tissue that is diseased, whether it be muscle, bone, blood vessel, nerve, etc., even which type of cell in that tissue is diseased, and more recently the intra-cellular changes that take place in the diseased cell.

In acupuncture the reverse to the ideas of cellular pathology often seems to apply. If, for example, someone has an insect bite on the elbow, this is best treated in acupuncture by stimulating the meridian which runs over that part of the elbow. If, for example, it was in the region of the lateral epicondyle of the humerus, the large intestine meridian would be treated, preferably on the opposite side. If, instead of having an insect bite on the elbow, that same patient

had muscular rheumatism, a painful wound, early arthritis, epicon-
dylitis, a localised skin disease or any other disease involving any of
the cellular elements in that region of the body, the treatment would
be exactly the same, namely by treating the meridian of the large
intestine on the opposite side.

From this it may be seen that the cellular pathology does not
necessarily dictate any difference in treatment by acupuncture.

It would therefore seem that the meridians are the controlling
factor in the various regions of the body, and that they control the
body more in a regional way, irrespective of what type of tissue or
cell may be there. In addition to having this regional effect the
meridians have an effect on the whole body, and this appears to
operate via the mediation of the internal organs with which the
meridians are connected.

A knowledge of histology and cellular pathology is nevertheless
important in acupuncture in a more general way, in helping to
decide which disease can or cannot be treated. For instance, a
duodenal ulcer may be treated successfully, as the cells lining the
duodenum are of a type which regenerate easily. Diseases of the
nervous system can be treated only to a limited extent, for the
neurones of the brain and spinal cord do not regenerate.

CHAPTER II

LUNGS

Traditional Chinese and Western Scientific Conceptions

The Lungs Control Qi

'The lungs control Qi.' This has two meanings, for Qi in Chinese means both energy and breath, much as the Prana of the Hindus.

The Jing Qi of 'liquid and solid food', which is produced as the result of digestion in the stomach and upper digestive tract, passes first to the lungs, where it combines with the Qi of the air, and thus the true Qi of the human being is formed. This is also called the upright Qi of health, as opposed to the evil Qi of disease.

'True Qi is that which is received from Heaven, combined with the Qi of nourishment. It fills the whole body.'

(Ling Shu, zijie zhenxie lun)

'Man's breathing connects the Jing Qi of Heaven and Earth in order to form the true Qi of the body.'

(Zangshi, leijing)

A deficiency of Qi results, therefore, amongst other things in a general fatigue of the body and also air-hunger. As far as the respiratory function is concerned, J. Barcroft writes: 'Acute anoxia simulates drunkness, chronic anoxia simulates fatigue.'

The Lungs and Heart

The Chinese call the lungs the Complementary Official, recognising an association in function between the lungs and the heart. This is something that is well known by clinical experience and can also be explained by the theories of Western medicine. It may be seen in the dyspnoea caused by cardiac failure, or the tachycardia caused by pulmonary insufficiency.

From the Chinese point of view, the lungs control Qi, while the heart controls Blood.

'Qi is the commander of the Blood: if Qi moves, then Blood moves. Blood is the mother of Qi: if Blood reaches a place, then Qi also reaches it.'

There is even an embryological relationship between the heart and the lungs in-so-far as the one makes room for the development of the other: the heart being mainly on the left where there are two lobes of the lung, while the right side on which the heart encroaches to a lesser extent has three lobes. What would be the third bronchus on the left side (equivalent to the right apical bronchus) is only vestigal and fails to induce the formation of a separate lobe from the surrounding mesenchyme, supposedly because of the relative caudal recession of the aortic arch or the rotation of the heart. The space not taken up by the heart (and pulmonary vein) on the right, is partially filled by the cardiac lobe, which is a branch of the lower lobe, and only appears on the right.

The chemoreceptors of the carotid bodies (IX cranial nerve) and the aortic body (X cranial nerve) respond to a decrease in the concentration of oxygen or an increase in the concentration of carbon dioxide, both largely dependent on pulmonary function. Via this reflex the sino-auricular node is affected, thus altering the rate of the heart. In this case the interaction of the lungs and heart is not direct, but indirect via the gases (largely dependent on pulmonary function) dissolved in the arterial blood on the one hand, and the carotid and aortic bodies associated with the heart on the other.

As is well known, the inspired air and the blood are in intimate contact in the alveolar sacs, being separated from one another by a membrane only one cell thick, usually consisting of nothing but capillary endothelium.

Not infrequently dysfunction of the lung and heart affects the external configuration, as may be seen in the person who has a long narrow flat chest, with dyspnoea and palpitations on slight exertion. In this type of patient pulse diagnosis shows that both the lung and the heart are under-active.

Case History. A girl of twelve was seen with extreme fatigue; wishing to go to bed at 6 p.m. and unable to concentrate well at school. On slight exertion she became breathless with occasional retrosternal pain. She had ulcers on the tip and sides of her tongue—see section on heart for explanation of this last symptom. Her chest was long, narrow and flat.

Pulse diagnosis showed an underactivity of both lung and heart. She was cured after four treatments at L9 and H7.

The Lungs, Skin and Hair

The lungs are related to the skin and the body hair for Qi controls the exterior of the body, while Blood controls the interior.

Normally in cold weather the pores of the skin close and perspiration ceases, while in warm weather the pores open and there is perspiration.

If there is a deficiency of lung Qi, this impairs the ability of the skin to adapt itself to change in external circumstances, such as cold and heat, dryness and damp, so that colds, influenza or pneumonia are more easily contracted. In severe cases, the patient will suffer from spontaneous sweating, or sweating from the slightest exertion.

If on the other hand there is an excess of lung Qi, so that the exterior, *i.e.*, the skin, is over full, the patient may easily contract diseases of the lungs, with coughing and dyspnoea, but with a sweatless fever. If drugs or acupuncture are used to cause perspiration, the breathing will become normal and the fever will subside.

The Chinese conception of an association of the lungs and skin was well known in European mediaeval medicine. In many animals the skin performs an important respiratory function:

The loach, Misgurnus, excretes up to 92% of its carbon dioxide through the skin. In the loach, 63% of the oxygen is obtained through the skin, and 37% through the gills. If the gills are occluded (by tying the pharynx and gills) the consumption of oxygen through the skin increases to 85%. The remainder is obtained through the intestine.*

The eel, Anguilla, and the mud-skipper, Periophthalmus, use the skin to absorb oxygen. The frog breathes both through its lungs and through its skin, the main pulmonary artery being divided into two branches, one going to the lung, the other to the skin, *i.e.*, the vascularisation of the skin belongs to the pulmonary circulation.

Pulmonary diseases may often be recognised by the texture or colour of the skin: the dry flaking skin of certain asthmatics or the discolouration of the skin in negroes with tuberculosis (E. Cochrane).

Case History. A patient was seen with asthma and a dry scaling skin. He had the dry skin from childhood, while the asthma was of more recent onset.

Pulse diagnosis showed a weak pulse of the lung. The lungs were treated by acupuncture which quickly cured the asthma. The skin responded more slowly, improving, though not being completely cured.

The Lungs Open the Nostrils

The nose is part of the respiratory system, and as such is associated with the lungs.

*G. V. Nikolsky. The Ecology of Fishes. Academic Press.

'Lung Qi penetrates to the nose; if the lungs are harmonious, then the nose is able to distinguish odours.'

(Ling Shu, modu pian)

Thus, when the lung Qi is invaded by wind and cold, there may be the symptoms of a clear nasal discharge and anosmia. If in addition it is affected by heat, the discharge will become purulent. If the lung is excessively hot, and this cannot be dissipated, this results in coughing, dyspnoea and anxious breathing, there may be irritation of the nose, and movement of the alar nasae.

Embryologically, the nose is only secondarily adapted to the respiratory system, being originally the mouth—the cephalic end of the primitive gut.

Case History. A patient was seen at the very beginning of a cold, with sneezing and a clear nasal discharge. The associated point of the lungs, B13, was stimulated, which cured all symptoms within a few minutes. (This particular technique is only occasionally effective in the earliest stages of the common cold.)

The Lungs, Trachea and Larynx

The larynx being part of the respiratory system, it follows that timbre of the voice reflects the state of the true Qi of the body.

Not infrequently, the timbre of the voice is affected by other organs which have a direct or indirect effect on the lung, which in turn affects the larynx. In addition, the three lower Yang meridians pass through the neck alongside the larynx on their way to the feet, and can thus influence speech.

That part of the larynx which is below the vocal cords is formed in the embryo from the lung bud; while the part above the vocal cords is formed from the pharynx. From this point of view one would expect the lower part of the larynx to respond to the lung meridian and the upper part to respond to the stomach meridian.

Case History. A patient had a weak voice, a slightly breathless manner of speech and looked as if he could easily be blown over by the slightest breath of wind.

Pulse diagnosis showed an underactive lung. Stimulation of the lung meridian, S9 locally, and Cv17 the alarm point of the lung, cured the condition.

The Lungs in Relation to Anguish and Claustrophobia

From the psycho-somatic point of view, the mind can affect the body and the body the mind. Certain mental diseases cause or are caused by a dysfunction of the lungs.

The type of mild fear and anguish, which one may experience when holding one's breath, is a lung symptom.

Case History. A patient was suffering from a mixture of anguish, fear and depression for no obvious reason, *i.e.*, there was no external cause. I therefore assumed the mental state was the result of an internal dysfunction. I tried various treatments without success. Then, going over the history again more thoroughly, I found that the patient disliked small rooms, a condition amounting to a mild claustrophobia. The lung was stimulated at L8 and within minutes the patient felt better and was cured with a further three treatments.

Case History. Over a period of a few weeks a patient developed an extreme dislike of crowds, particularly parties held in small over-crowded rooms, something which she had adored before. She thought she was going mad, even though she did not feel mad. A psychiatrist was consulted to no avail. A chance chest X-ray at a mass radiography unit showed pulmonary tuberculosis. Chemotherapy cured the tuberculosis and the mental symptoms.

The above two histories show that apart from an anguish-fear complex, claustrophobia is also a lung symptom. Claustrophobia, being only the mental counterpart of physical air hunger, can be successfully treated in this way in a certain proportion of patients. It should not be forgotten though that all symptoms or diseases, though seeming identical, may have different causes and therefore require an entirely different treatment.

Mucous

Mucous being the secretion of the lungs, is dependent on them. Sometimes the spleen (the lung and spleen are greater Yin organs) is more effective in the treatment of the viscid mucous of the asthmatic.

Sobbing

Sobbing, in which one's respiration becomes violent and jerking (not just crying), is a pulmonary symptom.

Autumn

Autumn is the season when the lungs are most easily affected.

Dryness

Dryness frequently makes lung diseases worse. A steam kettle in the room of children with pneumonia and bronchitis, may assist recovery. Occasionally dryness is beneficial.

White

A white discolouration of a particular quality, especially of the face, may be a pulmonary symptom.

The Lungs, Kidney and Bladder

'*The lungs give life to the skin, which in its turn nourishes the kidney.*'

The lungs excrete 500 cc of water, as vapour in the expired air, under average conditions in a day. Under similar conditions the skin loses about 1,000 cc as perspiration.

Some types of oedema may be cured by treating the lungs. I have not as yet been able to clearly define this group however.

Case History. For over ten years, a patient had a skin disease with marked hyperkeratosis, especially of the wrists and ankles. He was unable to perspire however hot he became.

Pulse diagnosis showed an underactivity of the lungs and kidneys. These were stimulated at L9 and K5. Two weeks later he suddenly woke up in the middle of the night, bathed in perspiration so that he had to change his pyjamas and sheets. This excessive perspiration, which was accompanied by a desquamation of the hyperkeratotic areas, continued for three months, thereafter dying down to normal.

Heat Loss

Heat loss takes place largely via the skin.

The skin loses 87.5% by evaporation, radiation and conduction. 7% is lost by evaporation from the lungs. Warming the expired air accounts for 3.5%. 2% is lost via the urine and faeces. (Vass, Short, Pratt.)

Dogs lose relatively more via the lungs directly (and the mucus membrane of the mouth), for they pant when they are too hot. Their skin loss is concentrated in the pads of their feet.

Clinically I find the above of little importance, at least as far as the lung-skin relationship is concerned. Patients who feel too hot or too cold, or where a part of the body is subjectively too hot or too cold, may have a hyper or hypoactivity of any of the twelve basic organs; other symptoms and signs are normally a better guide.

The thermoregulatory function of the kidney should not be forgotten.

Symptomatology

Main Meridian Symptoms

The chest is distended, dyspnoea, coughing, pain in the supra-clavicular fossa going down to the thumb or index finger. When severe, blurred vision, palms of hands hot, palpitations, polydipsia.

SYMPTOMS OF EXCESS

Upper part of the back and shoulder ache, the patient feels superficially cold, perspiration and fainting, micturition frequent but in small amounts.

SYMPTOMS OF INSUFFICIENCY

Upper part of back and shoulders painful and cold, gasping for breath, colour of urine changes.

Lung Cold Symptoms

If the lungs are invaded by cold evil, this may cause the lungs to lose the function of Qi transformation, with the result that fluids are not transformed and digested.

This causes coughing, dyspnoea, excessive phlegm, lack of thirst. Possibly the chest is distended, with constant coughing, inability to lie down, and oedema of the whole body including the face and round the eyes.

The pulse is floating and wiry, possibly wiry and slippery.

The tongue is white and slippery.

Lung Hot Symptoms

May be caused by dry evil or dry heat, or cold which has become extreme and therefore has changed to fire, producing heat symptoms.

The symptoms of lung heat are fever with a red face, both cheeks red, mental agitation, thirsty even after drinking, throat red and painful, stools dry hard and dense, urine dark, nose slightly red, epistaxis, coughing and vomiting of thick mucous, possibly the mucous is streaked with blood, pain in chest and back during coughing, throat feels blocked and constricted, possibly tonsillitis.

The pulse is slippery and rapid.
The tongue is dry and yellow.

Lung Empty Symptoms

The condition lung empty may entail either lung Qi empty or lung Yin empty.

The main symptoms of lung Qi empty are:—breathing light, voice weak, sweating, throat and head dry, face shiny and white, skin dry, hair on head comes out easily, frequent micturition, body fears the cold, easily catches colds, influenza, pneumonia, etc. In addition there may be long periods of coughing and dyspnoea, difficult breathing and the patient may lack strength.

The pulse is empty and fine, the right inch pulse being particularly weak.

The tongue substance is pale red.

The principal symptoms of lung Yin empty are:—flushing and spontaneous sweating, both cheeks red, throat dry and mouth parched, violent coughing, slow and heavy coughing. In some cases the throat may be painful and the voice very weak; there may be haemoptysis, and the body may become increasingly emaciated.

The pulse is empty, fine and rapid, or hollow and rapid.

The tongue substance is deep red.

Lung Full Symptoms

If wind cold full evil blocks and restricts the lungs, then the lung Qi is obstructed and does not penetrate, causing dyspnoea and distension of the chest. The pulse is slippery and full.

If lung Qi is abundant, then there is coughing and Qi rises, the shoulders and back are painful, and there is sweating.

If fluid is stopped, then there is dry coughing and shortness of breath, pain in chest whilst coughing.

If phlegm is hot, then there will be continuous coughing and Qi rises. In severe cases, there is purulent phlegm with a foul smell, and distension of the chest. The pulse is rapid and full.

Connecting Meridian (Luo) Symptoms

SYMPTOMS OF EXCESS

Lower end of radius and palm of hands both hot.

Coughing, yawning with mouth wide open, constant desire to urinate.

Muscle Meridian Symptoms

Muscular spasm, pain and dysfunction along the course of the meridian. Haemoptysis with pains in the sides.

Course of Meridians

Lung Main Meridian

Principal Course

From L1 below the clavicle, the meridian arches over the front of the shoulder, to descend along the embryologically anterior and outer surface of the arm, terminating at the end of the thumb at L11.

Special Details

The meridian starts in the middle warmer stomach area, deep to Cv12. It descends to loop around the transverse colon, with which it is connected at the level of Cv9; ascends again to Cv13, passing the pylorus and the cardia of the stomach. It penetrates the diaphragm and enters the lungs to which it belongs (?represented by Cv17), rising to the level of the larynx. Here it passes horizontally to emerge at L1, and thence goes down the arm to L11.

A branch goes from L7 along the outer side of the index finger to L11.

Lung Connecting Meridian (Luo)—L7

This meridian follows the course of the main meridian and enters the palm of the hand. From L7 it diverges to connect with the Luo of the large intestine.

Lung Muscle Meridian

The meridian begins at the end of the thumb, unites at the wrist; ascends the forearm, unites at the elbow; ascends the upper arm, enters the chest, emerging at the sterno-clavicular joint where it unites; goes across the clavicle to unite at the front of the shoulder. It descends and unites inside the chest, and is dispersed as far as the diaphragm.

Important Points

Wood	L11	
Fire	L10	
Earth	L9	Tonification
Metal	L8	Metal point of Yin metal meridian
Water	L5	Sedation
Source	L9	
Luo	L7	
Xi	L6	
Alarm	L1	
Associated	B13	

CHAPTER III

LARGE INTESTINE

Traditional Chinese and Western Scientific Conceptions

'The Large Intestine Controls the Transmitting and Drainage of the Dregs'

According to Chinese conceptions:

The stomach controls the receiving, rotting and ripening (digestion) of liquid and solid food.

The spleen controls the moving, transforming and distribution of the pure essence of the already rotted and ripened liquid and solid food, to all parts of the body, in order to nourish it.

The small intestine takes the waste materials of the liquid digestate and via the bladder expels them through the urethra.

The large intestine takes the remaining solid dregs and expels them via the anus. The large intestine takes the surplus of the solid matter and expels it at the appropriate time, having the functions of: transmission, drainage of dregs and control of defaecation.

Thus the small intestine has the function of dividing the food and water into the 'pure and impure', *i.e.*, the relationship of micturition defaecation. It can quite often be observed that patients who have diarrhoea pass little urine, while those who are constipated pass more urine. It follows from this that one type of diarrhoea may be treated either by stimulating the large intestine or by increasing the flow of urine.

The Lung and Large Intestine

The lung and large intestine have coupled meridians and thus influence one another. In pneumonia there is usually constipation, though occasionally diarrhoea. Conversely, with constipation there is often dyspnoea with distension of the chest, which is cured when the constipation is cured. That the lung and large intestine are coupled organs, or as the Chinese say, have an interior-exterior relationship, both under the jurisdiction of the element metal, may seem a little peculiar to the Westerner. The astute observer will notice clinical correlations, such as those mentioned in the above sentences. The following examples from embryology and comparative anatomy shed some light on the problem.

The large intestine and lungs are both derived from entoderm: The large intestine is formed from the caudal part of the primitive gut; the lung bud, which develops into the bronchial system, is a ventral evagination of the primitive foregut.

In fish the inner portion of the gill clefts (pulmonary function) is also formed from the primitive gut—albeit the opposite end to the colon.

In many larvae and embryos of fish, before the definitive gills have developed as an organ for the assimilation of oxygen from the water, this function is performed by the blood vessels in the yolk sac (which is the external part of the primitive gut) and the fin folds (fin folds are skin, which comes under the metal organs). The more favourable the respiratory conditions under which the embryos and larvae develop, the less strongly developed is their capillary respiratory system. As the yolk sac is absorbed and its respiratory blood vessel network is reduced, there is a corresponding increase in the blood vessel network in the fin folds. (Nikolsky and Soin, 1954.) This fin fold respiration is part of the lung/large intestine, skin and respiration complex, partly discussed in the section on the lungs.

There is intestinal respiration among Cuprinoids (sheat-fish, loaches) and Symbranchidae. In these the length of the intestine is increased with the capillary network nearer the internal mucosal surface. In some parts of the gut there is complete absence of digestive function and intestinal villi.

In the tropical sheat-fish, Otocinchus, there is a special blind outgrowth from the stomach, usually full of air, which performs a respiratory function.

Swallowed air in the fish loses about 5% of its oxygen and acquires about 3% of carbon dioxide. Human pulmonary respiration is more effective as about 25% of the inspired oxygen is absorbed and the exhaled air contains about 4% carbon dioxide (dry air at sea level contains 0.04 volumes per cent). The used air in the fish leaves, either through the mouth as in many sheat-fish, or through the anus as in the loach.

The Nose, Throat and Teeth

The nose, throat and the teeth are to some extent controlled by the large intestine, particularly those regions covered by the meridian.

Case History. A patient had a clear nasal discharge. This was cured by stimulating the large intestine at Li4. In other patients Li20 gives a better result.

Haemorrhage

According to Soulié de Morant, there is an increased tendency to bleed when the large intestine is under-active. This could possibly be explained by the biosynthesis of vitamin K in the colon. Supposedly menorrhagia can for this reason be treated by stimulating the large intestine.

In my experience pernicious anaemia cannot be treated via the large intestine, despite the fact that vitamin B12 is made there by bacterial action.

Symptomatology

Main Meridian Symptoms

Toothache, swelling of the neck, diseases associated with Fluid which this meridian controls, discolouration of the eyes, dry mouth, clear flow of mucus from the nose, epistaxis, sore throat, pain in shoulder arm thumb and forefinger.

SYMPTOMS OF EXCESS

Warmth or swelling along the course of the meridian.

SYMPTOMS OF INSUFFICIENCY

Cold, shivering with difficulty in getting warm again.

Large Intestine Cold Symptoms

If the large intestine is cold then the waste products that it expels will be cold, with relatively little smell. Abdomen painful with borborygmi, urine clear, diarrhoea, hands and feet cold.

The pulse is deep and slow.

The tongue fur is white and slippery.

Large Intestine Hot Symptoms

If the large intestine is hot, then the mouth is dry and the lips are scorched, with constipation, rectal pain and a feeling of swelling. If there is damp heat, then the stools are often loose and foul smelling. If the condition is severe, they are reddish-brown, and dark urine is passed in small quantities. If the disease persists for a long time, it may result in Zang intoxication. If the blood is hot and the blood vessels are injured, there will be blood in the stools.

The pulse is rapid.

The tongue fur is yellow and dry.

Large Intestine Empty Symptoms

If the large intestine Qi is empty, there is prolapse of the rectum. This occurs more easily in women if they exert too much pressure during labour, or it may occur if the Qi is weak after prolonged dysentery. In each case the limbs are cold.

The pulse is fine and minute.

Large Intestine Full Symptoms

If the stomach is full and hot, and this moves into the large intestine, then there will be constipation, painful abdomen, thirst, incoherent speech.

The pulse is deep and full.

The tongue fur is dry, yellow and greasy.

If damp poison and heat combine in the large intestine, then the lower abdomen is painful, which is worse when pressed, stools moist and bloody, alternately cold and hot, with sweating.

The pulse is slippery and rapid.

If summer heat and damp evils combine and form a blockage together with food and drink in the large intestine and this becomes dysentery, then the abdomen is painful, with a great desire to defaecate.

Connecting Meridian (Luo) Symptoms

SYMPTOMS OF EXCESS

Dental caries, deafness.

SYMPTOMS OF INSUFFICIENCY

Teeth cold, diaphragmatic area feels as if it is blocked.

Muscle Meridian Symptoms

Muscular spasm, pain and dysfunction along the course of the meridian muscle. Cannot raise shoulders, cannot turn head.

Course of Meridians

Large Intestine Main Meridian

Principal Course

The meridian starts on the index finger at Li1. It goes up the embryologically posterior and outer surface of the arm, over the shoulder neck and jaw, to end at the side of the nose at Li20.

Special Details

From Li14 to T13.

From Li16 the meridian goes (? via Si12) to Gv14 and thence over the shoulder to S12. From here it passes through the lungs, with which it is connected, penetrates the diaphragm and enters the large intestine, to which it belongs, at S25.

The branch meridian leaves S12 to go to Li17, Li18 (? via S7), Gv26 and then across the midline to Li19 and Li20 on the opposite side.

From the region of S7 through the lower jaws and teeth to the region of Cv24.

(? From Li20 to S4 and G14.)

Large Intestine Connecting Meridian (Luo)—Li6

The meridian begins above the wrist at Li6, runs along the arm, goes over the shoulder and jaw and connects with the teeth and ears. It combines with the ?Zong Mo in this region. It links with the lung meridian Luo.

Large Intestine Muscle Meridian

The meridian begins at the end of the index finger, unites at the wrist; ascends the arm, unites at the elbow; ascends the upper arm, unites at the shoulder. A branch goes over the shoulder blade then going up and down the spine. The main muscle meridian ascends over the shoulder and neck in front of the small intestine muscle meridian, then up the lateral side of the forehead and temple, over the summit of the head, to descend on the opposite side as far as the jaw. A branch from the neck ascends the jaw, to unite at the side of the nose.

Large Intestine and Lung Divergent Meridians

Large Intestine Divergent Meridian

The large intestine divergent meridian leaves the large intestine main meridian at the outer tip of the shoulder. It goes to the spinal column and thence over the shoulder, thorax and upper abdomen to the large intestine to which it belongs and also to the lungs. It emerges at the supra-clavicular fossa, going along the throat to the large intestine meridian.

Lung Divergent Meridian

The lung divergent meridian leaves the lung main meridian at the armpit, whence it enters the lungs and scatters in the large intestine. Above this, it emerges from the supra-clavicular fossa, follows the throat and again meets the large intestine meridian.

Important Points

Metal	Li1	Metal point of Yang metal meridian
Water	Li2	Sedation
Wood	Li3	
Fire	Li5	
Earth	Li11	Tonification
Source	Li4	
Luo	Li6	
Xi	Li7	
Alarm	S25	
Associated	B25	

CHAPTER IV

STOMACH

Traditional Chinese and Western Scientific Conceptions

The Digestive Function of the Stomach

The Stomach is called 'the sea of water and nourishment and the controller of the rotting and ripening of liquid and solid food'. The Jing Qi which is required to nourish the organs of the body is produced by the 'rotting and ripening' of food and liquid in the stomach. Without the nourishing action of the Jing Qi, the other organs of the body could not function.

'The stomach is the sea of the five Zang and six Fu; liquid and solid food enter the stomach and the five Zang and six Fu are endowed with Qi from the stomach.'

(Ling Shu, wuwei pian)

The Jing Qi produced in the stomach and distributed to the other organs is stored in the kidney. This stored Jing can be used to nourish the organs and can also be transformed to the Jing of sexual power and semen. It is therefore said:

'The kidneys are the root of the former heaven (pre-natal). The spleen and stomach are the root of latter heaven (post-natal).'

The kidney semen-Jing gives the stimulus to birth. The stomach-Jing is required for growth.

The digestive function of gastric juice, particularly pepsinogen, is well known. The stomach may even digest itself in a healthy person who dies suddenly after a meal.

The Stomach and Spleen

The stomach and spleen are coupled organs, and as such their function is mutually interdependent. While the stomach controls the rotting and ripening of food and water, the spleen controls the 'moving and transforming' of food and water, and transports and distributes Jing Qi and fluid.

The spleen is a Yin Zang, the stomach is a Yang Fu. The spleen is damp earth, dislikes damp and likes dryness. The stomach is dry earth, dislikes dryness and likes moisture. For the spleen, the ascent of Qi is normal; for the stomach, the descent of Qi is normal.

If the spleen does not move and transform, then the stomach cannot digest; if the stomach does not rot and ripen water and food, the spleen cannot move and transform. If the spleen is empty and accumulates damp, then this can distress and check stomach Yang, and can produce a distended abdomen with anorexia. If the stomach is dry and hot, this will dry up the spleen's fluid, and can produce the symptoms of dry mouth and lips, owing to the spleen's fluid not having the means of ascending and moistening the mouth.

Vomiting may be caused by a malfuntion of stomach Qi which has lost its normal function of descending, and instead rebels upwards. In diarrhoea, the spleen has lost its strength and movement and power to ascend, thereby allowing descent and diarrhoea.

The stomach is influenced by abnormal hunger or satiation, or by an excess of cold or hot foods.

From the point of view of Western medicine there is no association in function between the stomach and spleen. They are though in intimate contact, not only in man but also in most fishes, amphibians, birds and mammals. In the dogfish the spleen is attached by a membrane to the hinder end of the stomach as a triangular lobe with a forward prolongation along the right side of the pyloric division. In the pigeon the spleen is attached to the right side of the proventriculus. In the rabbit the spleen is a narrow, crescentic body lying on the convex side of the stomach.

The Salivary Glands

The salivary glands are influenced by stimulation of the stomach meridian, which passes over the parotid gland between S2 and S3, and over the submaxillary gland between S8 and S9.

Saliva assists the stomach, by the digestion of starches with ptyalin, by the lubrication of food, and by making it possible to taste food, which is only possible if the tongue is moist.

In poisonous snakes the action of saliva goes beyond digestion to that of killing its prospective meal, for the poison glands are modified parotid glands.

The Tongue

The tongue is used as an important diagnostic criterion in Chinese

Traditional Medicine, whole books being entirely devoted to this subject.

The fur on the tongue principally reflects the condition of the stomach or, indirectly, the effect of other organs such as the liver on the stomach.

The mucous membrane covering the tongue is derived from entoderm, just as the lining of the whole of the gastro-intestinal tract. The oral membrane divides the tongue of the embryo into an internal and external portion in front of the row of vallate papillae, the former being covered by entoderm, the latter by ectoderm. At a later stage of embryonic development though, the entoderm covering the root of the tongue slips forward to coat the whole of the body as well.

Case History. A patient was seen whose tongue was covered with a white greasy fur. She was able to eat only small amounts of food at a time and had frequent epigastric pain or discomfort.

Pulse diagnosis showed a dysfunction of the stomach and this was cured by treating S36.

Symptomatology

Main Meridian Symptoms

Shivering with cold, constant yawning, dark complexion. When the disease is serious, the patient hates other people, is alarmed when hearing the sound of leaves rustling, has palpitations, and wishes to close the doors and windows and live by himself in the house. In severe cases, he may ascend to high places and sing, take off his clothes and run away. Abdomen distended, intermittent fevers, warm diseases, Shen confused, leading to madness, followed by fever. Spontaneous sweating, clear nasal discharge, epistaxis, mouth awry, mouth and lips develop dry sores, swelling of neck, ascites, pain or disturbance of function along the course of the meridian, especially the second and third toe.

SYMPTOMS OF EXCESS

Front of body hot. The heat in the stomach dissolves the liquid and solid food causing hunger and thirst. Yellow urine.

SYMPTOMS OF INSUFFICIENCY

The front of the body is cold and shivering. When the stomach is cold, the abdomen will be swollen and full.

Stomach Cold Symptoms

If the stomach Yang is deficient and cold Qi is dominant, this may cause the stomach to become distended and painful, the pain being continuous, with heartburn and waterbrash. When more severe, there will be vomiting and hiccoughs. Possibly there is very severe pain, with a desire for heat and pressure on the stomach. Possibly the limbs are cold.

The pulse of the right 2nd position is deep and slow.

The tongue has white and slippery fur.

Stomach Hot Symptoms

If the stomach fire is excessive, then the fluid in the stomach is easily destroyed, giving rise to a parched mouth, polydipsia, a feeling of hunger and discomfort, foul smell from mouth, bleeding from gums, gingivitis, vomiting immediately after meals. If the stomach heat moves down into the large intestine, then defaecation is often difficult, and if severe the stools become dry, and there is constipation.

Stomach Empty Symptoms

If the stomach Qi is empty, then the upper abdomen and lower chest feel blocked and melancholic or painful; there is no desire to eat and possibly belching; food is not digested, and there may be diarrhoea. If the condition is severe, then undigested food is passed and lips and tongue become pale white. If the fluid in the stomach is deficient, this can produce chocking or inability to swallow food.

The pulse in the 2nd position right is weak and pliable.

Stomach Full Symptoms

Stomach full symptoms are usually produced in externally contracted diseases and are Fu full symptoms. As the stomach and intestines are full and hot, there is pain in the abdomen and constipation; if the food is not digested, then there is abdominal distension and pain, sour and putrid vomitus, constipation, or possibly mild diarrhoea.

The pulse is full and large.

The tongue is thickly covered with yellow fur.

Connecting Meridian (Luo) Symptoms

SYMPTOMS OF EXCESS

Sudden loss of speech, insanity.

SYMPTOMS OF INSUFFICIENCY

Feet flaccid and weak, flesh and skin on shins withered and shrunken.

Muscle Meridian Symptoms

Spasm of the middle three toes and along the tibia, front of thigh swollen, herniae, muscular spasm of abdominal muscles or of the jaw, facial paralysis. If the muscles affecting the jaw are cold, there is muscular spasm extending from the jaw to the mouth. If they are hot, then the muscles are flaccid and cannot contract, therefore the mouth droops. According to circumstances it may be impossible to open or close the eyes.

Course of Meridians

Stomach Main Meridian

Principal Course

The meridian starts at S1, going over the face and the forehead, over the chest, and along the embryologically posterior and outer surface of the leg to end at the tip of the second toe at S45. According to some accounts the meridian starts at S1, going to S2, S3 (angle of jaw), S4 (below the eye), S5, S6, S7 (angle of mouth), S8 (jaw), S9 (larynx), etc. According to other accounts the meridian starts at S4 (below the eye) going to S5, S6, S7 (angle of mouth), S8, S3, S2, S1 (angle of forehead), the main meridian continuing downward to the larynx at S9 from a point slightly anterior to S8.

Special Details

The meridian starts at the side of the nose at Li20, goes to the midline just below the bridge of the nose to meet its companion from the other side, and then goes on to B1, S4, S5, S6, Gv26, S7, Cv24, S8, S3, S2, G3, G6, G5, G4, S1, (? via G14) to Gv24.

From S8 to S9, S10, S11 (? over the shoulders to Gv14 and thence forward again) to S12. Thence over the chest and abdomen to S30, and down the leg to end at the lateral tip of the second toe at S45.

A branch leaves S12, descends to the diaphragm, and enters the stomach, to which it belongs, at Cv13, and connects with the spleen.

A branch leaves Cv12 at the pylorus and moves inside the abdomen down to S30.

A branch leaves S36 going lateral to the main meridian, to end at the lateral tip of the third toe.

A branch leaves S42 going to Sp1.

According to classical accounts, the whole of the main meridian below S8 is described as a branch.

Stomach Connecting Meridian (Luo)—S40

The meridian begins in the lower leg at S40, ascends to reach the head and nape of neck where it combines with the meridian Qi of all the other meridians and descends to connect with the throat. It links with the spleen meridian Luo.

Stomach Muscle Meridian

The meridian begins at the 3rd toe (possible also 2nd and 4th toe), unites at the ankle; ascends the lower leg and unites at the outer side of the knee; continues up to unit at the hip joint; crosses the ribs and joins the spinal column to which it belongs. The main muscle meridian ascends from the ankle to unite at the antero-lateral side of the knee. A branch from here goes laterally to unite with the gall-bladder muscle meridian. The main muscle meridian ascends past S32 to unite at the top of the thigh; accumulates in the genitalia; ascends and scatters in the abdomen; and unites in the supra-clavicular fossa. It ascends at the side of the neck and mouth to meet at the side of the nose and then unites at the nose. It ascends to meet the bladder muscle meridian; the bladder muscle meridian running supra-orbitally, and the stomach muscle meridian mainly infra-orbitally. A branch from the jaw unites in front of the ear.

Stomach and Spleen Divergent Meridians

Stomach Divergent Meridian

The stomach divergent meridian leaves the main stomach meridian at the middle of the thigh; thereafter it enters the abdomen and goes to the stomach to which it belongs, and thence disperses in the spleen. Thereafter it ascends further to penetrate the heart and continues along the throat to emerge at the mouth. Thence it goes round the ala of the nose to the bridge of the nose between the eyes, with which it is linked, and there it meets the main stomach meridian.

Spleen Divergent Meridian

The spleen divergent meridian leaves the spleen main meridian at the middle of the thigh, thereafter it follows the course of the stomach divergent meridian to the throat, where it penetrates the middle of the tongue.

Important Points

Metal	S45	Sedation
Water	S44	
Wood	S43	
Fire	S41	Tonification
Earth	S36	Earth point of Yang earth meridian
Source	S42	
Luo	S40	
Xi	S34	
Alarm	Cv12	
Associated	B21	

CHAPTER V

SPLEEN

Traditional Chinese and Western Scientific Conceptions

The Spleen's Function of Distributing Nourishment

The principal function of the spleen is to move and transport the Jing Qi of liquid and solid food, and to distribute the Jing Qi around the whole body.

'Drink enters the stomach, the Jing Qi overflows, and it is transported to the spleen. The Spleen Qi scatters the Jing.'

(Su Wen, jingmo bielun)

'The spleen controls the movement of fluid in the stomach.'

(Su Wen, juelun)

Jing Qi and fluid are the two essential nourishing substances and, although they are first processed in the stomach, they are further transformed and also distributed by the spleen.

'The spleen meridian is earth, and only this Zang irrigates the four sides.'

(Su Wen, yuji zhenzang lun)

This is the phenomenon of 'earth creates the myriad things' applied to the function of the spleen.

If the moving and transforming ability of the spleen is deficient, the refined parts of the food cannot be transported to each part of the body, and the symptoms of fullness of the abdomen, borborygmi, diarrhoea, non-digestion of food, and possibly loss of appetite will appear. There will also be the symptoms which arise from these, such as emaciation of flesh, Jing Shen weary, etc.

The spleen moves and transforms not only the fine parts of the food, but also those of liquid. If the spleen Qi is empty and weak and loses its moving and transforming ability, this can lead to disease. For example, if the water in the stomach and intestines is not absorbed, this will cause diarrhoea and oliguria. If the water in the flesh and skin does not escape, then the body will be heavy and the skin swollen.

Case History. A patient had generalised subcutaneous oedema; it was not more marked in one part of the body than another. Her abdomen felt distended, she was depressed and lethargic, she sometimes had symptoms similar to those of a deep vein thrombosis of the leg. All symptoms and signs were helped by giving diuretics. The results though were only temporary.

Pulse diagnosis showed an underactive spleen. She was considerably improved, though not completely cured, by stimulating Sp3.

The Spleen Governs the Blood

Many blood diseases are related in one way or another to the spleen, *e.g.*, continuous defaecation of blood (?), polymenorrhoea, dysmenorrhoea,' etc. In these cases, one should 'lead the blood back to the spleen, and tonify the spleen so that it unites the blood'.

As is well known, there is a splenomegaly in certain anaemias. The spleen also takes part in the destruction of erythrocytes, the regulation of blood flow in the portal system, the function of a blood reservoir, the conversion of haemoglobin to ferritin and bilirubin-globin, the formation of lymphocytes and monocytes, and haematopoiesis in the embryo.

The Spleen, Flesh, and Lips

'*Now if the spleen is diseased, it cannot move the fluid on behalf of the stomach. The four limbs are thus not able to obtain the Qi of liquid and solid food. Hence the Qi decays gradually. The meridian cannot function correctly and the muscles, bones, skin and flesh have no Qi with which to grow, and therefore they do not function.*'

(Su Wen, taiyin yangmin lun)

The above quotation explains, via the theories of traditional Chinese medicine, why weakness or emaciation of the skin, flesh or limbs are diseases that are dependent upon the spleen.

Likewise, the redness and the moisture of the lips and mouth is also dependent upon the spleen. Patients who have a weak digestion due to an under-activity of the spleen usually have pale red and dry lips, and the mucous membrane lining of their mouth has a greyish tinge.

Yin earth likes dryness and hates damp. If the spleen is empty, water and dampness are not transformed. If there is an abundance of dampness, the spleen earth will suffer, producing amongst other symptoms large loose stools that float on water.

The Spleen and Pancreas

From the above, mainly translations of Chinese texts, it is obvious that many of the functions ascribed to the spleen really belong to the pancreas. For this reason many French doctors call this the Spleen-Pancreas meridian.

The external secretions of the pancreas—trypsin, chymotrypsin, carboxypeptidase, amylase, maltase, lipase—account for many of the previously mentioned symptoms. The internal secretion of the pancreas—insulin—may probably account for the other symptoms, such as wasting of the flesh.

Anatomically the spleen and pancreas are closer together than one might think, for both are developed in the dorsal mesogastrium, a connection that is virtually lost in the adult. Accessory spleens or pancreases occur in much the same region.

I do not know of any digestive function of the spleen, or even one concerning the distribution of the products of digestion, though this may one day be found. At least the spleen is distended after a meal and it belongs to the portal circulation, as do other organs associated with digestion.

Obsession and Concentration

The spleen seems occasionally to be connected with obsessions. The person who goes back twice to see if he has locked his front door, or who always insists on doing something in a certain way, may have a splenic dysfunction.

Excessive sympathy or over-concentration may be associated with the spleen or the stomach, as seen in one type of duodenal ulcer.

Symptomatology

Main Meridian Symptoms

Root of tongue stiff and hard, vomiting on eating, epigastrium tender, abdomen distended, continuous belching, difficulty in swallowing food, feels great relief and contentment on defaecating or breaking wind, dysentery, stools thin and watery, ascites, jaundice, body aching and heavy, cannot lie down peacefully, inner side of knees and thighs become swollen and cold if forced to stand for a long time, difficulty in moving big toe, palpitations, cardiac pain, cold intermittent fevers, feeling of oppression in chest, sharp pain below the heart, abdomen distended due to constipation, oliguria.

Pain in abdomen.

Abdomen distended and taut like a drum.

Spleen Cold Symptoms

If the spleen Yang is deficient and cannot move and transform water and damp, thus causing Yin cold to become dominant, then clinically one may see continuous pain in the abdomen, clear cold diarrhoea, inability to digest food and drink, cold limbs, heavy body. The skin may be yellow-black, the whole body may be swollen and puffy; oliguria may be present.

The pulse is deep and slow, particularly the right 2nd position.

The tongue is furred white and is greasy.

Spleen Hot Symptoms

The spleen is basically damp earth; if heat is associated with it, then damp and heat contend with each other, and the face becomes swollen and red and bloated. The body is heavy, there is a feeling of melancholy in the chest, and some anorexia, it is relatively easy to become jaundiced, urine is dark and in small amounts; there may be hot dysentery with abdominal pain that is not constant, lips may be red, and the mouth may have a sweet sticky and dirty taste.

Spleen Empty Symptoms

If spleen earth is empty and weak, and its transporting function is impaired, there will be a concomitant decrease in the desire to eat and drink, or there will be difficulty in digestion after eating. There is vomiting with a swollen abdomen, borborygmi and loose stools, four limbs cold, weariness and fondness for lying down, abdomen painful with a desire to press it, possibly emaciation and at the same time oedema.

The pulse is empty and slowed down, specially so in the right connecting position.

The tongue substance is pale, with white and slippery fur.

Spleen Full Symptoms

If the spleen is full, then there are usually diseases caused by damp evil remaining, and the symptoms are opposite to those of spleen empty symptoms.

If damp obstructs and blocks communication, then the upper abdomen is full and distended; if damp remains in the skin and flesh, then the body will feel heavy; if damp obstructs Qi, there will be oligura and constipation, weak respiration, with a melancholic feeling in the chest, and a feeling of fullness, pain, and possibly swelling in the abdomen.

Connecting Meridian (Luo) Symptoms

SYMPTOMS OF EXCESS
Sharp pain in intestines.

SYMPTOMS OF INSUFFICIENCY
Ascites.

Great Luo of the Spleen—Sp21—Symptoms

SYMPTOMS OF EXCESS
Whole body painful.

SYMPTOMS OF INSUFFICIENCY
Bones and joints of the whole body flaccid and weak and without strength.

Muscle Meridian Symptoms

Pain or muscular spasm in big toe, inner side of knee, inner side of thigh, genitalia, navel and ribs. Pain along the spine extending to the breast.

Course of Meridians

Spleen Main Meridian

Principal Course

Starting at Sp1 on the big toe, the meridian goes up the embryological anterior and outer surface of the leg, over the abdomen and chest to the axilla at Sp20, and then down a little to Sp21.

Special Details

The meridian starts at Sp1 and goes up the leg to the groin at Sp13. From Sp13 via Cv3 and Cv4 to Sp14.
From Sp15 via Cv10 to Sp16.

From Sp16 via G24 and Liv14 to Sp17, and thence on to Sp21.
From Sp21 via L1, up the throat to end on the under surface of the tongue.

A branch leaves Cv10, penetrates the diaphragm and goes to the heart and heart meridian.

Traditionally, from Sp13 the meridian is described as entering the abdomen, going to the spleen to which it belongs, and connecting with the stomach.

Spleen Connecting Meridian (Luo)—Sp4

The meridian begins near the root of the big toe at Sp4 and ascends to enter the abdomen, connecting with the intestines and stomach. It links with the stomach meridian Luo.

Great Luo of the Spleen—Sp21

The meridian begins on the side of the chest below the axilla at Sp21, and then divides and disperses throughout the chest and ribs.

This connecting meridian unites all the Yin and Yang Luo like a net and if there is any 'extravasated blood' it should be treated at Sp21.

Spleen Muscle Meridian

The meridian begins on the medial side of the end of the big toe, unites at the internal malleolus; ascends to unite at the medial side of the knee; ascends the medial surface of the thigh to unite at its upper end; accumulates in the genitalia; ascends the abdomen to unite at the navel; crosses the abdomen to unite at the ribs, and scatters in the chest. An inner branch ascends the spine.

Important Points

Wood	Sp1	
Fire	Sp2	Tonification
Earth	Sp3	Earth point of Yin earth meridian
Metal	Sp5	Sedation
Water	Sp9	
Source	Sp3	
Luo	Sp4	
Xi	Sp8	
Alarm	Liv13	
Associated	B20	

CHAPTER VI

HEART

Traditional Chinese and Western Scientific Conceptions

'The Heart is the Ruling Organ and Controller of the Shen Ming'

The heart is the controller of life and movement in the body, and occupies the first place among the Zang and Fu. All Jing Shen, consciousness and thought are connected with the function of the heart; it is called therefore the 'ruling official (or organ)'.

'The heart is the supreme controller of the five Zang and the six Fu, and is the dwelling place of the Jing Shen.'

(Ling Shu, xieke pian)

'The heart is the root of life, and the location of change of Shen.'

(Su Wen, liujie zangziang lun)

These quotations explain that the heart includes the function of Shen, leads the movement of the Zang and Fu, and is the controller of life and movement; the ancients thus stressed the importance of the function of the heart. Clinical experience shows that, if the heart becomes diseased, one may have the symptoms of palpitations, nervousness, insomnia, delirium, incoherent speech, confused Shen Zhi, liability to sorrow, incessant laughter, etc. The causes of these conditions have two aspects; inner injury and outer suffering. Inner injury is present if the heart itself is not strong, or when excessive emotions (happiness, melancholy, fear, worry) cause disease. Outer suffering is present if the 'six excess disease evils' invade, if evil heat rebels and is transmitted to the pericardium, etc. However, the principal cause is still that the heart's action has lost its control.

Since the heart is 'the great controller' of the Zang and Fu, it can 'unite and lead the division of work, and the working together of the Zang and Fu; moreover it can reciprocally obtain harmony and produce the functional co-ordination of the whole body.' If each organ honours its office, the health of the body will be maintained. Conversely, if the heart is diseased, then the movement of the other Zang and Fu will be in disorder, and thus the health of the whole body is affected, and at all times there is the possibility of disease.

'Thus if the controller is bright, there is peace . . . if the controller is not bright, then the twelve organs are in danger.'

(Su Wen, linglan midian lun)

Case History. A patient had variable symptoms one day in one part of the body, another day in another part.

Pulse diagnosis showed a different disturbance every time the pulse was felt. The overall quality of the pulse was always the same; the specific abnormalities shifting from one pulse position to another. The pulse position of the heart did not show any greater abnormality than any other position. This variable symptomatology nevertheless suggested the heart as the main culprit, and when this was treated the condition was largely cured.

The Heart Controls the Blood Vessels, its Exterior Reflexion is in the Face

The blood vessels are one of the 'five substances', and their function is to enclose the blood and cause it to circulate constantly round the whole body. This circulation, though, is controlled by the heart.

'The heart is the root of life . . . its exterior reflection is in the face, its interior reflection is in the blood vessels.'

(Su Wen, zangziang lun)

If the heart and blood vessels are 'bloodless', the face has a grey ashen colour.

'If the arm lesser Yin (heart) Qi is interrupted, then the blood vessels will not function; if the vessels do not function, then the blood does not flow; if the blood does not flow, then the hair and skin are not moistened. Thus the face will be black like lacquer wood and the blood will die.'

(Ling Shu, jingmo pian)

The phylogenetic and ontogenetic development of the heart as a specialisation of the blood vessels need hardly be mentioned. In fish the heart is little more than the hypertrophied muscular wall of the aorta. In the human embryo primitive blood vessels appear first— and these are only later modified to form a heart.

Case History. A patient of 28 had mitral incompetence. The heart was enlarged; the apex beat could easily be seen, let alone felt; he could only walk a few hundred yards and then stopped because of tingling in his hands and dyspnoea. He perspired profusely.

Pulse diagnosis showed an abnormality not only of the heart but also of the liver and kidney. After eight treatments the patient went without

349

my knowledge on the C.N.D. Aldermaston march to London (30 miles). He did this with no more difficulty than any of the other marchers of his age.

Presumably the effect of acupuncture was to increase the function of the heart so that it was able to compensate for the mitral incompetence. It should be stressed that such a good result, in an irreparable structural lesion, can only be obtained in a small proportion of patients.

The Relationship Between the Heart and the Tongue

A red or a deep red tongue generally indicates that the heart is hot, and that fire Qi has a surplus. A pale red tongue shows that blood is empty, and that the heart Qi is deficient. If the Shen of the heart receives disease, this can cause a feeble tongue and inability to speak.

'(Heart) its influence reaches to the tongue.'

(Su Wen, yinyang yingxiang dalun)

'The heart Qi communicates with the tongue; if the heart is harmonious, then the tongue is able to recognise the five tastes.'

(Ling Shu, modu pian)

The tongue and heart are much nearer to one another in the embryo than in the adult, the heart being more or less in the neck.

In the embryo the heart is connected with the region of the base of the tongue by the dorsal mesocardium, a proximity which is probably not fortuitous.

Case History. A patient was seen whose leading symptom was tingling at the tip of the tongue, which had been constant and unremittant for many years. On close questioning she had slight retrosternal discomfort and dyspnoea on extention.

Pulse diagnosis showed an underactivity of the heart. She was cured by stimulating various points on the heart meridian.

The Thyroid and Heart

In Chinese pulse diagnosis, hyperthyroidism is shown by the pulse of the heart (position 1, deep, left) becoming distended and hard. The all too frequent over-dosage of thyroxin which physicians give their patients, in an attempt to 'pep them up', may in this way be diagnosed. The sinus tachycardia, systolic murmur, vasodilation, raised pulse pressure and paroxysmal fibrillation, which are the well-known Western cardiovasular symptoms of thyrotoxicosis, only occur at a much later stage than that noted by the more sensitive Chinese pulse diagnosis.

The endocrine glands were not known to the ancient Chinese and were therefore not considered. In view of the above though, I think the thyroid should be classified as belonging to the heart in the system of classification under twelve organs. (Likewise, as mentioned further on, the adrenal belongs to the kidney.)

Embryologically the thyroid is connected with the tongue, via the thyroglossal duct, whose remnant may be seen as the foramen caecum at the junction of the base and body of the tongue. As mentioned in the previous section the tongue is likewise connected with the heart: physiologically in the adult, anatomically in the embryo. Sometimes even the thyroid, or more frequently, aberrant parts of the thyroid, migrate downwards to lie over the pericardium.

Mild thyrotoxicos may thus be treated acupuncturally via the heart.

The Menopause

The majority of symptoms accompanying the menopause are dependent on the heart, even though Western science attaches prime importance to the oyarian hormones. Possibly one day a cardiac ovarian hormone will be discovered.

The menopause is heralded by the cessation of menstruation. Blood, which in the menopause is retained, is in the Chinese view most often classified with the heart.

The most frequent symptom of the menopause is hot flushes. Heat is traditionally classified under the heart. Palpitations and other nervous symptoms of a cardiac type may also be noted.

Patients with menopausal symptoms normally have an underactive pulse of the heart and possibly lung.

Case History. A patient was seen with severe hot flushes of several years' duration.

Pulse diagnosis showed an underactive heart and lung. She was cured in four treatments, using H7 and L9.

General

As the heart 'stores Shen' and 'controls blood', therefore it is also affected by Shen Zhi and blood. This is associated with symptoms such as palpitations, nervousness, confused Shen, delirium, haemoptysis, epistaxis, spontaneous sweating, night sweats.

Case History. A patient had pain in the region of the 5th thoracic vertebra for twenty years. Most doctors he had previously consulted thought it was a vertebral lesion, for slight arthritic changes could be seen on X-ray. On closer questioning the patient said that he felt dead elbow the level of the fifth thoracic vertebra—including his genitalia. Certainly the lower part of his body was pale while his face was bright red. There was a funnel-shaped depression over the lower part of the sternum, which was also the area where he perspired more easily than anywhere else.

Pulse diagnosis showed an overflowing heart. Treatment included H7, H5, H3, B15, B39, Gvii—all heart points. The patient was nearly, though not completely, cured.

Symptomatology

Main Meridian Symptoms

Throat dry, mouth parched, desire to drink, cardiac pain, pain in chest, pain stiffness or insensitivity down the arm along the course of the meridian, eyes yellow, palms of hands hot.

SYMPTOMS OF EXCESS

Dreams of fright, fear and anxiety.

SYMPTOMS OF INSUFFICIENCY

Inability to speak, dreams of smoke and fire.

Heart Hot Symptoms

Face red, tongue dry, tip of tongue red, pulse rapid, mouth parched, thirsty, eyes painful, under surface of tongue swollen and protruding (heavy tongue), possibly tongue swollen and hard (wooden tongue), haemoptysis, epistaxis, heart agitated and feels hot, insomnia, delirious speech, laughs incessantly, chest feels hot and melancholic, pain like a needle stab. If the heart heat moves into the small intestine, the urine becomes dark, possibly even haematuria.

Heart Empty Symptoms

Pulse generally fine and weak, tongue pale red, poor memory, nervous and not at ease often resulting in insomnia, much dreaming, dreaming that one is falling down, palpitations not only during physical exertion but even with mental effort, hurried breathing, heart seems 'noisy and hungry', violent pain below heart, pain round the lower border of the chest front and back, face withered and pale, root of tongue stiff, often sad and miserable.

A person whose heart is excessively empty is prone to sudden loss of consciousness. Other symptoms such as sweating and spermatorrhoea are also produced by the heart being empty. However, spontaneous sweating and nocturnal sweating are divided into Yin empty and Yang empty, and loss of sperm is frequently related to the kidneys, the cause being known as 'heart and kidney deficient'.

Connecting Meridian (Luo) Symptoms

SYMPTOMS OF EXCESS

Chest and diaphragmatic area feel as though they are bearing a heavy weight and are uncomfortable.

SYMPTOMS OF INSUFFICIENCY

Inability to speak.

Muscle Meridian Symptoms

Muscular spasm, pain and dysfunction along the course of the meridian. Haemoptysis.

Course of Meridians

Heart Main Meridian

Principal Course

The meridian starts in the axilla at H1, and passes along the anterior and inner surface of the arm, to end near the nail of the little finger at H9.

Special Details

The meridian emerges from the heart, to which it belongs, connects with the great vessels entering and leaving the heart, penetrates the diaphragm, and connects with the small intestine.

The main meridian leaves the heart, transversing the lung, to emerge at the armpit at H1, from where it goes down the arm to H9.

A branch from the heart goes up through the throat to the eye and contents of the orbit.

Heart Connecting Meridian (Luo)—H5

The meridian begins at H5 above the wrist, ascends alongside its main meridian and enters the heart, ascending again to link up with the root of the tongue and further to connect with the eye. It diverges and connects with the Luo of the small intestine.

Heart Muscle Meridian

The meridian begins on the little finger, unites at the wrist; ascends the forearm, unites at the elbow; ascends the upper arm, crosses the axilla where it joins the lung muscle meridian and across the anterior surface of the thorax, to unite in the middle of the chest; it runs downwards to link with the navel.

Important Points

Wood	H9	Tonification
Fire	H8	Fire point of Yin Sovereign fire meridian
Earth	H7	Sedation
Metal	H4	
Water	H3	
Source	H7	
Luo	H5	
Xi	H6	
Alarm	Cv14	
Associated	B15	

CHAPTER VII

SMALL INTESTINE

Traditional Chinese and Western Scientific Conceptions

The Small Intestine Controls the Transformation of Matter and the Separating of the Pure and Impure

'The small intestine is the official who receives abundance and is concerned with the transforming of matter.'

(Su Wen, linglan midian lun)

This explains that the function of the small intestine is to 'receive the water and food already rotted and ripened and sent down from the stomach, and to advance the work of separating it into the pure and impure'. It causes the Jing Qi to return to the spleen and to be distributed to the five Zang so that it may be stored there. It also causes the fluid in the 'dregs' to return to the bladder, and the solid matter to go to the large intestine, thence to be expelled from the body, thus completing the function of 'transforming matter'. Accordingly, if the function of the small intestine is not strong, it can influence micturition and defaecation.

'Small intestine disease causes water and food to go through and appear in the stools, with oliguria or haematuria . . .'

(Zhangfu biaoben yongyao shi)

From the above it may be seen that the Chinese conception agrees to some extent with that of the West, particularly in regard to the digestive function of the small intestine. The Chinese consider however that the main part of the process of 'rotting and ripening' takes place in the stomach, while we in the West would probably consider the small intestine, with its many enzymes (enterokinase, lipase, amylase, sucrase, lactase, maltase, polypeptidases, alkaline phosphatase) to be of greater importance in this respect. This relative contradiction may be explained by the difference between the anatomical stomach, and what is felt on the pulse of the stomach by Chinese pulse diagnosis. As may be seen from their old drawings, the Chinese knew the anatomical position and configuration of the stomach. On pulse diagnosis, however, the pulse of the stomach also includes the first part of the duodenum, for duodenal ulcers show on the pulse of the stomach and not on that of the small intestine. Possibly for this reason the Chinese assign to the stomach some of the functions which we ascribe to the small intestine.

The idea that the small intestine divides the 'pure' from the 'impure', should be taken to mean that the 'impure' passes on from the small intestine to the large intestine as faeces, while the 'pure' is absorbed by the small intestine, and after having passed through the body, is excreted by the kidneys into the bladder as urine. Although this is not new to us, it does present the problem from an unaccustomed angle, from which we can derive new clinical insight, namely, that the small intestine controls the proportion of urine to faeces. Most of the water from the gastro-intestinal tract is absorbed in the small intestine—up to ten litres per day; the colon absorbs normally only 350 cc and the stomach minimal amounts in a day.

The Relationship between the Small Intestine and the Heart

This is the relationship of coupled organs, or as the Chinese say, mutually exterior and interior.

A red tongue with wasting of its substance belongs to heart fire, violent and abundant; together with this, however, there are often the symptoms of small quantities of dark urine, and sometimes there may be haematuria.

'*The heart controls blood and unites with the small intestine. If someone has a cardiac disease caused by heat, the heat will converge into the small intestine. Thus one will urinate blood.*'

(Chaoshi bingyuan)

With these conditions, if one uses the methods of purifying the heart and benefiting micturition, then one can cause the fire of the heart and small intestine to drain downwards with the urine.

A physiological relationship between the small intestine and heart, is far from obvious. There are nevertheless a few clues:—

In congestive cardiac failure, little urine is passed. This is supposed to be due to a reduced glomerular filtration, consequent on a diminished circulation. On the other hand the small intestinal absorption of water may perhaps play a part.

In the majority of fevers (fire disease), with tachycardia (fire symptom), the patient passes dark urine. The Chinese say this is due to the heart and small intestine; we would say it is due to dehydration and increased metabolism. This is not entirely contradictory for dehydration and increased metabolism are both fire symptoms.

Anatomically there is only a vague connection, in so far as in the embryo, the pericardial and peritoneal cavities intercommunicate via the pleural canal.

Symptomatology

Main Meridian Symptoms

Throat and pharynx ache, swelling below the jaw prevents the patient from turning his head, shoulders ache as though they are being pulled, upper arm hurts as though it were broken, deafness, tinnitus, area around ear becomes hot or cold, discolouration of the eyes, eyes water, cannot bend waist, abdomen distended, bradycardia.

SYMPTOMS OF EXCESS

Hyper-relaxation of joints, elbows useless.

SYMPTOMS OF INSUFFICIENCY

Formation of swellings or nodules.

Small Intestine Empty and Cold Symptoms

Urine colourless and in big quantities, oliguria, low abdominal pain, diarrhoea, borborygmi.

The pulse is fine and weak, the left pulse being extremely so.
The tongue is thinly furred white.

Small Intestine Full and Hot Symptoms

The navel and abdomen are swollen, only comfortable after flatus has been passed, small intestine painful. If severe then includes base of spine and texticles, urine dark, dysuria, sometimes alternately hot and cold. If excessively hot then an intestinal ulcer may form.

The pulse is slippery and rapid, the left pulse particularly so.
The tongue is thickly furred yellow, the sides and point of tongue may be red.

Connecting Meridian (Luo) Symptoms

SYMPTOMS OF EXCESS

Bones and joints flaccid and weak, elbow joint cannot move.

SYMPTOMS OF INSUFFICIENCY

Nodules between the fingers.

Muscle Meridian Symptoms

Pain, muscular spasm and dysfunction along the course of the muscle. meridian Tinnitus and pain in ear extending to the jaws. Weak eyesight.

Course of Meridians

Small Intestine Main Meridian

Principal Course

The meridian starts at the little finger at Si1, goes along the embryological posterior and inner surface of the arm, over the side of the neck and face, to end in front of the ear at Si19.

Special Details

The meridian begins at Si1 at the end of the little finger, goes up the arm and over the scapula (? from Si13 via B36 to Si14 and ? from Si14 via B11 to Si15) and thence to Gv14.

From Gv14 over the shoulder to S12.

From S12 down the chest to connect with the heart at Cv17. It penetrates the diaphragm to reach the stomach at Cv13 and Cv12, and continues downward to end at the small intestine, to which it belongs.

From S12 a branch goes over the throat and jaw to the outer corner of the eye, and then enters the ear, following the course Si16, Si17, G1, (?T22), Si19 to (?T20).

Another branch starts from the jaw just above Si17, going across the cheek to the inner corner of the eye at B1, and thence on to Si18.

Small Intestine Connecting Meridian (Luo)—Si7

The meridian begins above the wrist at Si7, ascending along the arm to the tip of the shoulder. It links with the heart Luo.

Small Intestine Muscle Meridian

The meridian begins at the end of the little finger, and unites at the wrist; ascends the forearm to unite on the medial side of the olecranon; ascends and unites posterior to the armpit. Goes over the shoulder to unite at the mastoid process, whence a branch enters the ear. Another branch continues over the ear and descends anteriorly to unite at the jaw; whence it ascends to the outer corner of the eye.

The original branch goes over the jaw in front of the ear to the outer corner of the eye, whence it ascends to the forehead and unites at the temple.

Small Intestine and Heart Divergent Meridians

Small Intestine Divergent Meridian

The small intestine divergent meridian leaves the small intestine main meridian behind the shoulder in the axilla, whence it moves across the chest to the heart and then down the abdomen to link with the small intestine.

Heart Divergent Meridian

The heart divergent meridian leaves the heart main meridian in the axilla; it goes to the heart to which it belongs, thereafter ascending the throat and face to the inner corner of the eye.

Important Points

Metal	Si1	
Water	Si2	
Wood	Si3	Tonification
Fire	Si5	Fire point of Yang Sovereign fire meridian
Earth	Si8	Sedation
Source	Si4	
Luo	Si7	
Xi	Si6	
Alarm	Cv4	
Associated	B27	

CHAPTER VIII

BLADDER

Traditional Chinese and Western Scientific Conceptions

The Bladder Controls the Storing of Fluid

'*The bladder is the official of a region, and fluid is stored in it.*'

(Su Wen, linglan midian lun)

In the above quotation fluid means urine. After food and drink have been turned into fluid (other meaning) by the stomach and spleen, this is transported to the whole body in order to nourish it. But the Fluid essential to the body has a normal level. The remainder, apart from a small part which is expelled to the exterior of the body as sweat, passes through the triple warmer water path, and is transported down to the bladder as urine.

'*Urine is the surplus of the body's fluid.*'

(Chaoshi bingyuan)

Therefore fluid, urine and sweat have a close relationship in waxing and waning, fullness and emptiness. If there is an excess of urine, then the fluid within the body will decrease; conversely, if sweating is excessive, or violent vomiting or diarrhoea cause the level of fluid to decrease, the volume of urine will also decrease, and in extreme cases there will be no micturition. Again, in hot weather there is much sweating, and therefore little micturition. In cold weather there is little sweating, but much micturition.

The Relationship between the Bladder and the Kidneys

The bladder (leg greater Yang meridian) and the kidney (leg lesser Yin meridian) have a reciprocal relationship of exterior and interior, *i.e.*, they are coupled meridians and organs.

'*The kidneys unite the bladder, the bladder is the Fu of Fluid.*'

(Ling Shu, benshu pian)

The ability of Fluid to become urine is also closely connected with the Qi transformation action of the kidneys.

'*The bladder is the official of a region, Fluid is stored in it; if the Qi moves, then one can urinate.*'

(Su Wan, linglan midian lun)

Thus, although retention and incontinence of urine are principally an abnormality of the bladder, sometimes deficiency of kidney Qi or deficiency of fire of destiny, can also produce these symptoms. In treatment, one should increase the kidney Qi or tonify the fire of destiny.

Case History. A male patient had to urinate about fifteen times a day. The pulse of the kidney and bladder were weak.

Stimulation at K5 made him better; stimulation at K3 made him worse. After twelve treatments he urinated four times a day.

Case History. A female patient suffered from headache and general fatigue over a period of many years. There were no bladder symptoms. Various points were stimulated, amongst them K5. This caused the patient 'to disappear behind every bush on the way home' to her house in the country, to the amusement of her friends in the car with her. This excessive urination stopped after one day, with the improvement of her headaches and fatigue. She was cured after repeated treatments.

It should be noted that in the first case history mentioned above K5 diminished bladder irritation, while in the second case history K5 increased bladder irritation.

General

The kidneys 'open the holes in the ears', control the loins and lumbar region, the sacral area, and to some extent the whole back. They also rule the bones. Therefore when the kidneys are diseased there are frequently symptoms in these areas.

Case History. A patient had mild tinnitus of four months' duration. The pulse of the kidney was weak.

Stimulation at K1 cured the condition. It should be noted though that tinnitus of longer duration (over six months) can only rarely be cured by acupuncture—unless it is catarrhal.

The Bladder, Associated Points and Metamerism

The bladder meridian differs from all others, as there are on it the associated points (Yu) of all other meridians. The associated points have a more or less segmental distribution, the only acupuncture points that have a distribution reminiscent of lower animals such as the earth worm, in which most structures are metamerically arranged.

In the human embryo the kidney is the only internal organ with a metameric arrangement similar to that of the associated points of the bladder. The pronephros, mesonephros and metanephros are of course kidneys and not bladders, but I think the function in the embryo is close enough for a comparison to be drawn; the external glomerulus of the pronephros opening into the coelonic cavity, for there is no bladder.

The pronephros originates from the 2nd to the 14th somite, the mesonephros from the 9th to the 26th, and the metanephros the 26th to 28th; i.e., all the associated points alongside the vertebral column are within this range.

The bladder meridian probably goes along the back, as the pronephric duct runs dorsal to the nephrotome, between this and the ectoderm, to reach the cloaca.

Diseases along the Course of the Bladder Meridian

Points on the bladder meridian seem to have a greater effect on diseases of the spinal cord, than points on other meridians. Possibly this is because the bladder meridian runs paravertebrally, and a meridian always controls all structures in its neighbhourhood. In the embryo the nephrotome and the neural tube are likewise near one another.

Case Histories. I have treated several patients with disseminated sclerosis at an early stage of the disease, by stimulating point B62, or the paravertebral bladder points. The majority noticed a remarkable improvement within a few minutes or hours of treatment, the effect usually lasting several days. I do not think I have ever achieved a permanent improvement or cure, even with repeated treatments.

Haemorrhoids are likewise partially affected by the bladder meridian (see also the section on the liver), for the bladder meridian and meridian divergence run alongside the anus.

Certain types of occiptial neuralgia or pain at the medial end of the eyebrows may be cured by treating the bladder or kidney meridians. Care should be taken to differentiate these from the nearby gall bladder meridian.

Case History. A patient had unilateral supra-orbital neuralgia over the middle and medial part of the eyebrows. Stimulation of the liver at Liv8 on the opposite side removed the pain over the middle of the eyebrow —which had been in the region of and below point G14—within minutes. The pain at the medial end of the eyebrow—in the region of B2— remained, but was later removed by stimulating B60 on the same side.

Sciatica and lumbago may also be treated via the bladder meridian, in so far as the pain follows the distribution of this meridian. Sometimes points on the feet are best, sometimes those in the lumbar or sacral region. Choosing exactly the right point decides whether the patient will be cured in a few, or in many treatments, or even at all. Other types of lumbago or sciatica have to be treated via other meridians.

Symptomatology

Main Meridian Symptoms

Qi rushes upwards causing headache, pupils of eyes appear as though about to come out, nape of neck hurts as though being dragged and pulled, spine is painful, waist feels as if it is broken, lumbago, sciatica, hip joint cannot move, spasm of muscles in popliteal fossa calf and ankle, haemorrhoids, intermittent fevers, madness, insanity, yellowish discolouration of eyes, excessive lachrymation, clear or bloody nasal discharge.

SYMPTOMS OF EXCESS

Anosmia, headache, pain along spine.

SYMPTOMS OF INSUFFICIENCY

Epistaxis.

Bladder Full and Hot Symptoms

If damp and heat are congealed and bladder Qi transforms but does not motivate, then urine is passed in small quantities, is yellow-red in colour, is possibly turbid, and there is dysuria with a hot burning feeling during micturition and an abnormal smell; if severe there may be urinary incontinence and pain that is difficult to bear, the urine possibly being thick and bloody. There are also cases of a fusion of damp and heat, collecting to form a stone or gravel. Other organs may also influence micturition, for example, if damp and heat enter the bladder from the small intestine, the urine may become yellow-red, or there may be retention of urine.

Bladder Empty and Cold Symptoms

If the kidney Yang is deficient and there is a deficiency of the function of warming and transforming water and Qi, this may induce empty cold symptoms of the bladder, resulting in frequency of micturition, the urine being clear and light in colour, or in retention or urine, the face being blackish or oedematous. If the orthodox Qi is empty and weak, the bladder often loses its normal receiving action and causes incontinence of urine, or frequency of micturition. Although they are in the bladder, these diseases in fact concern the whole body, because the bladder is the Fu of the kidneys. The lungs also have the function of regulating water and Qi, therefore the disease signs are all the result of kidney Qi being deficient or lung Qi being weak.

Connecting Meridian (Luo) Symptoms

SYMPTOMS OF EXCESS

Clear nasal discharge, blocked nose, cold nose, pain in cervical spine.

SYMPTOMS OF INSUFFICIENCY

Clear nasal discharge, epistaxis.

Muscle Meridian Symptoms

Little toe and heel swollen and painful, cramp at back of knee, pain in back, muscular cramp at the back of the neck, inability to raise shoulders, upper arm and shoulder stiff and painful, inability to move shoulder girdle from side to side.

Course of Meridians

Bladder Main Meridian

Principal Course

The meridian starts at the inner corner of the eye at B1, then goes over the head to the neck, where it divides into two parallel meridians which rejoin at the buttock or the knee, according to interpretation. Thence it goes along the embryologically posterior and inner surface of the leg, to terminate at the little toe at B67.

Special Details

The meridian starts at the inner corner of the eye at B1, goes to B2, and thence via Gv24 to B3.

A branch goes from B7 (? via G7) to G8, G9, G10, G11, G12.
The main meridian, apart from going over the cranium along the
course of the bladder meridian, also goes from B7 to Gv20, whence
it enters the brain and emerges at the nape of the neck.

From B9 via Gv17 (? and Gv16) to B10.

From B10 via Gv14 (? and Gv13) to B11.

From B11 alongside the spinal column to B23, where it connects
with the kidneys, and enters the bladder to which it belongs.

A branch continues downwards, making a zigzag on the inner
surface of the buttocks to B50, and then goes down the thigh to
B54.

Another branch leaves B10, going lateral to the main meridian to
B49, thence via G30 it crosses the other branch between B51 and
B52, to join it at B54.

From B54 it goes down the leg to end at the little toe at B67.

Bladder Connecting Meridian (Luo)—B58

This meridian begins above the ankle at B58 and links with the
kidney meridian Luo.

Bladder Muscle Meridian

This meridian begins in the little toe, unites in the external
malleolus; ascends and unites at the lateral corner of the popliteal
fossa. From the external malleolus it goes to and unites in the heel;
ascends the calf and unites at the back of the knee. The divergence
from the external malleolus to the back of the knee unites in the calf.
The main meridian muscle ascends to the buttocks where it unites;
and then ascends para-vertebrally to the nape of the neck. A branch
goes across the neck to unite in the root of the tongue. The main
meridian muscle continues up to unite in the occiput; going over the
cranium to unite in the nose. A branch arches over the eyebrows to
unite over the cheek. A branch from the upper part of the shoulders
goes to the tip of the shoulders where it unites. Another branch
continues below the armpit to the supra-clavicular fossa where it
ascends to unite over the mastoid process. Another branch from
the supra-clavicular fossa ascends from the supra-clavicular fossa to
unite in the cheek joining the circum-orbital branch.

Bladder and Kidney Divergent Meridians

Bladder Divergent Meridian

The bladder divergent meridian leaves the main bladder meridian behind the knee, whence it ascends the back of the thigh to the inferior gluteal fold where it divides into two. The one part goes to the bladder and then enters and is dispersed in the kidney. The other part ascends para-vertebrally to the heart, in which it is dispersed, and then continues to ascend to the nape of the neck, where it joins its parent main bladder meridian.

Kidney Divergent Meridian

The kidney divergent meridian leaves the kidney main meridian behind the knee, whence it ascends up the posterior surface of the thigh and then para-vertebrally to the kidney at the level of the 2nd lumbar vertebra. Here it is associated with the Dai mo and then ascends over the abdomen and thorax to link with the root of the tongue. Thereafter it passes laterally to the nape of the neck where it meets the bladder main meridian.

Important Points

Metal	B67	Tonification
Water	B66	Water point of Yang water meridian
Wood	B65	Sedation
Fire	B60	
Earth	B54	
Source	B64	
Luo	B58	
Xi	B63	
Alarm	Cv3	
Associated	B28	

CHAPTER IX

KIDNEY

Traditional Chinese and Western Scientific Conceptions

The Kidneys Store Jing

The kidneys store two types of Jing; firstly the Jing of the five Zang and six Fu, and secondly the Jing of reproduction.

The Jing of the Zang and Fu originates from the ingested water and food; it is a basic nourishing substance which maintains the life and movement of the body. It is stored in the kidneys and is distributed from there to the rest of the body when required.

'The kidneys control water, receive the Jing of the Zang and Fu and store it.'

(Su Wen, shango tianzhen lun)

The Jing of reproduction is the Jing of sexual fertilisation possessed by both male and female; it is the basic substance which enables man to reproduce. From the time of conception to birth the Jing Qi is in abundance and is able to nourish the embryo.

This type of Jing is formed from the transformation of the combined kidney Qi of Former Heaven (pre-natal) and the Jing Qi of the five Zang of Latter Heaven (post-natal), and it is stored in the kidney. The development and decline of Jing is controlled by the kidneys; hence diseases such as spermatorrhoea, nocturnal emissions, deficiency of semen or infertility, are all controlled by the kidneys.

Case History. A man in his forties had become impotent during the previous year. He also had slight lumbago.

He was cured by stimulating K5 and Gv4. (Governing vessel points in the lumbar and sacral area have an effect on the kidney.)

The Relationship between Kidney Qi and Birth and Growth

Kidney Qi is endowed with the Jing Qi of the Former Heaven of the mother and father. After the mother has become pregnant it is the basis for the development of the foetus. After birth the kidney Qi is nourished by the Jing Qi of water and food, and is thus able to promote the growth of the body.

'When a female reaches the age of 7 the kidney Qi is abundant, the teeth change and the hair grows long. At the age of 14 menstruation arrives, the vessel of conception communicates, the Dai mo and the Chong mo are abundant, menstruation occurs at the proper time, therefore there are children. At 21 the kidney Qi is balanced, thus the true teeth grow and develop. . . . At 49 the vessel of conception is empty, the Dai mo and Chong mo are decayed and small, menstruation is exhausted, the Dao (Tao or Path) of earth does not penetrate, therefore form is destroyed and there are no children.'

'When a man reaches the age of 8 the kidney Qi is full, the teeth change and the hair grows long. At the age of 16 the kidney Qi is abundant, sexual substance (Tienkui occurs in males and females) arrives, Jing Qi flows out, Yin and Yang harmonise, therefore it is possible to have children. At 24 the kidney Qi is balanced, and muscles and bones are strong, therefore true teeth grow and develop; . . . At 40 the kidney Qi decays, the teeth wither and the hair falls; . . . At 56 the liver Qi decays, the muscles cannot move, sexual substance is exhausted, there is little Jing, the kidney Zang decays, form and substance are all at their limits. At 64 the teeth and hair have gone. . . . Now that the five Zang are decayed, the muscles and bones have decayed, sexual substance is finished; therefore the hair becomes white, the body is heavy, walking is not upright and there are no children.'

'If people have children in old age this means that their normal span of life exceeds the normal limits, their Qi and blood vessels continue to penetrate normally, and the kidney Qi has a surplus.'

(Su Wen, shango tian zhen lun)

From the above quotations it can be seen that sexual ability and production of Jing, together with the growing processes of the whole body, are closely connected with the kidneys. Thus there is a saying: 'The kidneys are the root of Former Heaven.'

Case History. A woman of thirty had tried to become pregnant for five years. Tubal insufflation and the normal gynaecological tests were negative. Hormones and psychiatry had failed. She had slight lumbago, was slightly tense during intercourse and the kidney pulse was weak.

She was stimulated at K5 and several ancillary points, and became pregnant within one month. The tension during intercourse had also stopped but the lumbago remained.

The Kidneys Control the Fire of the Gate of Life

The fire of the Gate of Life is also called Minister Fire. The Gate of Life has the meaning of "the basis of life". Minister Fire is spoken of in referring to the Sovereign Fire controlled by the heart, and has the function of benefiting the Sovereign Fire. The kidney Zang controls water and stores Jing, and also controls the fire of the Gate of Life, and is the dwelling place of the original Yin and original Yang Qi (also called true Yin, true Yang or kidney Yin and kidney Yang). As a consequence all the functioning of the Zang and growth, together with conception and birth, all depend on the mutual assistance of kidney water, and fire of destiny.

'The Gate of Life is the sea of Jing and blood; spleen and stomach are the sea of water and nourishment; together they are the root of the five Zang and six Fu. Moreover the Gate of Life is the origin of original Qi and the dwelling place of water and fire; without this the Yin Qi of the five Zang cannot nourish and the Yang Qi of the five Zang cannot begin. The spleen and stomach use the earth of the middle region, and without fire they cannot create. . . . The spleen and stomach are the root of irrigation and obtain the Qi of Latter Heaven; the Gate of Life is the source of transformation and obtains the Qi of Former Heaven.'

'The Gate of Life has the strength of fire, called original Yang, and this is the fire of living things.'

(Jingyue quanshu)

The above view can be applied pathologically. In a person whose kidney Yin is deficient the deficiency may produce the Empty Yang Violent Above symptoms of dizziness in the head and eyes, caused by liver Yin being deficient. Alternatively, kidney Yin deficiency can cause the heart Yin to be deficient, producing heart Fire Violent and Vigorous symptoms such as palpitations, insomnia, etc. In severe cases it may cause the lung Yin to be deficient, producing the symptoms of dry cough, haemoptysis and spontaneous sweating.

Case History. A patient had palpitations for no apparent reason and had suffered from insomnia over a period of two years.

Pulse diagnosis showed an underactivity of the kidney and not an overactivity of the heart as expected.

Stimulation at K2 cured the condition.

Deficiency of kidney Yang may cause spleen Yang to be deficient, producing various types of diarrhoea. Or it may cause heart Qi to be empty and weak causing palpitations. In severe cases it results in an emptiness and weakness of lung Qi and produces dyspnoea and Yang empty with spontaneous sweating.

In all these cases one must nourish the kidney Yin or stimulate the kidney fire. On the other hand if the fire of the Gate of Life is deficient, this can cause a decrease of sexual desire or even impotence; conversely, if the minister fire is moving recklessly this can cause excessive sexual desire. In the first case one must warm and tonify the kidney Yang, and in the second strengthen water to regulate fire. This is consistant with the view that the fire of the Gate of Life of the kidney Zang is directly related to the function of reproduction.

The Kidneys Control the Bone and Marrow and Communicate with the Brain

The growth and development of the bones and marrow have a definite connection with the kidneys; for example the Su Wen recognises that 'bone paralysis disease' is due to 'kidney Qi hot'. When the kidneys receive heat which injures the kidney Yin, this causes the bones to wither and the marrow to decline, so that the loins and back cannot move and turn, and both legs are paralysed and wasted, and one cannot stand up straight.

'*The kidneys create bone and marrow.*'

(Su Wen, yinyang yingziang dalun)

'*If the kidneys do not create then the marrow cannot be full.*'

(Su Wen, nitiao lun)

The meeting and unifying of the marrow is in the brain.

'*The brain is the sea of marrow.*'

(Ling Shu, hailun)

'*All marrow belongs to the brain.*'

(Su Wen, wuzang shengcheng lun)

Since the brain is the meeting point of all marrow, and marrow is also formed by transformation of the kidney Jing, the kidney Zang is not only the basis of the Zang and Fu, but is also connected to the functioning of the bones, marrow and brain.

'*The kidneys are the official who does energetic work and excels by his ability and cleverness.*'

(Su Wen, linglan midian lun)

Thus if the kidneys are strong and full, then the Jing strength of the body is full and copious, physical energy is great, and at the same time the brain feels that it is strong, is clever and able. On the other hand if the kidney Qi is deficient, not only can it cause aching loins and painful bones, along with body weakness, but so also can it cause amnesia, insomnia, mental confusion, tinnitus, etc. To cure all these conditions one must tonify the kidneys to increase Jing and restore the kidney Qi.

Case History. A ten-year-old boy was near the bottom of his class. Previously he had been reasonably bright, but now his mind wandered and he was unable to concentrate.
He was cured after two treatments at K8.

This type of disturbance can only be cured if it is physiological. If the boy's laziness were due to his innate nature or to faulty upbringing, it would not have been cured by acupuncture. An astute clinical judgement is required to differentiate these different types, so as to decide which may be successfully treated.

The Kidneys Open the Holes in the Ears and the Two Yin

In the upper part of the body the kidneys open the holes in the ears, in the lower part they open the front and rear Yin (urethra and anus).

'The kidney Qi penetrates to the ears; if the kidney is harmonious then the five sounds can be heard.'

(Ling Shu, modu pian)

Clinically this means that those with an empty kidney often have tinnitus, in severe cases deafness; in early cases this may be treated by tonifying the kidneys.

The opening of the two Yin holes means chiefly the connection between the kidneys with micturition on the one hand and defaecation on the other; the kidneys are the water Zang and thus have the function of managing all the fluid in the body. This function however requires the collaboration of both kidney water and kidney fire, *i.e.,* the fire of the Gate of Life. Thus the correct functioning of micturition and defaecation, although related to the spleen, stomach, large intestine, bladder, etc., is also related to the fire of the Gate of Life. If kidney water is deficient it may cause dry stools and constipation or oliguria. If the fire of the Gate of Life is deficient it may cause diarrhoea, urinary incontinence or polyuria. If the kidney Zang's function is abnormal, Qi does not transform water, and this may cause the fluids to remain inside the body, causing retention of urine, oedema and ascites.

'The kidney is the gateway to the stomach; if the gateway is not functioning, water accumulates and acts according to its class. Above and below it overflows into the skin and causes swelling.'

(Su Wen, shuirexue lun)

This type of water retention caused by the kidney's loss of normal function may often be treated by stimulating the kidney Yin and kidney Yang.

371

Case History. A patient thought there might be something wrong as she urinated only twice a day. She also had extreme fatigue which nearly made me think of Addison's disease. (Kidney and adrenal cortex are related in acupuncture.)

The fatigue was reduced and the urination increased to nearer normal frequency by treatment of a large number of acupuncture points for a long time, using mainly kidney points.

The Kidneys, Adrenal Cortex and Gonads

The majority of diseases of the kidneys, adrenal cortex or gonads, are revealed by pulse diagnosis at the pulse of the kidney. If an underactivity of the pulse is found at this position, no more can be told than that there is a disturbance which has its most probable seat in one or other of these three organs. Further elucidation of the history or examination is required to differentiate the one affected.

I think the best explanation for the close relationship between these three organs lies in embryology, for all are derived, at least partially, from the urogenital ridge:

The testis is formed from the urogenital ridge, utilising both the pronephric duct and mesonephric tubules as excretory duct.

The ovary is likewise formed from the urogenital ridge. Its excretory duct of Müller is induced to arise by the presence of the pronephric duct, not forming if this is absent. In sharks the Müllerian duct arises by a longitudinal splitting of the pronephric duct.

The adrenal cortex also arises from the urogenital ridge, dorsal and medial to the gonad. The medulla arises separately from the same tissues as the sympathetic. Abberant adrenals may accompany the gonads or may be found buried within the kidneys.

The definitive mammalian kidney, the metanephros, is formed partly (ureter, renal pelvis, calyces, collecting tubules) from the pronephric or mesonephric duct, and partly from the nephrogenic cord (secretory tubules and Bowman's capsule), a specialisation of the urogenetial fold.

The above close embryological inter-relationship between the kidneys, adrenal cortex and gonads, is also reflected in their physiological function:

The adrenal cortex not only produces the cortisone-like hormones but also (*a*) the sex hormones—androgens, oestrogens and progesterone, and (*b*) influences water metabolism with either retention of urine or an excessive diuresis.

The sexual (gonad) effect of hyperadrenocortism, especially if due to a tumour, may be seen in the foetus as a pseudohermaphrodite, in prepubertal boys as pubertus praecox, in girls and women as masculinisation, and in the adult male as adrenal feminism.

The pulse diagnosis seems to record the primitive condition, that is when all three organs and functions were probably more or less the same.

The Kidneys and Bones

The bones, particularly the vertebral column, seem to be dependent on the kidney—or what might be called the kidney complex.

Any disturbance in the lumbar or sacral area is always found in the pulse of the kidney and bladder. This can perhaps be partly explained by the dorsal position of the kidneys and the close connection between the developing metanephros and the notochord.

From the above an association between the parathyroids and the kidney would be expected. This is in fact the case, as hyperparathyroidism with acidosis and phosphate retention, may be caused by advanced renal disease. Likewise hypoparathyroidism may be caused by chronic nephritis. The reverse may also be seen as primary hyperparathyroidism may cause nephrocalcinosis. Primary hypoparathyroidism though has no obvious renal symptoms. The above are of course advanced pathological states, but I am sure that investigation would show that the stimulation of points on the kidney meridian influences the production and circulation of parathormone.

Symptomatology

Main Meridian Symptoms

Hungry and yet no appetite for food, dark complexion like lacquered ash, rusty sputum, severe dyspnoea, wishing to stand when sitting and then the eyes blur as if blind, vision blurred, fondness for lying down and sleeping, frightened, nocturnal enuresis, hot lips, hot dry tongue, swollen pharynx, heart and chest feel oppressed, palpitations, heart suspended as though hungry, jaundice, abdominal distension, diarrhoea, bones ache, difficulty in walking, soles of feet hot and painful, extremely cold.

SYMPTOMS OF EXCESS

Intestinal blockage?, depression.

SYMPTOMS OF INSUFFICIENCY

Lumbago, sciatica.

Kidney Empty Symptoms

In kidney diseases the principal symptoms if Yin is empty, are spermatorrhoea, tinnitus, dental neuralgia, lumbago, sciatica, weakness and aching of the legs; if the condition is severe there can be paralysis.

At times this may affect other organs.

If kidney Yin is deficient and liver fire becomes vigorous and abundant, there will be: dry mouth, dry throat, dizziness in head and eyes, red face and ears, ears with a noise in them similar to that when covered by a sea-shell, also deafness.

If the lungs are affected then there may be coughing, night sweats, haemoptysis and emaciation. This is caused by deficient Yin and vigorous fire, which ascends and burns the lung metal.

Kidney and Heart

The kidneys belong to water, the heart belongs to fire, water and fire must contend. If kidney Yin is empty and heart fire blazes upwards, this can cause the Shen in the heart to be ill at ease, causing insomnia, etc. Conversely, if the heart Shen is ill at ease, or if Shen Qi is decayed and weak, this easily becomes a kidney disease, causing spermatorrhoea, tinnitus and lumbago.

Kidney Yang Empty Symptoms

If the kidney Yang is empty then Jing Qi cannot collect, and there is always Jing cold slippery leakage, *i.e.*, involuntary loss of seminal fluid, impotence, feeling of cold in waist and legs, numb and weak feet. If kidney Yang is deficient and cannot transform water, this can cause the water Qi to remain collected in the body, causing oliguria and pale lips; if the condition is severe there may be superficial oedema, heaviness of the body and ascites. Apart from this, the five types of diarrhoea are due to the kidney Yang being too empty and weak to warm and move the spleen Earth, thus causing diminution of the spleen's functions of transporting and transforming water and Qi, and of moving and transforming food and drink. Other symptoms caused by kidney Yang being empty and not being able to disseminate water fluid, include dryness of the mouth associated with drinking of much fluid, increased micturition, and a desire to urinate immediately after drinking. If the kidneys are empty and cannot receive Qi, then Qi rebels and escapes upwards producing numb and cold feet and Qi rebellious dyspnoea. If the condition is severe there is perspiration of the forehead and the pulse is deep, and there is oedema of the feet, in which case the disease has already become dangerous.

Connecting Meridian (Luo) Symptoms

SYMPTOMS OF EXCESS

Feeling of depression in the region of the heart, oliguria, constiptation.

SYMPTOMS OF INSUFFICIENCY

Pain at the waist.

Muscle Meridian Symptoms

Spasm or pain in the sole of the foot and those places passed by the muscle meridian. There may also be epilepsy, convulsions and generalised muscular spasms. If the disease occurs posteriorly the patient cannot bend forward. If it occurs anteriorly the patient cannot lean back or look up, i.e., if the Yang is diseased there is difficulty in flexion, if the Yin is diseased there is difficulty in extension.

Course of Meridians

Kidney Main Meridian

Principal Course

The meridian starts on the sole of the foot at K1, goes up the embryologically anterior and inner surface of the leg, over the abdomen and chest near the midline, to end near the sterno-clavicular joint at K27.

Special Details

The meridian begins under the little toe and then goes to K1. (According to some descriptions the points round the internal malleolus are in the following order: K2, K3, K4, K5, K6, K7.

In other books K2, K6, K5, K4, K3, K7. Occasionally there are other variations.)

From K8 to Sp6 to K9.

From the inside of the thigh, the main meridian goes to Gv1, then up the spine to the kidneys to which it belongs, thereafter connecting with the bladder.

From the bladder it goes to Cv4, Cv3, K11 and thence over the abdomen and chest to K27.

The direct meridian goes from the kidney through the liver and diaphragm to ramify in the lungs, whence it follows the trachea to enter the root of the tongue.

From the lungs a branch goes to the heart, spreads over the chest, thence going to Cv17. This branch joins the circulation-sex meridian, which may be taken to be the branch from K22 to Cx1.

Kidney Connecting Meridian (Luo)—K6

The meridian begins at the ankle at K6, and ascends with the meridian to the pericardium and thence penetrates to the back. It links with the bladder meridian Luo.

Kidney Muscle Meridian

The meridian begins under the little toe, follows the course of the spleen meridian for a short part of the foot, and then unites at the heel; ascends the lower leg and unites at the medial corner of the popliteal fossa where it meets the bladder muscle meridian; ascends the inner side of the thigh together with the spleen muscle meridian to unite at the genitalia; ascends the spine to unite at the occiput where it meets the bladder muscle meridian.

Important Points

Wood	K1	Sedation
Fire	K2	
Earth	K5	
Metal	K7	Tonification
Water	K10	Water point of Yin water meridian
Source	K5	
Luo	K6	
Xi	K4	
Alarm	G25	
Associated	B23	

CHAPTER X

CIRCULATION-SEX

(Envelope of the Heart or Pericardium)

Traditional Chinese and Western Scientific Conceptions

The Chinese characters for this meridian mean, literally, 'envelope of the heart'. In modern Chinese the same characters are used to denote the pericardium, something which was not known in the early days of acupuncture. I have used the word circulation-sex, as it is used by several other European doctors. The function of the meridian is partially concerned with the circulation. However the pulse position of this meridian (3rd position right deep) represents both this meridian and the kidney meridian, particularly the Mingmen, which is concerned with the sexual function of the kidney. Hence the name circulation-sex.

This meridian is the external protector of the heart and has the function of guarding the heart Zang. At the same time it has the function of administering the controlling action of the heart.

'The pericardium is the organ from which the feeling of happiness comes.'

(Su Wen, linglan midian lun)

'The heart is the great controller of the Zang and Fu . . . if an evil enters the heart it will injure it as the heart cannot withstand it; if the heart is injured then the Shen will leave and if the Shen leaves then one will die. Thus the presence of evil in the heart depends on the pericardium.'

(Ling Shu, xieke pian)

Thus it was recognised that the pericardium can receive evils on behalf of the heart. For example, symptoms such as confused Shen, trismus, incoherent speech, etc., are all 'evil entering the pericardium', and from the point of view of treatment one uses the method of purifying the heart and sedating fire, or purifying the heart and pacifying Shen.

Case History. A patient in her thirties had recurrent bouts of severe depression, during several of which she had unsuccessfully tried to commit suicide. She thought the cause of her depressions lay in her upbringing as a child, which involved more abstract psychology than common sense. During the previous fifteen years she had visited many psychiatrists and had tried several drugs—both of which had helped, though only to a minimal extent.

Chinese pulse diagnosis and symptomatology were inconclusive at least to me. The first four treatments, during which several meridians were used, had no effect. The fifth treatment in which I stimulated the circulation-sex meridian at Cx7 for the first time, caused her to feel nearly normal by the next day, the cure being complete with one further treatment. As this was a long standing history, a few booster treatments were required for a further two years to prevent recurrence.

What is precisely governed by this (and the triple warmer) meridian is less specifically stated in Chinese texts than the influence of the other ten meridians. Clinically it is also harder to define its effect in terms of understandable anatomy or physiology. Amongst its functions are cardiac, circulatory, renal and mental.

The pericardium itself seems hardly worth considering amongst the important organs, though it should be remembered that in the human embryo the pericardium is as big as the head and is separated from it only by the pharyngeal membrane. Presumably the size of an organ has at least a little to do with its importance.

Symptomatology

Main Meridian Symptoms

Heart feels hot, forearm and elbow stiffen and feel constrained, axilla becomes swollen, chest and ribs feel oppressed, thumping and lurching of the heart, cardiac pain going into throat, face flushed, pyrexia, vision blurred, eyes discoloured, wild laughter without ceasing, hot palm of hand.

SYMPTOMS OF EXCESS

Cardiac pain.

SYMPTOMS OF INSUFFICIENCY

Head and neck stiff.

I have not been able to find in Chinese texts a systematic classification into HOT, COLD, FULL, EMPTY, as for the other meridians. These may though be calculated from basic principles.

Connecting Meridian (Luo) Symptoms

SYMPTOMS OF EXCESS

Painful heart.

SYMPTOMS OF INSUFFICIENCY

Stiffness and inability to turn the head.

Muscle Meridian Symptoms

Muscular spasm, pain and dysfunction along the course of the meridian. Haemoptysis with pain in the chest.

Course of Meridians

Circulation-Sex Main Meridian

Principal Course

Starting lateral to the nipple at Cx1, the meridian arches over the axilla, to go down the middle of the anterior surface of the arm between the other two arm Yin meridians and ends at the middle finger at Cx9.

Special Details

The meridian begins in the middle of the chest, emerging from the pericardium to which it belongs, and represented by Cv17. It penetrates the diaphragm and passes through the abdomen being connected with the upper middle and lower divisions of the triple warmer; this part of its course is represented by the points Cv12 and Cv7.

A branch from Cv17 goes across the chest to Cx1 and thence down the arm to Cx9.

A branch leaves Cx8 to go to T1.

Circulation-Sex Connecting Meridian (Luo)—Cx6

The meridian begins above the wrist at Cx6 and ascends with its meridian. Links with the circulation-sex meridian Luo.

Circulation-Sex Muscle Meridian

The meridian begins at the middle finger and goes up the forearm to unite at the elbow; continuing along the upper arm to unite below the armpit; thereafter dispersing through the front and back of the chest.

A branch from the axilla disperses in the chest and unites at the cardia.

Important Points

Wood	Cx9	Tonification
Fire	Cx8	Fire point of Yin Ministerial fire meridian
Earth	Cx7	Sedation
Metal	Cx5	
Water	Cx3	
Source	Cx7	
Luo	Cx6	
Xi	Cx4	
Alarm	?Cv17 or ?Cv15	
Associated	B14	

CHAPTER XI

TRIPLE WARMER

Traditional Chinese and Western Scientific Conceptions

The Division of the Three Warmers According to their Position

The Triple Warmer is one of the six Fu, but there are differences between it and the other Fu. The body is divided into the Upper Warmer, the Middle Warmer, and the Lower Warmer. From the cardia of the stomach to the base of the tongue, including the chest, and in particular the heart and lungs, is the region of the Upper Warmer. From the cardia to the pylorus of the stomach, including the upper abdomen, and in particular the spleen and stomach, is the region of the Middle Warmer. From the pylorus to the two Yin (urethra and anus), including the lower abdomen and in particular the liver, kidneys, large and small intestines and bladder, is the region of the Lower Warmer.

'*The Upper Warmer, from the lower diaphragm below the heart to the upper orifice of the stomach controls receiving and does not expel. The Middle Warmer, at the middle of the stomach, has a middle position, controls the rotting and ripening of food and water. The Lower Warmer, at the upper orifice of the bladder, controls the division of the pure and impure, controls expelling and not receiving in order to transmit.*'

(Nanjing sanshiyinan shuo)

The Functional Division of the Triple Warmer

In general terms the function of the Triple Warmer is to circulate Qi blood and fluid, to rot and ripen food and water, and to harmonise the digestion of solid and liquid food.

'*Water and food enter through the mouth; they have five tastes; each one flowing into its own sea; the fluids all move along their own paths; therefore the three Warmers emit Qi in order to warm the flesh; that which fills the skin is Jin, that which remains and does not move is Ye.*'

(Ling Shu, wulong jinyue bielun)

'*The Triple Warmer is the path of water and food, the beginning and end of Qi.*'

(Nanjing, sanshiyinan)

The above quotations explain that the function of the Triple Warmer is to cause the Qi, blood and fluid which come from water and food to circulate in the skin and flesh and between the Zang and Fu; the stomach and spleen on the one hand and the Middle Warmer on the other (both are in the same region) control the rotting and ripening of water and food.

'*The Triple Warmer is the middle draining Fu and the digestion comes from this. It belongs to the bladder.*'

(Ling Shu, benshu pian)

Thus the Triple Warmer also has the function of clearing the digestive tract. However, the functions of the separate warmers are in control of specific things, and are closely associated with the organs which they include.

Upper Warmer

'*The Upper Warmer is like mist (fog, mist, vapour etc.).*'

(Ling Shu, yingwei shenghui pian)

This means that the upper warmer is described as having much Qi (the lungs control Qi, the chest is the sea of Qi) and its function is similar to mist in its all pervading irrigation. The Qi of the Upper Warmer originates in the Middle Warmer.

'*The Upper Warmer is a prime mover, it distributes the five food tastes, vapourises into the skin, fills the body, moistens the hair on the body, is like the irrigation of mist and dew, and is called Qi.*'

(Ling Shu, jueqi pian)

'*The spleen scatters Jing, Qi is like a cloud, a mist, and returns to the lungs. This is called Upper Warmer like mist.*'

(Zhangshi leijing)

The Upper Warmer's function of circulating Qi around the whole body and moistening and vapourising the skin, filling the body, moistening the hair and the exterior skin of the body, obtains nourishment and so develops the function of protecting the outside— a function which is called Wei Qi. If the Upper Warmer loses its normal function, the circulation becomes blocked, the skin and the space between the skin and flesh cannot obtain the warmth of Wei Qi, the opening and closing of the sweat holes (pores) is not effective, and thus may produce the symptoms of cold or fever. Apart from this the Upper Warmer also has the function of 'controlling reception'. The so-called reception includes both that of air and food and drink. Because the lungs (which control breathing) and the stomach (which controls the receiving of food and water) both operate in (literally 'open holes in') the Upper Warmer, the Upper Warmer is said to have the function of 'controlling reception.'

Middle Warmer

'The Middle Warmer is like foam (froth, foam, bubbles etc.).'
(Ling Shu, yingwei shenghui pian)
This refers to the appearance of the food and drink that has been transformed by the spleen and stomach. From the point of view of the scope of the Middle Warmer and the function of the Zang and Fu, which it includes, the most important aspects are the moving and transforming of water and food and the distilling of Qi, blood and fluid, which then nourish the whole body. Within this process, the power of transformation and movement includes the functions of the spleen and stomach and also the Lower Warmer.

'The Middle Warmer also unites the middle of the stomach, and the Qi which is received there flushes the dregs, distils the fluid, transforms its essential and fine parts, and pours upwards into the lung meridian which then transforms it into blood.'
(Ling Shu, yingwei shenghui pian)
'The Middle Warmer receives Qi, extracts the juice and changes it into a substance. This is called blood.'
(Ling Shu, jueqi pian)
Thus the function of the Middle Warmer is principally to take water and food and transform it into Qi blood and fluid, all of which have the function of nourishing. The Middle Warmer's attribute of being 'like foam' is the result of its physiological movement of 'changing, transforming, distilling the flushing'. If the action of the Middle Warmer is blocked it will harm the process of digestion and the transformation of Qi and blood.

Lower Warmer

'The Lower Warmer is like a drain.'
(Ling Shu, yingwei shenghui pian)
'Drain means the flowing and draining of water. The Lower Warmer controls emitting and not receiving, departing and not returning.'
(Zhangshi leijing)
Thus the principal function of the Lower Warmer is the draining and flushing of the pure and impure, and also the expulsion of urine and faeces.

'*The Lower Warmer helps the function of separation and passes the dregs into the large intestine.*'

'*The Lower Warmer permeates the fluid, unites with the bladder, controls emitting and not entering, divides pure and impure.*'

One type of diarrhoea is due to the pure and the impure not being separated, with retention or incontinence of urine, the bladder Qi having lost its function. This may be due to a dysfunction of the Lower Warmer.

The Relationship between the Triple Warmer and the Pericardium

The Triple Warmer and the pericardium are coupled meridians. In Chinese parlance they have an exterior and interior mutual relationship.

'*The Triple Warmer is the external protector of the Zang and Fu, the pericardium is the external protector of the heart, like the great walls of the Imperial Palace; thus both belong to Yang, and both are called Minister Fire. Moreover the meridians communicate reciprocally and are mutually exterior and interior.*'

(Zhangshi leijing)

In the above context the pericardium is called Yang because it protects the heart, taking upon itself diseases which would otherwise affect the heart; thus it is like the wall protecting the Imperial Palace. In the interior-exterior relationship of Triple Warmer and pericardium, however, the pericardium is Yin.

The heart and small intestine are called Sovereign Fire (or sometimes Princely Fire) while the pericardium and Triple Warmer are called Minister Fire, because the Minister protects the Sovereign. In other words the triple warmer and pericardium have protective functions, protecting on the one hand the Zang and the Fu in general, and on the other hand the heart.

Case History. A patient was excessively tired, so tired that she usually returned to bed again after breakfast. Her skin was hot, the superficial veins were always dilated, she had migraine and was nervous. T1 cured her fatigue.

Symptomatology

Main Meridian Symptoms

Deafness, confused mind, pharyngitis, swollen jaws, pain in outer corner of eye, pain behind the ear and over mastoid, perspiring for no reason, distension of lower abdominal, inability to urinate, pain or loss of function along course of meridian.

SYMPTOMS OF EXCESS

Elbow in position of flexion.

SYMPTOMS OF INSUFFICIENCY

Elbow cannot be flexed.

Upper Warmer Symptoms

Includes principally the arm greater Yin lung meridian and the arm absolute Yin pericardium meridian.

The symptoms of the lung meridian are:—headache, slight dislike of wind and cold, body hot and spontaneous sweating, thirst, and possibly coughing with absence of thirst.

The pulse is neither slowed down nor tight, but moving and rapid.

If the condition is transmitted to the pericardium meridian, then the tongue is deep red, and there is agitation and thirst. If the condition is severe then the Shen is confused, causing incoherent speech, restless sleep, stiff tongue and cold limbs.

Middle Warmer Symptoms

Includes principally the leg Yang Ming stomach meridian and the leg greater Yin spleen meridian. Yang Ming controls dryness and the greater Yin controls damp.

The symptoms of the stomach meridian are:—no dislike of cold but dislike of heat, more severe in the afternoon, sweating, face and eyes red, harsh breathing, dense stools, dysuria, dry mouth and thirsty.

The pulse is large.

The tongue is furred old-yellow; if the condition is severe, it may be black and prickly.

The symptoms of the spleen meridian are:—moderate sensation of heat, comparatively heavy feeling after noon, mental dullness, head feels swollen and body heavy, melancholy feeling in chest and no appetite, dislike of all food and wish to vomit, micturition infrequent, defaecation sluggish, stools possibly very loose.

The pulse is slowed down.

The tongue has white and greasy fur.

Lower Warmer Symptoms

Includes principally the leg lesser Yin kidney meridian and the leg absolute Yin liver meridian. If the disease has reached this stage, then the fluid has withered and dried up.

The symptoms of the former (kidney) are:—comparative peace during day but agitation during night, dry mouth and no wish to drink, painful throat, inability to speak because of ulcers, the heart is agitated, oliguria, reddish urine.

The symptoms of the latter (liver) are:—alternating feelings of cold and heat, painful and hot heart, misery and melancholy, sometimes dry vomiting, perhaps headache and vomiting of saliva, heart feels hungry but unable to eat, emotions sometimes extremely depressed. If the symptoms are in upper part of body the mouth is dry and feels rotten; if in lower part of body then there may be diarrhoea and heaviness in rectum, perhaps wind-moving convulsions with feeling of cold, contracted testicles and painful abdomen, deafness.

Connecting Meridian (Luo) Symptoms

SYMPTOMS OF EXCESS

Restriction in movement of elbow joint.

SYMPTOMS OF INSUFFICIENCY

Elbow joint too flaccid, over-relaxed.

Muscle Meridian Symptoms

Muscular spasm, pain or dysfunction along the course of the meridian muscle.

Course of Meridians

Triple Warmer Main Meridian

Principal Course

The meridian starts at the end of the 4th finger at T1, goes up the posterior surface of the arm between the two other Yang meridians of the arms; thence it goes across the shoulders and neck, behind the ear, and over the face, to end at the lateral corner of the eyebrows at T23.

Special Details

The meridian begins at T1 at the tip of the 4th finger and goes up the arm to the shoulder at T14.

(? From T14 via Si12 to T15).

From T15 to G21, and over the shoulder to S12.

From here it descends to spread through the chest and is connected with the pericardium, going from S12 (?via Cx1) to Cv17.

From Cv17 it penetrates the diaphragm and goes to the three divisions of the triple warmer to which it belongs, represented by Cv17, Cv12 and Cv7.

A branch leaves S12 and goes (? via B11) to Gv14. From Gv14 to T16, T17, T18, T19, T20.

From T20 (? via G6) to G5, G4, G14, B1 down the naso-labial groove and lower jaw, to curl up the middle of the cheek and end at Si18. (Or possibly from T20 via an S shaped course to the eye at B1.)

From T17 a branch enters the ear to emerge in front of it at Si19, and thence goes via T21, T22 and T23 to end at G1. If the previously mentioned branch goes directly from T20 to B1, then this branch goes from T22 looping round the jaw, to Si18 and G1, to end at T23.

(? From T16 to G20 to G11.)

Triple Warmer Connecting Meridian (Luo)—T5

The meridian begins above the wrist at T5, goes up the outer surface of the arm and floods the chest. It links with the circulation-sex meridian Luo.

Triple Warmer Muscle Meridian

The meridian begins at the end of the fourth finger, unites at the wrist; goes up the forearm, unites at the elbow; ascends the upper arm goes over the shoulder, to the neck where it meets the small intestine muscle meridian. A branch goes to the jaw and links with the root of the tongue. The main muscle meridian ascends past the teeth to the ear, and then moves laterally to the outer corner of the eyes, whence it goes to the upper part of the temple, where it unites.

Triple Warmer and Circulation-Sex Divergent Meridians

Triple Warmer Divergent Meridian

The triple warmer divergent meridian leaves the triple warmer main meridian at the shoulder. One part goes to the crown of the head; the other part leaves the supra-clavicular fossa to disperse through the three divisions of the triple warmer in the chest and abdomen.

Circulation-Sex Divergent Meridian

The circulation-sex divergent meridian leaves the circulation-sex main meridian a little below the axilla. It enters the chest where it divides, the one part following the course of the triple warmer divergent meridian into the abdomen the other going to the throat, and thence behind the ear, where it meets the triple warmer meridian over the mastoid process.

Important Points

Metal	T1	
Water	T2	
Wood	T3	Tonification
Fire	T6	Fire point of Yang Ministerial fire meridian
Earth	T10	Sedation
Source	T4	
Luo	T5	
Xi	T7	
Alarm	Cv5 (Cv7, Cv12, Cv17)	
Associated	B22	

CHAPTER XII

GALL BLADDER

Traditional Chinese and Western Scientific Conceptions

The Gall-Bladder is a True and Upright Official: it Controls Judgements

'*The gall-bladder is the true and upright official who excels in making decisions.*'

(Su Wen, linglan midian lun)

'*All the other eleven Zang and Fu make their decisions in the gall-bladder.*'

(Su Wen, liujie zangxiang lun)

Case History. A man in his forties was unable to decide what he wanted to do, which country abroad he wished to visit for a holiday, which car he wanted to buy, etc. He was not like a spoilt child, though this could be suggested by the above symptoms. He had a few other gall-bladder/liver symptoms, such as weakness of the muscles and the inability to eat many of the richer foods.

Pulse diagnosis showed an under-activity of gall-bladder and liver. He was about half cured of all his mental and physical symptoms after a long course of treatment, involving the use of gall-bladder and liver points.

The Gall-Bladder is the Fu of Internal Purity

'*The gall-bladder is a true and upright official; it stores pure and clean fluid, therefore it is called the Fu of internal purity. That with which all the other Fu are filled is impure, and only the gall-bladder is filled with the pure.*'

(Zhangshi leijing)

Although the gall-bladder is one of the Fu, it is different from the rest. The other Fu either store or transport impure matter such as water and nourishment, faeces and urine; only the gall-bladder fluid, bile, is not impure.

The Reciprocal Relationship between the Liver and the Gall-Bladder

The ability to make plans and judgements is not only decided by the strength or weakness of the gall-bladder Qi, but is also connected with the liver, because the liver and gall-bladder are mutually exterior and interior.

'The gall-bladder is appended to the liver and they help one another. Even if the liver Qi is strong, without the gall-bladder there is no decision If the liver and gall-bladder mutually assist, bravery and courage are then created.'

(Zhangshi leijing)

Thus the idea that the liver controls planning and the gall-bladder controls deciding have a mutual connection. This may be seen clinically in those whose gall-bladder fire is vigorous and abundant, where there are often the symptoms of liver Yang partially violent, in which case the patient becomes agitated and easily enraged. If the gall-bladder Qi is deficient there is often a partial decaying of liver Qi and these patients are often timid and reluctant to speak. In treating these cases, liver-balancing medicine will usually sedate the spleen fire; and spleen-fire sedating medicine will usually balance the liver.

The exterior-interior relationship of the gall-bladder and liver is more intimate than that of other coupled organs so that at times it is impossible to distinguish between one and the other. Perhaps some of the functions ascribed to the liver should be classified under the gall-bladder and vice versa. For this reason both sections should be read together.

Case History. A man told me that his wife had been bad tempered, brooding and moody for a few years, and that the slightest thing would cause her to explode in an outburst of temper. Previously she had been quite different—it was as if she were now a different person. The lady in question was quite willing to be treated, for she had herself noticed that her personality had become changed, against her own wish, and she did not like being bad tempered. She felt there was something wrong which she could not control with her own will power.

Pulse diagnosis showed an over-activity of the liver and gall-bladder. Her face, forehead and neck, were slightly purple, as may sometimes be noticed in this condition. She was markedly better from the first treatment (Liv8 and G40), to the delight of her husband, children and herself.

She was cured in three treatments. To keep everything in check, I saw her for one treatment at half-yearly intervals afterwards.

Symptomatology

Main Meridian Symptoms

Bitter taste in mouth, deafness, frequent sighing, aching chest and ribs, inability to turn body easily, skin becoming pasty coloured, pain in temples, pain below jaws, pain in outer corner of eye, swelling of supra-clavicular fossa, swelling in front of neck, redness and swelling under armpits, pain under ribs, perspiration comes for no reason, pain or loss of function along course of meridian.

SYMPTOMS OF EXCESS

Limbs slightly cold, ? stupor.

SYMPTOMS OF INSUFFICIENCY

Weakness of the legs, difficulty in standing once seated.

Gall-Bladder Cold Symptoms

The gall-bladder has the function of purifying the Yang; if pure Yang cannot spread this can give rise to symptoms in the chest and stomach, a troubled feeling and melancholy, dizziness in the head and vomiting, insomnia, tongue furred slippery and greasy. The reasons for this are that pure Yang does not ascend and turbid phlegm is not transformed.

Gall-Bladder Hot Symptoms

Bitter mouth and proneness to anger, clear bitter fluid suddenly appears in mouth from the stomach, possibly alternating cold and heat, restless sleep at night, pulse wiry and rapid. At the same time there is often foggy vision, deafness, ribs are painful. The bitter mouth symptom is usually caused by liver heat influencing the gall-bladder. If gall-bladder heat includes damp this can cause yellow jaundice, and if severe, troubled heart and nervousness, inability to sit or lie down peacefully.

Gall-Bladder Empty Symptoms

The causes of gall-bladder empty and liver empty are basically the same, both being concerned with blood empty and deficient. Thus both liver and gall-bladder empty have the symptoms of dizziness of the head, susceptibility to fright, blurred vision. However gall-bladder empty also has the important symptom of insomnia, cowardliness, timidity, fondness of sighing.

Gall-Bladder Full Symptoms

If the gall-bladder is full then it is easy to become angry, the chest feels full and melancholy, and there may be swelling and pain below ribs. If the condition is severe then there may be pain and inability to turn the body, face coloured like dust, dry skin, fondess for sleep, and pain in sides of head, forehead and corners of eyes.

The pulse is wiry and full.

Connecting Meridian (Luo) Symptoms

SYMPTOMS OF EXCESS

Cold in extremities.

SYMPTOMS OF INSUFFICIENCY

Legs weak, and inability to walk, or to rise after sitting down.

Muscle Meridian Symptoms

Muscular cramp of the fourth toe, of the outer side of the knee, the knee cannot be bent, cramp in the muscles at the back of the knee. Muscular pain at front and side of thigh, buttocks and anal region, lateral side of the abdomen and thorax, lateral side of the neck and face.

The left and right sides of the meridian are linked via the summit of the cranium and also partly follow the course of the Yin and Yang qiao mo, hence if there is an injury to the left temple there may be paralysis of the right leg.

Course of Meridians

Lung Main Meridian

Principal Course

The meridian starts at the outer corner of the eye at G1, zig-zags over the side of the head, goes down the lateral side of the body and embryologically posterior (external) surface of the leg, between the other two Yang meridians, to end at the fourth toe at G44.

Special Details

The meridian starts at the outer corner of the eye at G1 and then covers a zig-zag course over the side of the head and neck to G21.

From G21 the meridian goes over the shoulder to Gv14, B11, (?T15), Si12 to S12.

From S12 to G22, G23 (? via Cx1 and Liv14) to G24 and thence down the side of the abdomen to G29.

From G29 over the sacrum to B31, B33, Gv1 to G30.

From G30, down the outside of the leg to G44.

Sometimes the position of G35 and G36 are reversed.

A branch from G1 goes to S8, Si18, S3 to S12 where it meets the main meridian. The branch then continues over the chest to G24 (possibly Cx1 and Liv14 are on this branch).

From G24 the branch continues over the abdomen via Liv13 (or possibly Liv13 is on the main meridian between G24 and G25) to S30 and thence joins the main meridian at G30.

A branch leaves G20, goes to T17, penetrates the ear to emerge at Si19 (with possibly a continuation to S2 and thence T22).

From G7 a branch goes to T20 (or possibly T20 lies on the main meridian between G7 and G8).

A branch goes from G14 to B1.

(? From G3 to S1 to G4.)

A branch goes from G41 to Liv1.

Gall Bladder connecting Meridian (Luo)—G37

The meridian begins above the external malleolus at G37, and descends to the dorsum of the foot. It links with the liver meridian Luo.

Gall-Bladder Muscle Meridian

The meridian begins on the lateral side of the end of the fourth toe, unites at the external malleolus; ascends the lower leg and unites at the lateral side of the knee. Another part of the meridian continues up the lateral side of the leg and unites on the anterior surface of the thigh at S32. The main meridian muscle continues upwards and sends a branch to unite at the anus. It continues over the lateral side of the body and front of the shoulder joint to unite at the supraclavicular fossa. A separate course runs anteriorly to link with the breast. The main meridian muscle ascends behind the ear to the top of the cranium where it meets the division from the other side of the body; it descends at the side of the jaw, and then ascends to unite at the side of the nose. A branch ascends to unite at the outer corner of the eye.

Gall-Bladder and Liver Divergent Meridians

Gall-Bladder Divergent Meridian

The gall-bladder divergent meridian leaves the gall-bladder main meridian at the buttocks, which it encircles, to enter the pubic area, where it meets the liver meridian. The divergence ascends to the lower border of the ribs whence it enters the gall bladder, to which it belongs, and disperses in the liver. It ascends to penetrate the heart and thence goes along the side of the neck, jaw and cheek, to the outer corner of the eye where it meets the main gall-bladder meridian.

Liver Divergent Meridian

The liver divergent meridian leaves the main liver meridian on the dorsum of the foot; it ascends up the inside of the leg to the pubic area where it meets the gall-bladder divergent meridian, whose course it then follows to the outer corner of the eye.

Important Points

Metal	G44	
Water	G43	Tonification
Wood	G41	Wood point of Yang wood meridian
Fire	G38	Sedation
Earth	G34	
Source	G40	
Luo	G37	
Xi	G36	
Alarm	G24	
Associated	B19	

CHAPTER XIII

LIVER

Traditional Chinese and Western Scientific Conceptions

The Storing of Blood by the Liver

'*The liver stores blood.*'

(Ling Shu, bian shen pian)

'*Thus when men lie down the blood returns to the liver.*'

(Su Wen, wuzang shengcheng lun)

Wang Bing's commentary to the above says 'When man moves the blood travels to several meridians; when man is still the blood returns to the liver Zang.'

These extracts explain that the liver has the function of storing the blood and regulating the amount of blood. Clinically, vomiting of blood may be caused by violent anger, and can be cured by treating the liver; the theory is expressed as 'anger injures the liver', and 'the liver stores blood'. At a time of great anger the Jing Shen receives a violent stimulus and this affects the normal functioning of the liver, causing the liver Qi to rebel upwards, so that it cannot maintain the function of storing the blood; the blood then rises with the Qi and flows out of the body. Thus the liver must be balanced before this complaint can be cured.

'The storing of blood by the liver,' probably refers to the portal circulation, which acts as a blood reservoir as outlined in the above three quotations. In dogs there is even an involuntary sphincter muscle at the junction of the hepatic vein and the inferior vena cava. Haemoptysis may be the result of oesophageal varices consequent on portal obstruction.

Haemorrhoids are at least partially associated with the liver, presumably because the portal circulation passes through the liver. Patients who have had mild haemorrhoids, which did not bother them so that they forgot to mention it when I treated some other condition, have frequently noticed an improvement in their haemorrhoids if I treated their liver (either because of their other condition or because of the pulse and other methods of diagnosis).

Sometimes haemorrhoids are better treated via the bladder meridian for the bladder divergent meridian passes alongside the anus. B56, B57, B58 may be used. Gvɪ or other points in the sacral area may also help. Gv20, at the opposite end of the body to the anus is useful, working via the law of polarity.

Patients who bruise easily normally have a dysfunction of their liver. This is frequently the case with women who may bruise with the slightest pressure on their skin, or even spontaneously for no apparent reason. Such conditions can presumably be at least partially explained by the fact that the clotting factors in the blood, such as prothrombin, fibrinogen and heparin are manufactured in the liver. This symptom is very marked in those who are jaundiced, making surgery with adequate haemostasis difficult.

Case History. A lady bruised so easily that one had the incorrect impression her husband had maltreated her. She was improved, but not completely cured, by treating the liver.

In general, at least in my experience, this condition of bruising easily can usually be improved by treating the liver, though sometimes it may be completely cured and sometimes this treatment has no effect at all.

The Liver as the General Official and Controller of Planning

The liver has the functions of guarding against insults from outside, considering plans, and resisting disease and evils.

The detoxification of drugs takes place mostly in the liver. Hence patients who have taken many drugs, which is often the case, will have to have their livers treated in addition to whatever other disease they have. Sometimes it may be difficult to distinguish the original disease from the drug induced disease.

The Relationship between the Liver and Muscles, and Finger and Toe Nails

The muscles are controlled by the liver.

If when examining a patient there are symptoms such as aching and pain of the muscles and bones, muscular spasm and cramp, spasms of the muscles of the tongue, it may be deduced that there is disease of the liver and muscles.

The strength and thickness of the finger nails and their colour and texture are also determined by the state of health of the liver. For instance, in patients whose liver (and blood) is deficient, the finger nails are often soft and thin, the colour underneath the nails is very pale, and in some cases the nails are cracked. Moreover the nails of old people may be withered when the liver and blood are no longer flourishing.

'*The liver* . . . *its external manifestation is in the nails.*'

(Su Wen, lu chie zhan zang lun)

'*Nails are the surplus of muscles.*'

(Zhubing yuanhou lun)

A patient whose liver is not functioning correctly normally finds that in the morning, when he feels worst, he is only able to run slowly; in the evening when he feels better, he can run faster. Other muscular activities follow the same hepatic pattern.

The above can perhaps be supported by the fact that parenteral bile salts cause skeletal muscular hyperactivity, twitching and spasm. (Ries and Still, 1930.)

The Relationship between the Liver and the Eyes

In general, red, swollen, painful and acute eye diseases belong to the liver fire ascending group; the symptoms of mild blurred vision, photophobia, spots in front of the eyes, weak eyesight, eyes dizzy, both eyes dry or night blindness, generally belong to the 'blood not nourishing the liver' group.

In clinical practice the liver is the organ most often associated with eye diseases. The local point which has the most effect on the eye is G20—a point that is the particular speciality of Dr Li Zhi-ming of Peking.

Why the eye and liver should be related to one another, as observed in clinical experience, and as recognised in the laws of acupuncture, is not clear. Possibly melanin is a partial bridge. On the one hand melanin is produced in the liver: tyrosin→tyrosinase→melanin; on the other hand the choroid of the eye is the only part of the body where melanin is stored in quantity. In jaundice melanin is also produced in the skin by melanoblasts.

Case History. A patient was only able to read a book for half an hour, after which his eyes were too tired to read any more. He had been to a good ophthalmologist and optician.

Pulse diagnosis showed an over-activity of the liver. He was cured in five treatments by using Liv8 and G20. He can now read for several hours at a time.

Psychology

The liver likes cheerfulness and reasonableness; anger and depression are the main causes of psychosomatic hepatic diseases.

In nearly all psychiatric diseases where depression or outbursts of anger are the leading symptom, the liver is most often the physical component of the disease. Once a psychiatric disorder has become so profound that the liver is actually affected, it would require extremely intensive psychotherapy to cure. My own experience is that the depression can more easily be cured by treating the liver.

Depression is a well-known complication of jaundice. For there to be a depression, however, it is not necessary for the hepatic damage to be of such a degree as to produce jaundice. Possibly different factors are involved from those which are invariably associated with jaundice. In German, if someone is bad tempered, one asks: 'Has a flea crawled across your liver?'

Case History. A patient was continuously depressed, took no interest in life and hardly did any work. He was cured by treating Liv6 and Liv13. At the same time he noticed that his appetite increased and that his bowel motions became darker.

The Liver and Water Retention

There are many causes of water retention, the more obvious being renal and cardiac. The liver however plays a dominant role in a certain type which is characterised by a very slight puffiness of the subcutaneous tissues, giving the skin a slightly thickened appearance. It is not a pitting oedema, nor does gravity play a role. Normally this puffiness of the skin is fairly generalised over the whole body. A localised form of this oedema occurs supraorbitally, as a puffy swelling between the eyebrows and eyelids.

Those women who gain or lose several pounds in weight during the course of a single day, or who gain more than the usual amount of weight premenstrually, usually have a dysfunction of the liver. In addition they often have premenstrual tension and depression, and this can be cured at the same time via the liver.

In a few women, the water retention is localised in the breasts, though in the reverse sense to the above example, for when there is a dysfunction of the liver the breasts become small; when the liver function has been normalised, the breasts enlarge to their normal size. There may be a difference by as much as four inches in the measurement round the bust. This association between liver and breast could be explained via the gall bladder muscle meridian, which goes to the breast.

Desoxycholic acid, one of the bile acids, exerts a mild diuretic action in patients with heart failure and oedema. (Modell & Gold, 1944.)

Case History. A patient gained four pounds whenever she did not feel well, with puffiness of the skin, supraorbital oedema, headache and spots before the eyes. She was cured by merely treating the liver at Liv8.

The Liver and Allergy

Most allergies can be cured at least partially, by treating the liver, though the treatment need not, of course, be by acupuncture; any effective method will suffice. Usually, to obtain the maximum benefit, there are additional localising factors, called target areas by Dr Richard Mackarness, and these should be treated in addition, though the liver itself will nearly always achieve the main response.

Amongst the allergies which may be treated there are:—one type of asthma, one type of hay fever, urticaria, angioneurotic oedema, the numerous food allergies, and contact dermatitis.

The milder and moderate allergies can normally be cured or considerably helped. I imagine the very severe cases, such as have anaphylactic shock from just the taste of an oyster, would be better but not cured, for their other concomitant symptoms such as migraine are undoubtedly better. I have considered it prudent however not to test them with another oyster. Contact dermatitis can, as a rule, be helped a little. Food allergies are alleviated a moderate amount, though only a few completely cured.

Case History. A patient had a rash, always on the same place on the lower leg, whenever he ate egg. Even one egg in a large cake was sufficient. Sometimes he had other allergic symptoms in addition.

After treating the liver, and to a slight extent the spleen and kidney, he was able to eat as much cake as he liked and, in addition, one egg a week, without symptoms. He was not cured for life though, and required a single booster treatment once or twice a year thereafter.

The Liver and Digestive System

Many digestive disturbances in which discomfort is felt in the upper abdomen are hepatic. There may be: swelling, discomfort, feeling of fullness, feeling as if food is lying undigested in stomach, one type of duodenal ulcer, etc. If there is insufficient bile the stools will be pale, at least intermittently. There may be spasm of the colon with ribbon stools, constipation, or a bitter taste in the mouth and a dry mouth—part of the liver meridian runs round the inside of the mouth.

Parenteral bile salts increase the motor activity of the gastro-intestinal tract.

The Liver and Life

A general sense of well-being and energy is more often dependent on the liver than any other organ in the body—at least in my experience.

Presumably this is because the liver is the centre of metabolism, which is after all the most important aspect of life. From the point of view of evolution the metabolism is what distinguishes the animate from the inanimate. Amoebae have a metabolism. Only at a later stage of evolution do supportive organs such as the heart, kidney or a nervous system, develop.

Symptomatology

Main Meridian Symptoms

Aching of waist, difficulty in looking up or down, distention of lower abdomen, dry throat, face looks as if it is covered with a layer of dust, asthma, dyspnoea, does not digest food, vomiting, diarrhoea, Qi rebels, loss of control of urination and defaecation—or no relief from these acts, depression, bad-temper, hernia.

SYMPTOMS OF EXCESS

Swelling of the penis, scrotal diseases, excessive erection.

SYMPTOMS OF INSUFFICIENCY

Pruritus.

Traditional Classification

The mother of liver wood is kidney water, and if kidney water is deficient it easily causes liver Yang violent diseases, and this is called 'water does not submerge wood'.

Among liver disease symptoms, the most prominent is a type which belongs to wind (inner wind, not the wind of the six excesses).

If, for example, there is dizziness, spasms, convulsions etc., it is what the Su Wen describes as 'all wind, collapsing and dizziness belong to the liver'.

Liver Cold Symptoms

The symptoms of liver cold generally appear in the Lower Warmer; if there is cold then the muscles and vessels contract and Qi and blood are congealed and blocked. This may cause contraction of the scrotum and pain in the testicles, pain and swelling in the lower abdomen.

The pulse is generally deep and wiry, but slow.

Liver Hot Symptoms

The cause of liver hot symptoms is generally 'wood vigorous creates fire'. Among them are the localised diseases such as pain in the sides, dizziness, proneness to anger, pain in the back, spasms and convulsions, 'extreme heat creates wind'. These are similar to liver full symptoms, but there are also many heat manifestations of liver fire burning upwards, such as swelling, pain and redness of eyes, excessive lachrymation, bitter mouth, red tongue, dry mouth, troubled and hot heart, restless sleep at night, being startled and agitated during sleep. It can also move downwards and become Yin internal pain, urethral discharge, haematuria, etc.

The pulse is wiry and rapid.

Liver Empty Symptoms

These generally arise from blood fluid being decayed and small in quantity, or from deficiency of kidney water and inability to submerge wood. The principle symptoms are tinnitus, dizziness, eyes dry, partial blindness.

The pulse is usually wiry, fine but weak.

If the liver is empty and there is little blood, it cannot nourish the muscles and vessels, so spasms and convulsions occur; possibly limbs and body numb, nails dried up and blue-green, desire to lie down. The cause of this is Yin empty, Yang vigorous, Yin and Yang are not of the same strength.

Liver Full Symptoms

If the liver Qi is excessive it causes people easily to become angry, Qi and blood are depressed and congealed, the chest is distended and painful and this distension and pain may extend to the abdomen, liver Qi rebels horizontally and may invade the stomach and spleen causing pain in the stomach and abdomen, vomiting sour-clear fluid, possibly painful diarrhoea. These are 'liver wood insulting earth'.

There is also liver Qi rebelling upwards and producing Qi blocked, dyspnoea and coughing, with haematemesis and haemoptysis in severe cases. If, in addition, there is movement of liver wind, then there can be spasms of arms and legs, rigidity, pain in the back.

The pulse is usually wiry and unyielding.

Connecting Meridian (Luo) Symptoms

SYMPTOMS OF EXCESS

Excessive erections, swelling of testicles.

SYMPTOMS OF INSUFFICIENCY

Genitalia itch violently.

Muscle Meridian Symptoms

Pain and muscular spasm along the course of the muscle meridian.

If there has been excessive sexual intercourse then there is impotence with inability to obtain an erection. If the patient suffers from cold then the penis shrivels in an inward direction; if the patient suffers from heat then the penis becomes relaxed and cannot tense.

Course of Meridians

Liver Main Meridian

Principal Course

The liver meridian originates on the big toe at Liv1. Thence it goes up the embryologically anterior surface of the leg, mostly between the other Yin meridians, then over the abdomen to end on the lower costal margin at Liv14.

Special Details

The meridian starts at the end of the big toe at Liv1, goes to Liv4, and then via Sp6 to Liv5, and thence up the leg to Liv11.

From Liv11 the meridian goes via Sp12 and Sp13 to Liv12.

From Liv12 the meridian loops around the genitalia going to Cv2, Cv3, Cv4 to Liv13, then on to Liv14.

From Liv13 it goes alongside the stomach (? going to Cv12), enters the liver, to which it belongs, and connects with the gall-bladder.

From Liv14 the meridian passes through the diaphragm, and is then scattered through the chest and ribs, going up the back of the throat, ascending through the jaw and cheek-bones to enter the eye.

From the eye the meridian goes over the forehead to the top of the head (? Gv20).

A branch leaves the eye, descends through the lower jaw and circles round the mouth inside the lips.

Another branch leaves Liv14, penetrates the diaphragm, pours into the lungs and joins the meridian of the lung (L1).

Liver Connecting Meridian (Luo)—Liv5

The meridian begins above the ankle at Liv5 and goes up the leg to the testicles and penis. It links with the gall-bladder meridian Luo.

Liver Muscle Meridian

The meridian begins at the big toe, unites in front of the internal malleolus; ascends along the tibia and unites at the inner side of the knee; ascends the thigh and unites at the genitalia and there collects with all the other meridian muscles.

Important Points

Wood	Liv1	Wood point of Yin wood meridian
Fire	Liv2	Sedation
Earth	Liv3	
Metal	Liv4	
Water	Liv8	Tonification
Source	Liv3	
Luo	Liv5	
Xi	Liv6	
Alarm	Liv14	
Associated	B18	

CHAPTER XIV

EIGHT EXTRA MERIDIANS

(also Conception and Governing Vessel Connecting Meridians)

Ren Mo

(Conception or pregnancy Vessel)

Course

Master point L7   *Coupled point* K3

The meridian arises at Cv1, going up the midline of the abdomen, thorax, neck and chin, and terminates below the lower lip at Cv24.

From Cv24 a branch goes round the lips, sending an off-shoot to S4, where it enters the eyes, thus joining the stomach and Yang qiao meridians.

Function and Symptomatology

The Ren mo is the 'sea' of the Yin meridians. The three lower Yin, the Yin qiao and Chong mo join the Ren mo. Therefore the Ren mo controls the Yin meridians of the body.

'The vessel of conception connects ⌄ through way . . . therefore the menses descend at the right time' '. . . controls pregnancy nourishment.' ' . . . the root of conception in the woman.'

The vertebral column belongs to Yang, the diaphragm to Yin, the lower abdomen is the Yin within the Yin. Diseases of the Ren mo therefore affect the lower abdomen and lower warmer. 'The male contracts the seven types of herniae; the female has red and white vaginal discharge or fibroids.' 'Distress in the lower abdomen, with pain encircling the navel going to the pubic bone with sharp pain in the genitalia.' 'If the abdomen is distressed there is Qi, like a finger, ascending to attack the heart. The patient can neither bend down nor straighten up.' There may be lumbago, pain at the back of the head and neck or abscesses of the mouth and tongue.

Cv4 may be used for menstrual disturbances, vaginal discharge, herniae and lunacy.

The individual points on this meridian have an effect on those organs which are roughly on the same segmental level: The lower points genito-urinary, the middle points digestive, the upper points thoracic.

Commoner Diseases

Asthma, bronchitis, pneumonia, pleurisy, asthenia, pulmonary T.B., laryngitis, cough, rhinitis, hay fever, emphysema, haemoptysis, influenza, sneezing, coryza, whooping cough, aphonia, hot flushes, meningitis of children, convulsions or epilepsy (or Yin wei mo), eczema, diabetes, dyspepsia, pharyngitis, mouth diseases (or Du mo), alimentary intoxication, menstrual disorders—not in virgins (or Dai mo), breast abscess, pain head and neck.

Vessel of Conception Connecting Meridian (Luo)—Cv15

The meridian begins at Cv15 and descends to scatter in the abdomen.

SYMPTOMS OF EXCESS

Skin of abdomen painful.

SYMPTOMS OF INSUFFICIENCY

Skin of abdomen itches.

Du Mo
(Governing Vessel)

Course

Master point Si3   *Coupled point* B62

The governing vessel begins at the tip of the coccyx at Gv1, sending a branch forward on the perineum to Cv1. The meridian continues up the spines of the vertebrae, at the same time uniting with them. At Gv16, below the occiput, it enters the brain, to reach the top of the head. It descends over the forehead and nose, to curl around the upper lip, and ends on the gum between the incisor teeth at Gv28.

A branch goes from Gv12, via B12 on both sides, to Gv13.

There are some additional points, apart from the 28 numbered points, on this meridian.

This meridian joins the Ren mo by sending a branch from Gv28 to Cv24, and also joins the stomach meridian.

Function and Symptomatology

The governing vessel unites the Yang Qi of the whole body. The three Yang meridians of the arms and the three Yang meridians of the legs join the Du mo, the most Yang of all the Yang meridians. The constitution is partly dependent on the Du mo, for it is connected with the kidney. From Cvi it ascends to the right kidney (fire), whereby Yin pertains to Yang. From XH3 (Tai Yang = Supreme Yang or the sun) it descends (? governing vessel connecting meridian) to the left kidney (water), whereby Yang pertains to Yin.

When the meridian is overactive, the spine becomes stiff, as the meridian Qi is blocked; there is also headache and pain in the eyes. When underactive, the head feels heavy, and the patient walks with rounded shoulders, as the pure Yang Qi is unable to rise.

In disease the Du mo unifies the Yang Qi of the whole body and unites with the Yin Qi, thus not only will there be stiffening of the spine at the waist but also 'insanity in adults and convulsions in children'. The above may also be due to the Du mo going to the brain. It may be treated via Gv20.

As the Du mo originates in the perineum, it may be associated with haemorrhoids, retention of urine, herniae and sterility.

The individual points on this meridian have an effect on the same organ as the associated points on the same level: e.g. Gv4 is on the same level as B23, both having an effect on the kidney; and Gvi2 is on the same level as B13, both having an effect on the lung.

All points in the lumbo-sacral region, whether they be on the governing vessel or the bladder meridian, have an effect on the kidney/bladder in addition to whatever other effect they may have.

Commoner Diseases

Headache (or Yang wei mo), pain in neck and back especially in the region of vertebra C7, neuralgia of forehead and eyebrows, lumbago, warm back, contraction of throat jaw and neck, torticollis, conjunctivitis, running eyes, over stimulation, hallucinations, dementia, epilepsy, vertigo, toothache (or Yang wei mo), tonsillitis, productive cough, mouth diseases (or Ren mo), deafness, cold extremities.

Governing Vessel Connecting Meridian (Luo)—Gvi

The meridian begins at Gvi, ascends paravertebrably to the nape of the neck, disperses over the occiput, descends and when it reaches the shoulders links with the bladder connecting meridian. It penetrates to pass through the inside of the spine.

SYMPTOMS OF EXCESS

Spine stiff and straight, cannot easily bend.

SYMPTOMS OF INSUFFICIENCY

Head heavy and shaking.

Chong Mo
(Penetrating vessel)

Course

Master point Sp4   *Coupled point* Cx6

This meridian together with the Ren mo arises in the uterus, represented by Cv1. It ascends the coccyx, sacrum and lower lumbar spine, where it acts as the 'sea' of the Jing and Luo. The superficial part goes over the groin at S30 and then up the kidney meridian from K11 to K21, there being a branch from K15 to Cv7. Thereafter it goes over the thorax and throat to encircle the mouth.

Function and Symptomatology

The Chong mo is called 'the sea of the twelve meridians' and 'the sea of blood'. In its upward course it connects all the Yang meridians, in its downward course all the Yin meridians.

The Chong mo is initially connected with the kidney and stomach meridians: the former regulating prenatal, the latter postnatal development. It is therefore said to store the True Qi.

'It restrains and regulates the sinews and meridians of the whole body.' 'Master of diseases of the heart, the abdomen and the five Zang.'

'Qi rebels upwards from the lower abdomen, abdomen swollen and extremely painful.' 'Pain in lower abdomen ascending to seize the heart.'

The Ren mo, Du mo and Chong mo all arise at Cv1, which is connected with the uterus. The Ren mo is the sea of the Yin meridians; the Du mo the sea of the Yang meridians; the Chong mo the sea of blood. 'When the Chong mo flourishes menstruation occurs at the right time.' 'When it is not regulated miscarriage occurs, (referring in one text to the Chong mo, and in another to Chong and Ren mo).'

'In a woman the Ren and Chong mo do not unite round the lips: hence she has no beard.' 'The Chong mo originates in the genitalia and goes round the lips. In a eunuch it is cut: hence he has no beard.'

Commoner Diseases

Digestive troubles in general, aerocolon, anorexia, hiccoughs, atonic gastritis, cholecystitis, atonic constipation, difficult digestion, 'tummy ache', hyperacidity, gastric ulcer, jaundice, vomiting, bradycardia, endo or myocarditis, palpitations, lumbago (or Yang qiao mo), malaria.

Dai Mo
(Girdle vessel)

Course

Master point G41   *Coupled point* T5

The meridian encircles the body at the level of the waist—G28, G27, G26 and possibly Liv13.

Function and Symptomatology

The gïrdle vessel binds all the meridians that course up and down the body. If it is in disorder the abdomen is bloated or there is 'sagging of the waist as when one is seated in water.' There may be aching and pain at the level of the waist.

Menstruation may be irregular, with red or white vaginal discharge. 'All the meridians go up and down creating heat between themselves and the Dai mo. Heat and cold contend with one another, white matter becomes over-full and leaks down in a constant stream.'

Commoner Diseases

Amenorrhoea, dysmenorrhoea, menstrual disturbance—not in virgins (or Ren mo), anaemia, weakness and general fatigue, fainting, trembling, pruritus (or Yang wei mo), contracture of hands and feet, pain in arm and shoulder, pain in knee, arthritis in general, pain in leg or foot or ankle, redness of wrists and ankles, articular rheumatism (or Yang qiao mo), spasms, abdominal pain (or Ren mo), lumbago, abdominal distension, vomiting (or Chong mo), inflammation of breasts, ovaritis, thinness.

Yin Qiao Mo
(*Yin heel vessel*)

Course

Master point K3   Coupled point B62

The meridian begins on the medial side of the foot near K2, goes to K3, K8 and up the leg, abdomen and thorax, to the supra-clavicular fossa near S12. Thence it goes in front of S9, to the medial corner of the eye at B1, where it meets the bladder, small intestine, stomach and Yang qiao meridians.

Function and Symptomatology

See section of Yang qiao mo.

Yang Qiao Mo
(*Yang heel vessel*)

Course

Master point B62   Coupled point K3

The meridian begins near the external malleolus at B62, then goes to B61, B59, up the leg to G29, over the lateral side of the body to Si10, Li15, Li16, over the neck and face via S7, S6, S4 to end at B1. An extension probably goes over the cranium to G20.

Function and Symptomatology of Yin and Yang Qiao Mo

These meridians are concerned with fluid, via their kidney and bladder master points (K3 and B62), therefore 'when the Qi has a free circulation the eye is moistened, and when the Qi is not in order, the eye is not in accord'.

'When the Yang Qi is over-full and glaring, "angry eyes" result; and when the Yin Qi is over-full then the vision is blurred.' 'If there is an excess of Yang, the eyes cannot be closed; if there is an excess of Yin, the eyes are always closed.' There may also be pain at the medial corner of the eye.

'When the Yang qiao sickens, the Yin relaxes and the Yang tenses. When the Yin qiao sickens, the Yang relaxes and the Yin tenses.' According to this sickness tenses and health relaxes. 'When the Yin qiao mo tenses, the medial side of the ankle and lower leg tenses, and the lateral side of the ankle and lower leg relaxes. When the Yang qiao mo tenses, the lateral side of the ankle and lower leg tenses, and the medial side of the ankle and lower leg relaxes.'

The above tension and relaxation occurs mostly in epilepsy and other types of convulsions in which there is muscle spasm. 'If the cause is not known treat K3 in females, B62 in males.' 'If epilepsy occurs during the day treat B62, during the night K3.'

Since the Yang qiao mo is connected to the bladder meridian, there may be lumbago. Since the Yin qiao mo is connected to the kidney meridian, there may be lower abdominal pain, backache, pain in the genitalia, herniae in men and abortions in women.

'When the Yang Qi is deficient, Yin Qi is abundant, and one is often very sleepy. When the Yin Qi is deficient, Yang Qi is abundant and there is often insomnia.'

Commoner Diseases (Yin qiao mo)

Absence of sexual pleasure, impotence, frigidity, sterility, habitual abortion, difficult delivery, post-partum pains, post-partum haemorrhages, toxic pregnancy, leukorrhea, metritis, metropathia, dysmenorrhoea of virgins, ovaritis, prostatitis, seminal loss, orchitis, albuminuria, anuria, cystitis, haematuria, nephritis, enuresis, urinary retention, bladder spasm or irritation or weakness, somnolence, constipation in women, pulmonary tuberculosis, oedema in general, weakness of women and the old.

Commoner Diseases (Yang qiao mo)

Cerebral congestion, apoplexy, hemiplegia, monoplegia, paraplegia, aphasia, contractures or cramps in general, facial paralysis, lumbago (or Chong mo), sciatica, torticollis (or Ren mo), articular rheumatism (or Dai mo), articular pains (or Yang wei mo), furunculosis (or Yang wei mo), obsessions.

Yin Wei Mo
(Yin linking vessel)

Course

Master point Cx6   *Coupled point* So4

The meridian starts on the medial side of the lower leg at K9, ascending the thigh and abdomen—Sp13, Sp15, Sp16, Liv14, and then over the chest to Cv22, to end at the larynx at Cv23.

Function and Symptomatology

'The Yin and Yang wei mo act as the binding network of all the vessels.' 'The Yin wei mo originates in the interchange of all the Yin.'

The meridian has interconnections with the Yin meridians, particularly the vessel of conception, heart and lung. 'When the Yin wei mo is diseased, the patient suffers from heart pains.' 'Yin wei mo moves all the Yin and controls Ying, Ying becomes blood, blood belongs to the heart, thus the heart is painful.' 'When the Yin wei mo is empty, the waist aches and there are pains in the genitalia'.

Commoner Diseases

Cardiac pain (or Chong mo), emotional states, unquietness, nervous laugh, failure to recall words, timidity, fear, apprehension, hypertension, mental depression, nightmares, delirium, sudden uncontrolled laughter, amnesia, agitation or epilepsy (or Ren mo), convulsions (or Ren mo), internal fullness, indigestion, abdominal pain (or Dai mo), haemorrhoids, spastic constipation, varicose veins and ulcers.

Yang Wei Mo
(Yang linking vessel)

Course

Master point T5   *Coupled point* G41

The meridian starts below the lateral malleolus at B63, then goes up the lateral side of the body to G35 and G24.

Then from G24 it passes behind the shoulder to Si10, T15, G21, Gv15, Gv16, G20, G19, G18, G17, G16, G15, G14 to end at G13. (The cranial course is possibly the other way round, going from G21 over the neck and side of the face to G13, and then on to G14, G15, G16, G17, G18, G19, G20, Gv16 to end at Gv15). (The part of the meridian which goes over the shoulder and neck is possibly more complex, going from G24 to Li14, T13, T15, G21, Si10, G20, Gv15, Gv16, G19 and over the cranium via the gall bladder meridian to G13.)

Function and Symptomatology

'The Yin and Yang wei mo act as the binding network of all the vessels.' 'The Yang wei mo originates at the meeting place of all the Yang.'

It has interconnections with the three Yang meridians of the legs and three Yang meridians of the arms, but most particularly with the leg greater Yang and lesser Yang—bladder and gall bladder. The former meridian controls the surface, the latter the sub-surface of the body, i.e. the protective layers of the body. Therefore 'when the Yang wei mo is diseased the patient suffers from colds and fevers.' 'Yang wei mo moves all the Yang and controls Wei, Wei becomes Qi, Qi dwells in the exterior of the body, therefore there is cold and heat.'

Commoner Diseases

Fevers in general, neuralgias in general, headache (or Du mo), pain in arms, toothache (or Du mo), pain in lower molars, pain in ears, otitis, tinnitus, arthritis of fingers and toes, articular pain (or Yang qiao mo), swelling of heel, abscess of head or mouth, furunculosis (or Yang qiao mo), acne, epistaxis, haematemesis, pruritus (or Du mo), general weakness, thinness (or Dai mo), mumps, pain and swellings of neck.

Technique for Use of Extra Meridians

1. Every extra meridian has its 'master point' and 'coupled point', as follows:

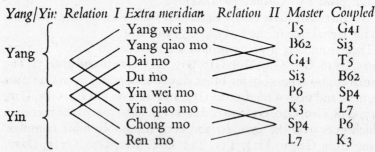

Yang/Yin Relation I	Extra meridian	Relation II	Master	Coupled
Yang	Yang wei mo		T5	G41
	Yang qiao mo		B62	Si3
	Dai mo		G41	T5
	Du mo		Si3	B62
Yin	Yin wei mo		P6	Sp4
	Yin qiao mo		K3	L7
	Chong mo		Sp4	P6
	Ren mo		L7	K3

An extra meridian may be emptied of its excess of energy by stimulating its master point. If this has not corrected the general Yin/Yang equilibrium of the pulse, the coupled point is stimulated. If this has still not given the desired result, the midline extra meridian (Ren mo or Du mo) of the opposite sign is used. This alternative rests on the fact that the excess energy of the one sign flows into the midline extra meridian of the opposite sign.

An example. A patient is suffering from obsessions. Since in this case there is no real emotional cause for the obsession, it may be regarded as a real illness—as real as any physical illness. The symptom index shows that the Yang qiao mo is affected. This is a Yang extra meridian, and as the pulse diagnosis reveals a general excess of Yang it is perfectly legitimate to use this extra meridian. The master point B62 is bilaterally stimulated, which achieves a slight diminution of the Yang quality of the pulse, but not enough. Therefore the coupled point Si3 is stimulated, which again achieves a reduction of Yang, but not enough. Therefore the third stage is employed and the master point of the midline Yin meridian of the opposite sign is used, i.e. L7, the master point of Ren mo.

It is not usually necessary to go through all three stages of treatment as in the above example—usually the first one suffices,

2. The extra meridians may also be emptied of their excess of energy by stimulating both ends of the meridian at the same time. Either the point at the extreme end, or the penultimate point should be used.

A further guide as to deciding which extra meridian should be used is given by a consideration of the pulse as a whole. If there is a predominance of Yang, a Yang extra meridian should be used, or if there is a predominance of Yin, a Yin extra meridian should be used.

If the pulses show a predominance of Yang and the symptom index suggests a Yin extra meridian, say Ren mo, the opposite Yang meridian should be used which, in this case, would be Du mo.

Case History. A patient had suffered from hyperacidity and symptoms of gastric ulcer for six years. The symptom index suggests the use of Chong mo, which was stimulated but did not alter the symptoms. Various other procedures not involving extra meridians were also tried, but made no difference. Cognizance was then taken of the fact that the overall pulse quality was Yang, so the opposite (i.e. Yang) extra meridian was used, Dai mo. From then onwards the patient started to improve.

ILLUSTRATIONS OF THE MERIDIANS

The continuous lines represent the course of the main, connecting, muscle, divergent or extra meridians.

The finely dotted lines represent the branches, or in some instances the deeper internal course of the meridians. They also represent the connection of coupled meridians.

The heavily dotted lines represent the main meridian in the illustrations of the divergent meridians.

The broken lines represent the continuation from one drawing to another of the various meridians.

The acupuncture points on the main meridians are numbered in heavy type at a few of their representative points. Where the main meridian or its branches go to acupuncture points on other meridians, this has been indicated in all instances by lettering and numbering in lighter type. The connecting points of the connecting meridians have also been lettered and numbered in light type.

The meeting points of the muscle meridians have not been labeled.

The words alongside the illustrations, indicate the course, described in greater detail in the text of this book, of some of the meridians.

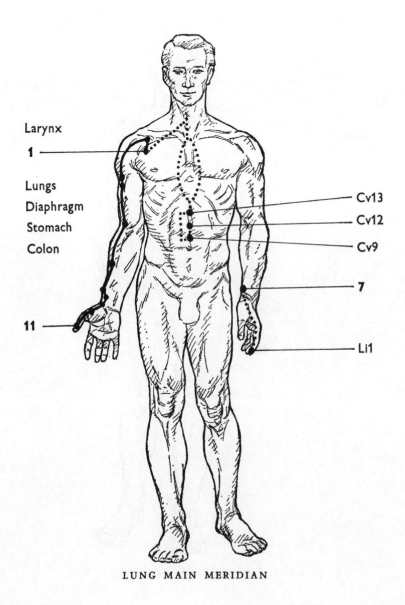

Larynx

1

Lungs
Diaphragm
Stomach
Colon

11

Cv13
Cv12
Cv9

7

Li1

LUNG MAIN MERIDIAN

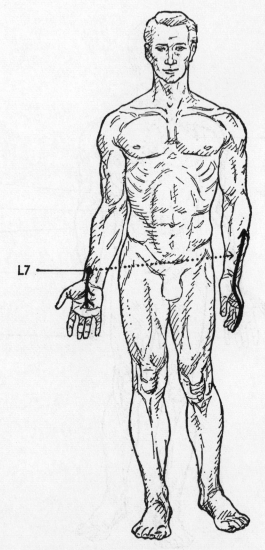

L7

LUNG CONNECTING MERIDIAN

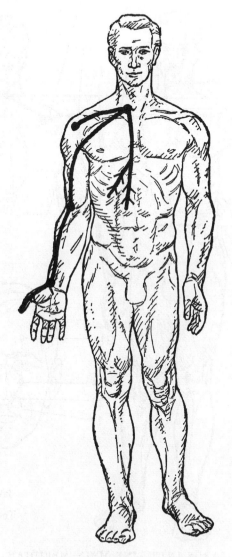

LUNG MUSCLE MERIDIAN

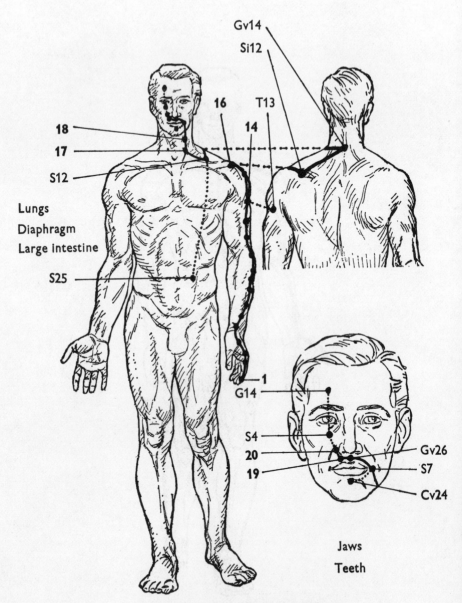

Gv14
Si12
16
T13
14
18
17
S12

Lungs
Diaphragm
Large intestine

S25

1
G14

S4
20
19

Gv26
S7
Cv24

Jaws
Teeth

LARGE INTESTINE MAIN MERIDIAN

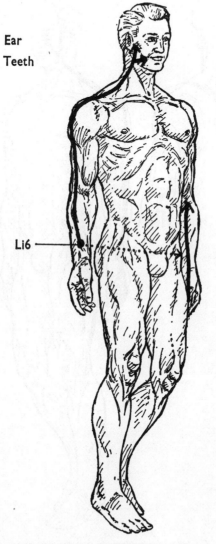

Ear
Teeth

Li6

LARGE INTESTINE CONNECTING MERIDIAN

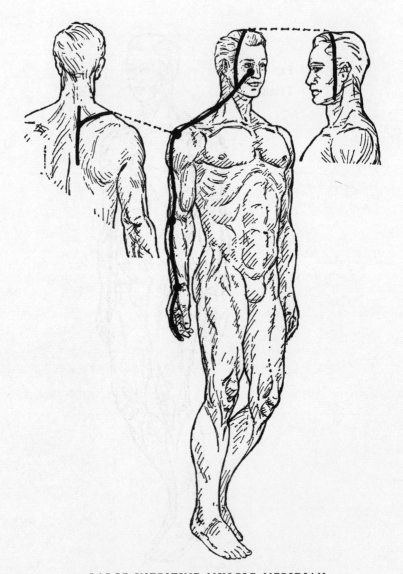

LARGE INTESTINE MUSCLE MERIDIAN

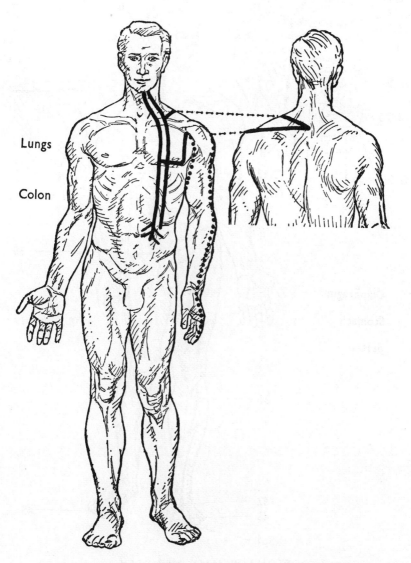

Lungs

Colon

LARGE INTESTINE AND LUNG DIVERGENT MERIDIANS

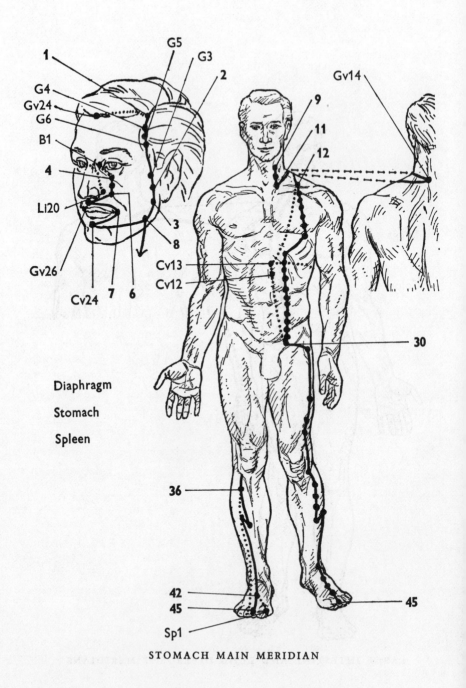

Diaphragm

Stomach

Spleen

STOMACH MAIN MERIDIAN

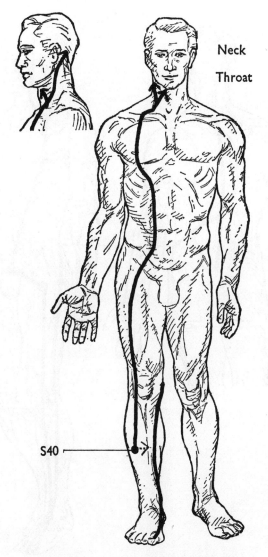

Neck

Throat

S40

STOMACH CONNECTING MERIDIAN

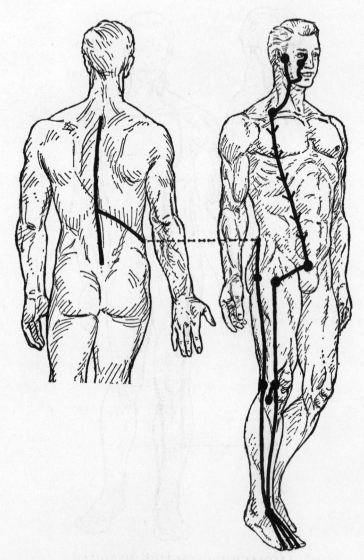

STOMACH MUSCLE MERIDIAN

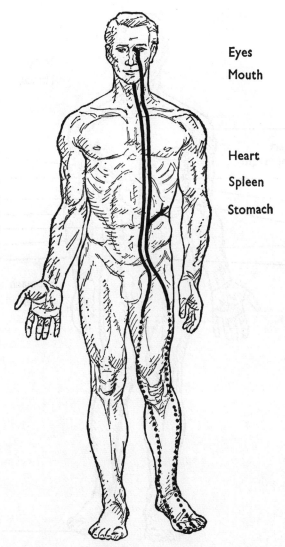

Eyes
Mouth

Heart

Spleen

Stomach

STOMACH AND SPLEEN DIVERGENT MERIDIANS

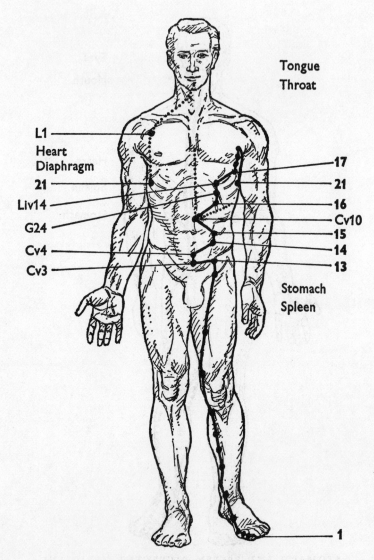

Tongue
Throat

L1

Heart
Diaphragm

21

Liv14

G24

Cv4

Cv3

17

21

16

Cv10

15

14

13

Stomach

Spleen

1

SPLEEN MAIN MERIDIAN

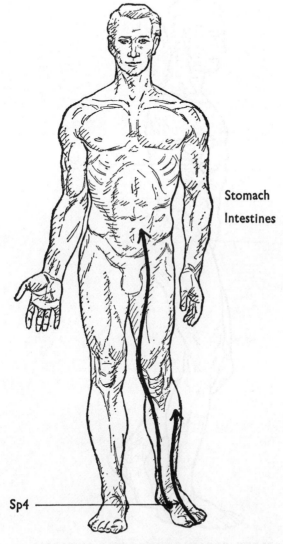

Stomach
Intestines

Sp4

SPLEEN CONNECTING MERIDIAN

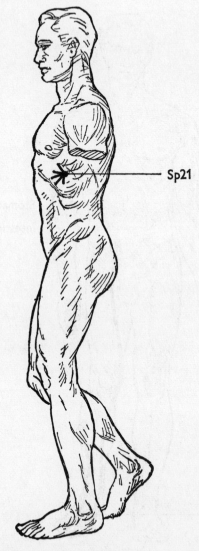

Sp21

SPLEEN GREAT CONNECTING MERIDIAN

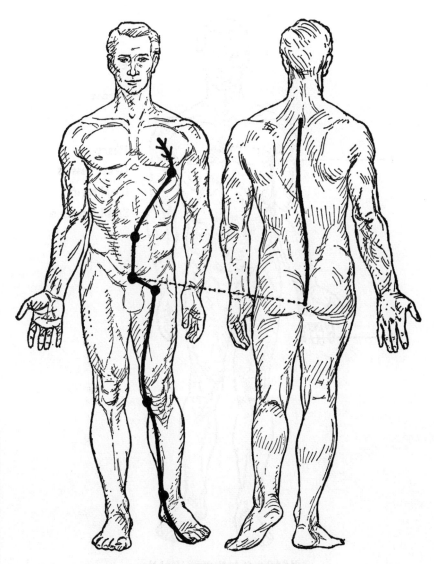

SPLEEN MUSCLE MERIDIAN

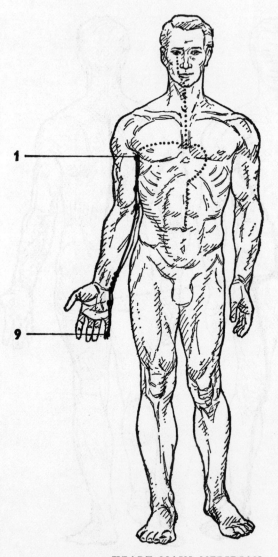

Eye

Throat

Heart
Great vessels
Diaphragm
Small intestine

1

9

HEART MAIN MERIDIAN

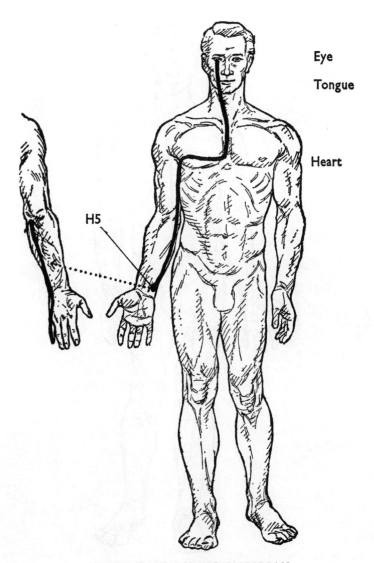

Eye

Tongue

Heart

H5

HEART CONNECTING MERIDIAN

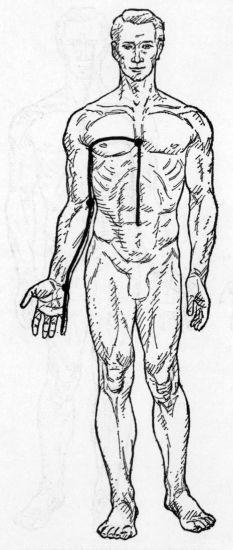

HEART MUSCLE MERIDIAN

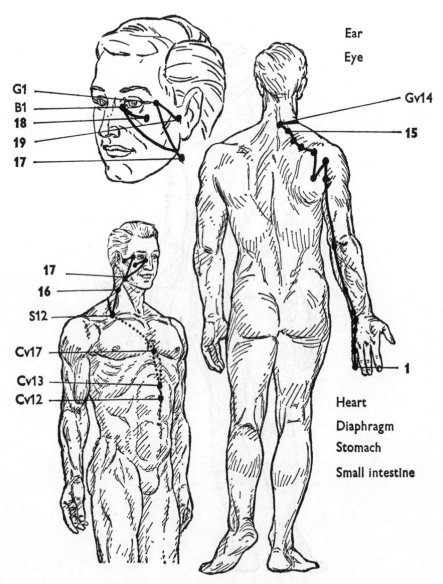

G1
B1
18
19
17

Ear
Eye

Gv14
15

17
16
S12
Cv17
Cv13
Cv12

1

Heart
Diaphragm
Stomach
Small intestine

SMALL INTESTINE MAIN MERIDIAN

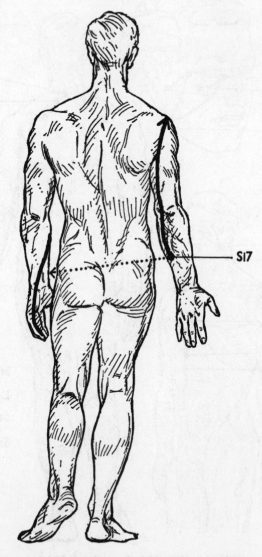

SI7

SMALL INTESTINE CONNECTING MERIDIAN

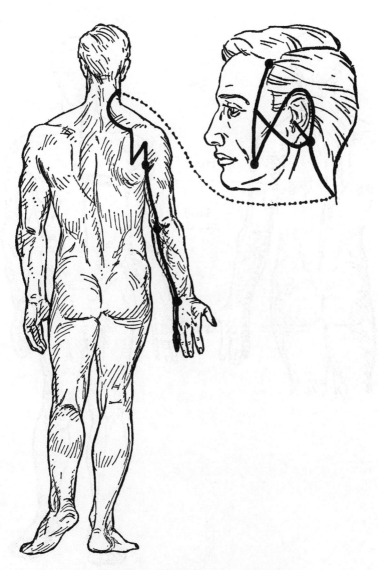

SMALL INTESTINE MUSCLE MERIDIAN

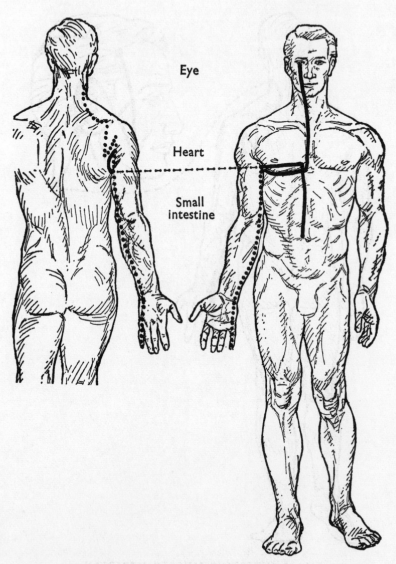

Eye

Heart

Small
intestine

SMALL INTESTINE AND HEART DIVERGENT MERIDIANS

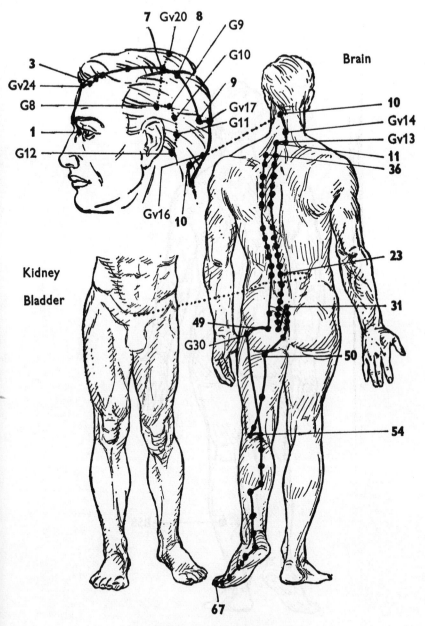

BLADDER MAIN MERIDIAN

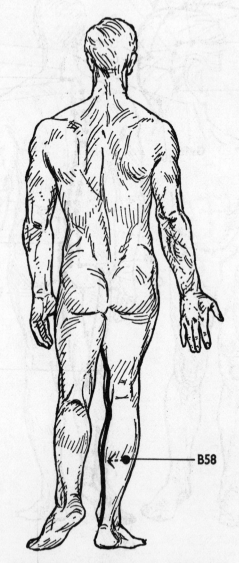

B58

BLADDER CONNECTING MERIDIAN

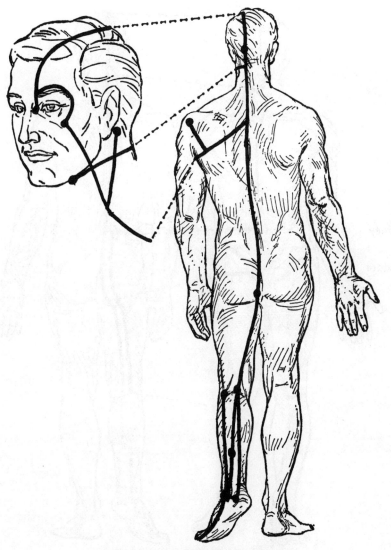

BLADDER MUSCLE MERIDIAN

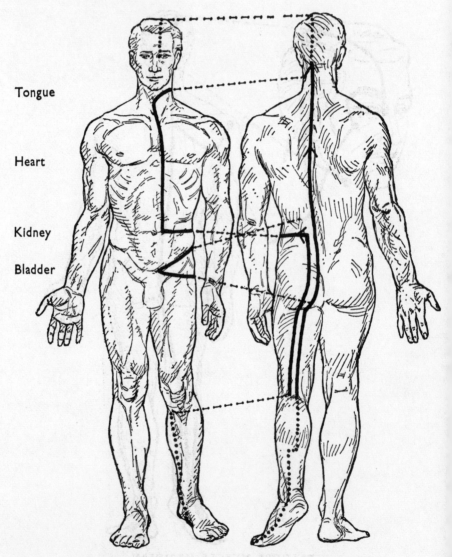

Tongue

Heart

Kidney

Bladder

BLADDER AND KIDNEY DIVERGENT MERIDIANS

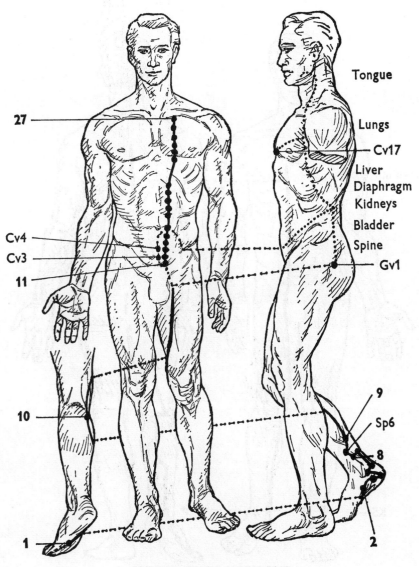

Tongue

Lungs

Cv17

Liver
Diaphragm
Kidneys

Bladder

Spine

Gv1

27

Cv4
Cv3
11

10

1

9

Sp6

8

2

KIDNEY MAIN MERIDIAN

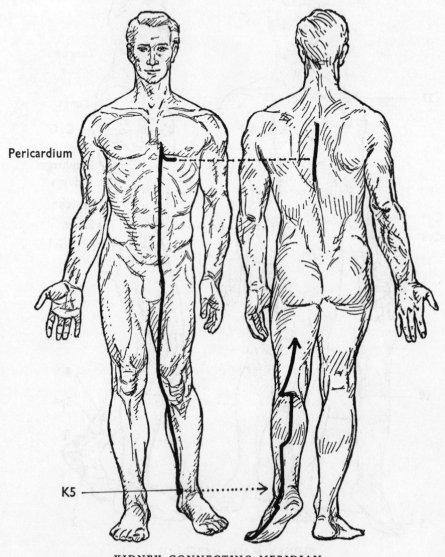

Pericardium

K5

KIDNEY CONNECTING MERIDIAN

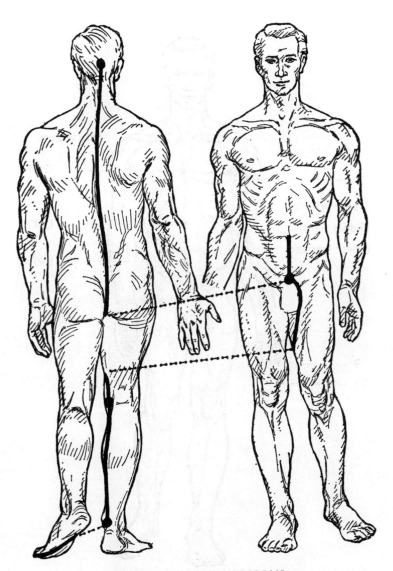

KIDNEY MUSCLE MERIDIAN

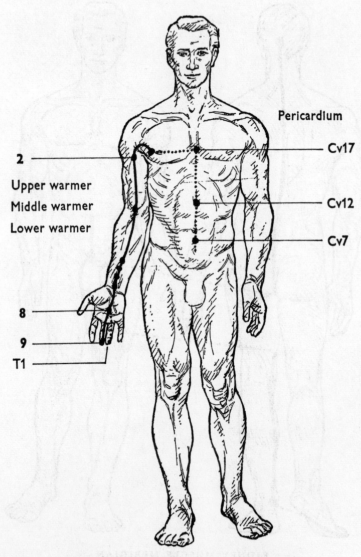

Pericardium

2

Upper warmer
Middle warmer
Lower warmer

Cv17

Cv12

Cv7

8

9

T1

CIRCULATION–SEX MAIN MERIDIAN

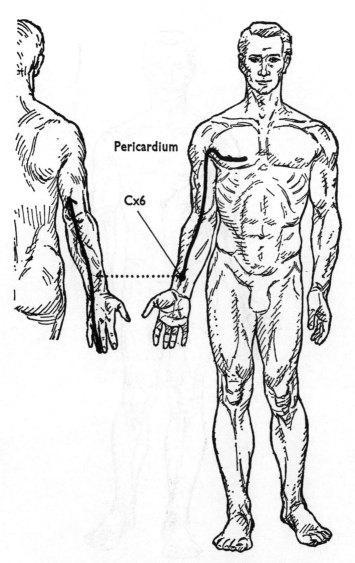

Pericardium

Cx6

CIRCULATION-SEX CONNECTING MERIDIAN

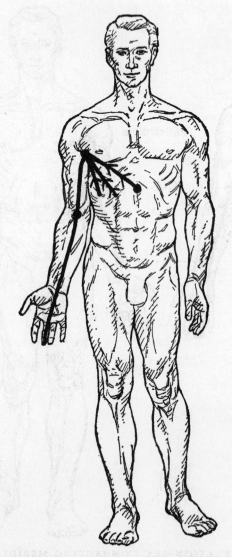

CIRCULATION-SEX MUSCLE MERIDIAN

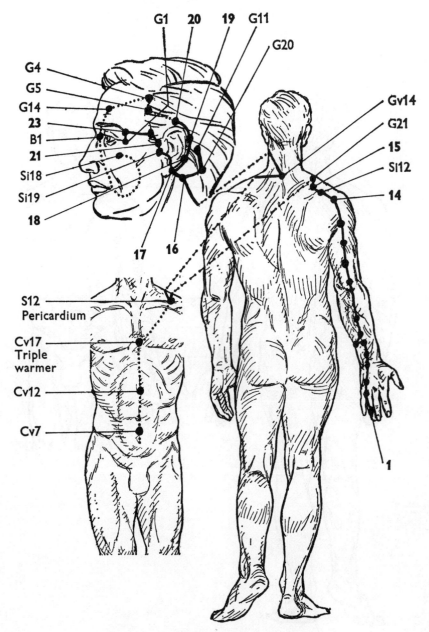

G1 20 19 G11

G20

G4
G5
G14
23
B1
21
Si18
Si19
18

Gv14
G21
15
Si12
14

17 16

S12
Pericardium

Cv17
Triple
warmer

Cv12

Cv7

1

TRIPLE WARMER MAIN MERIDIAN

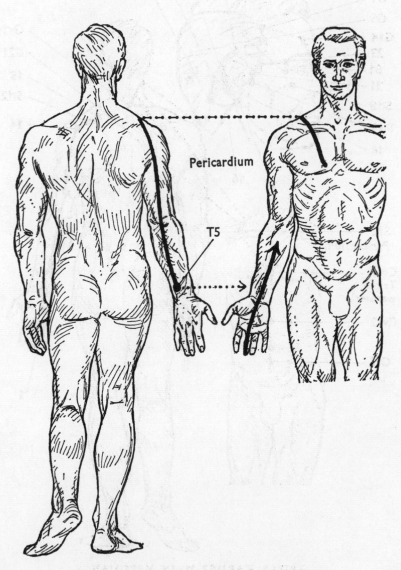

Pericardium

T5

TRIPLE WARMER CONNECTING MERIDIAN

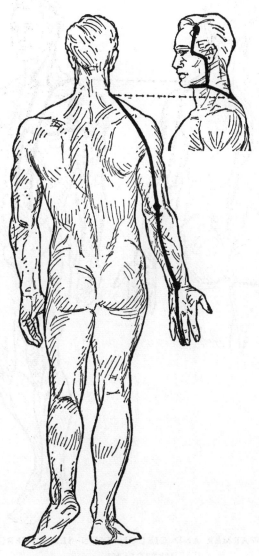

TRIPLE WARMER MUSCLE MERIDIAN

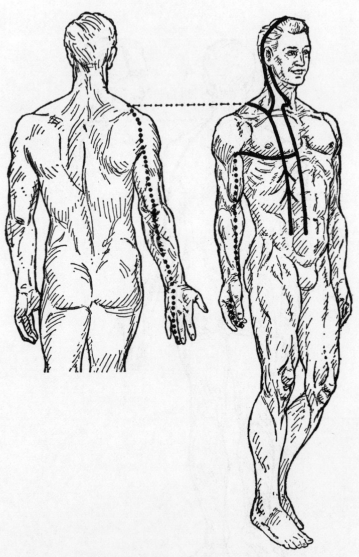

TRIPLE WARMER AND CIRCULATION-SEX DIVERGENT
MERIDIANS

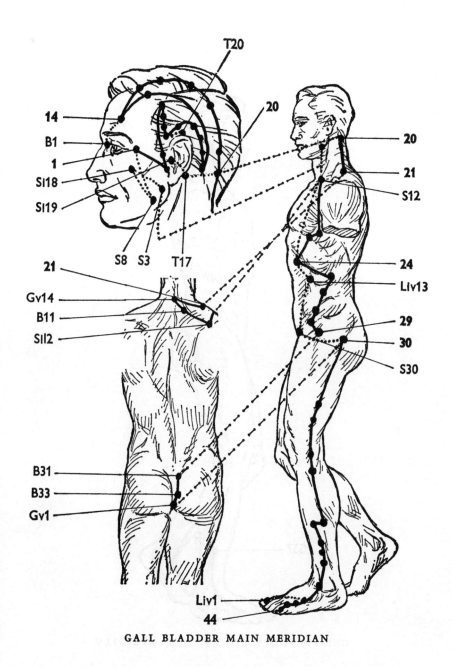

GALL BLADDER MAIN MERIDIAN

451

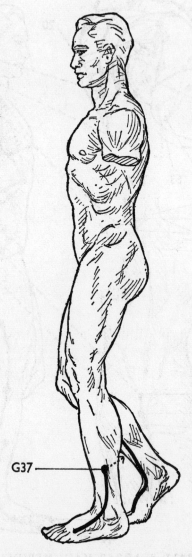

G37

GALL BLADDER CONNECTING MERIDIAN

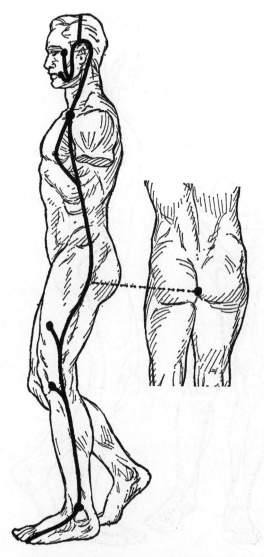

GALL BLADDER MUSCLE MERIDIAN

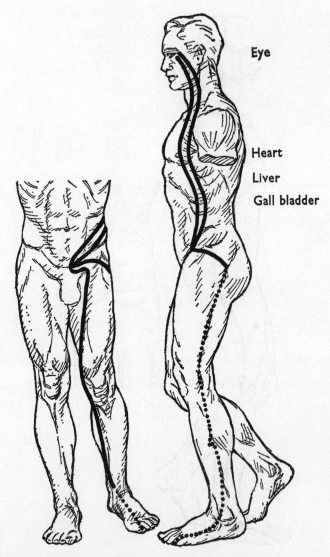

Eye

Heart

Liver

Gall bladder

GALL BLADDER AND LIVER DIVERGENT MERIDIANS

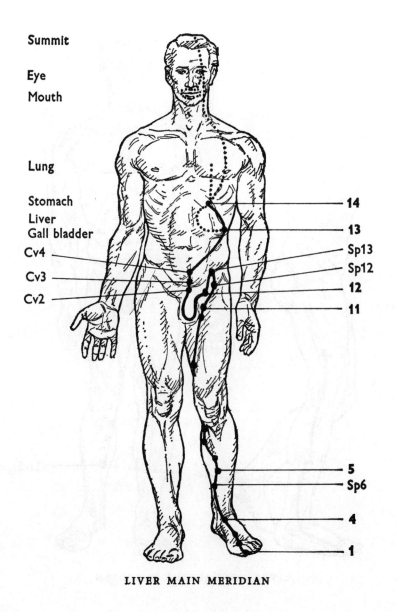

Summit

Eye
Mouth

Lung

Stomach
Liver
Gall bladder

Cv4
Cv3
Cv2

14
13
Sp13
Sp12
12
11

5
Sp6
4
1

LIVER MAIN MERIDIAN

455

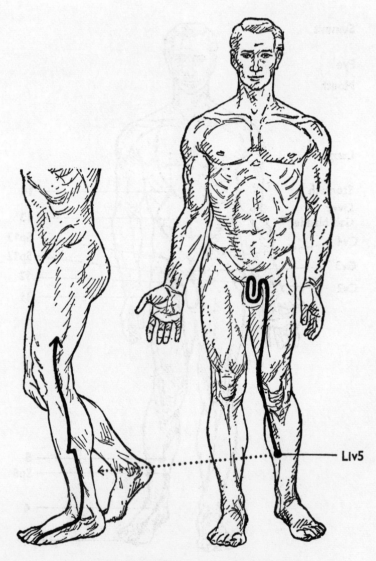

Liv5

LIVER CONNECTING MERIDIAN

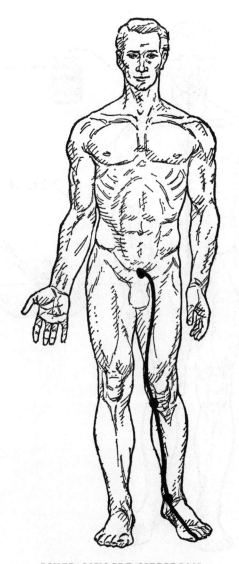

LIVER MUSCLE MERIDIAN

457

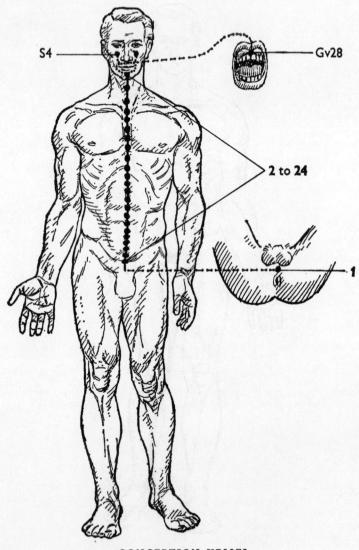

S4

Gv28

2 to 24

1

CONCEPTION VESSEL

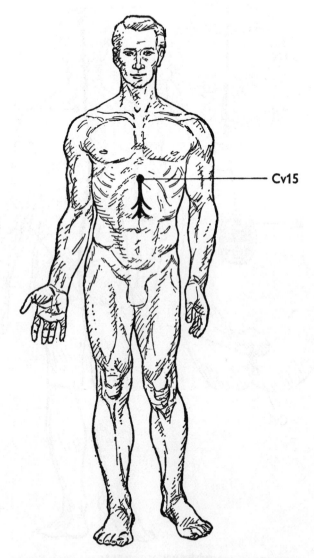

Cv15

CONCEPTION VESSEL CONNECTING MERIDIAN

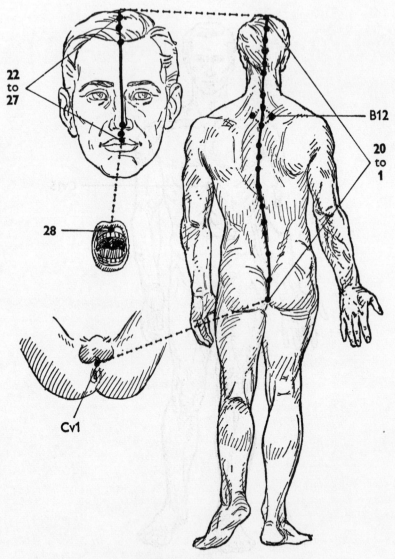

22
to
27

28

Cv1

B12

20
to
1

GOVERNING VESSEL

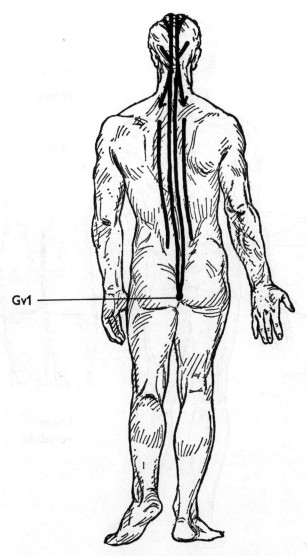

Gv1

GOVERNING VESSEL CONNECTING MERIDIAN

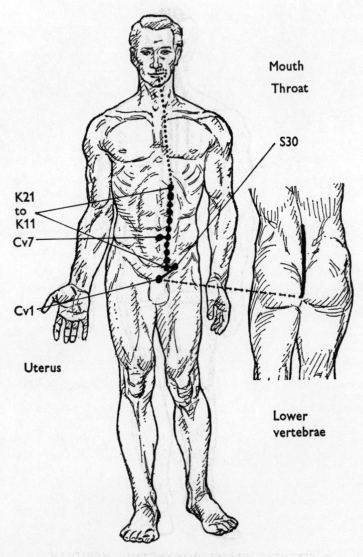

Mouth

Throat

S30

K21
to
K11

Cv7

Cv1

Uterus

Lower
vertebrae

PENETRATING VESSEL

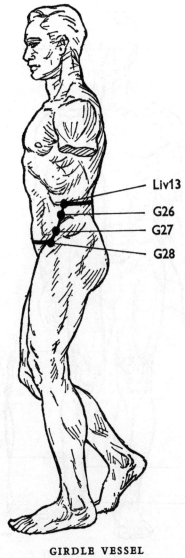

Liv13

G26

G27

G28

GIRDLE VESSEL

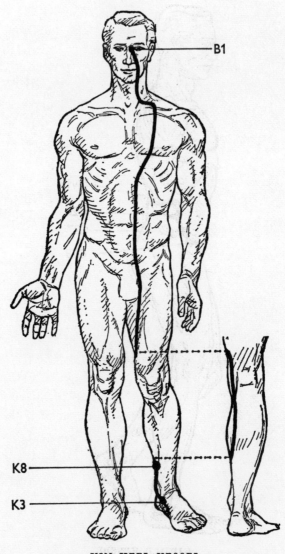

B1

K8

K3

YIN HEEL VESSEL

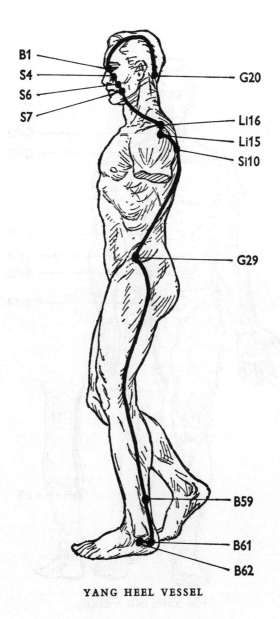

B1
S4
S6
S7

G20

Li16
Li15
Si10

G29

B59

B61
B62

YANG HEEL VESSEL

465

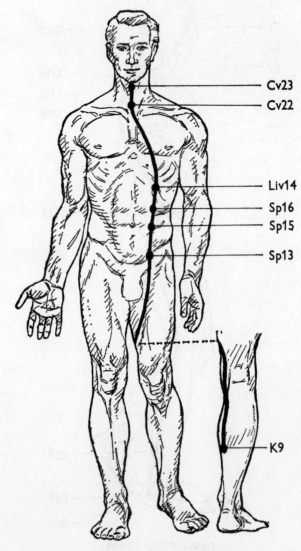

Cv23
Cv22

Liv14
Sp16
Sp15
Sp13

K9

YIN LINKING VESSEL

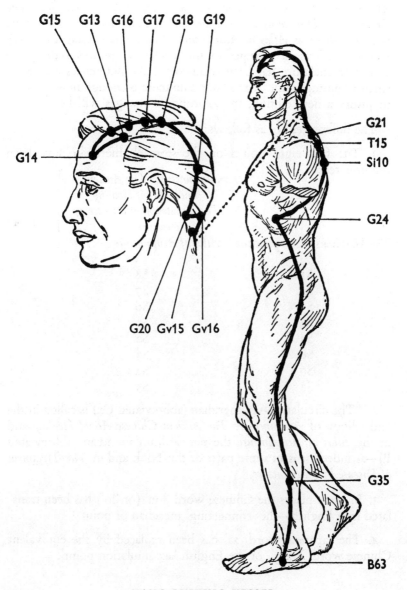

G15 G13 G16 G17 G18 G19

G14

G21
T15
Si10

G24

G20 Gv15 Gv16

G35

B63

YANG LINKING VESSEL

Nomenclature

Since this book was first published in 1964, there have been new editions of *Acupuncture: The Ancient Chinese Art of Healing*, *The Treatment of Disease by Acupuncture* and the *Acupuncture Charts* have been re-edited as *Atlas of Acupuncture*. In all three instances I have incorporated slight changes in nomenclature. In this reprint the 1964 nomenclature has been retained for the differences are either small or unimportant. If at a later date there is enough new material to justify a new edition, the appropriate changes will be made.

The differences are as follows:

1. The first eight points on the stomach meridian have been renumbered:

The Meridians of Acupuncture	*Acupuncture: The Ancient Chinese Art of Healing* *The Treatment of Disease by Acupuncture* *Atlas of Acupuncture*	New editions
S1	S8	
S2	S7	
S3	S6	
S4	S1	
S5	S2	
S6	S3	
S7	S4	
S8	S5	

2. The circulation-sex meridian (abbreviated Cx) is called in the 2nd edition of *Acupuncture: The Ancient Chinese Art of Healing* and in the *Atlas of Acupuncture* the pericardium meridian (abbreviated P)—as indeed it is in some parts of this book and in *The Treatment of Disease by Acupuncture*.

3. In some places the Chinese word 'lou' (or 'lo') has been translated into English—the 'connecting' meridian or point.

4. The Japanese word 'xi' has been replaced by the equivalent Chinese word 'hung', or the English 'accumulation point'.

SECTION 4

The Treatment of
Disease by Acupuncture

CONTENTS

PART I. FUNCTION OF ACUPUNCTURE POINTS:

Taken from ancient and modern sources (Chinese and European),
and the case histories of the author.

PART II. TREATMENT OF DISEASES.

SECTION 1 (CAPITALS) of each disease, is a translation of Changjian
Jibing Zhenjiu Zhiliao Bianlan.
SECTION 2 (ordinary print) of each disease, represents acupuncture
points taken from the case histories of the author, and other, mainly
European, sources.

Function of Acupuncture Points

TAKEN FROM ANCIENT AND MODERN SOURCES
(CHINESE AND EUROPEAN), AND THE CASE
HISTORIES OF THE AUTHOR

Lung

Lung 1
ZHONG FU   MIDDLE MANSION

Point of alarm
Point of entry
Meeting point (greater Yin)

Dyspnoea, fullness of chest, oppression, intermittent fever with cough, adenitis, purulent bronchitis, bronchiectasis or pneumonia, pleurisy, pain in chest on respiration, turbid phlegm, anorexia, rheumatism of neck chest and shoulder, tonsillitis, rhinorrhoea, stuttering, oedema of face and limbs, painful skin, acne, sweating at night, insomnia, sensation that energy rises to top of body, eyes red, urine has bad smell.

Lung 2
YUN MEN   CLOUD DOOR

'Harmful cold causing limbs to become hot', bouts of coughing, short of breath, feeling of oppression and pain in chest, asthma, fullness of chest, rheumatism and swelling of neck, tonsillitis, cannot raise arm, neuralgia of shoulder, sensation that energy rises, acne, general cardiac disease.

Lung 3
TIAN FU   HEAVENLY MANSION

Point 'Window of the sky'

Epistaxis, cerebral congestion, speaks to himself or does not speak at all, 'possessed by a devil', confused, forgetful, vertigo, depressed, very thirsty, vomiting, frog in throat, food sticks in throat, dyspnoea, bronchitis, likes to lie down, brachial neuralgia, intermittent fever, carbon monoxide poisoning.

Lung 4
XIA BAI   CHIVALRY WHITE

Rheumatic pains of the chest, cardiac pain, nausea, annoyed, melancholia, skin mottled red and white with excessive perspiration.

Lung 5
CHI ZE   FOOT MARSH

Water point
Category VI
Point of sedation

Cold and spasm of arm, bronchitis, pleurisy, cough with turbid mucus, haemoptysis, dyspnoea, sneezing, palpitations, body generally painful, rheumatism of throat and neck, tonsillitis, Wind disease of children, eyes not steady, fever of the five viscera, hemiplegia, quadriplegia, muscular spasm, rigidity of vertebral column, madness, renal pain, atony of the bladder.

Lung 6
KONG ZUI   SUPREME HOLE

Accumulation point

High fever with no perspiration, headache, migraine, fear-tension headaches, sore throat, loss of voice, cough, haemoptysis, pain in shoulder and arm.

Lung 7
LIE QUE   LISTING DEFICIENCY

Luo point
General Luo point
Point of exit
Master point of Ren mo

Pain on one side of head or face, trigeminal neuralgia, toothache, migraine, unable to open mouth or speak, tic douloureux, cough with thick mucus, influenza, cough, breathless, melancholic feeling in lower part of chest, trembling, petit mal, epilepsy, mad laughter, yawning, bad memory, middle of palm hot and painful, neuralgia of shoulder and arm with shaking of upper limb, hemiplegia, shivering, cold in the back, limbs ice cold, haematuria, spermatorrhea, pain in penis, haemorrhoids, stye, pruritis, dry skin.

Lung 8
JING QU   MERIDIAN GUTTER
Metal point of Yin
metal meridian
Category V
Cough, feeling that energy rises to top of body, intermittent fever, fever without perspiration, sudden onset of cardiac pain, rheumatism of neck, tonsillitis, pharyngitis, spasm of the oesophagus, palm of hand hot.

Lung 9
TAI YUAN   BIGGER ABYSS
Earth point
Category III & IV
Point of tonification
Source point
Reunion arteries and
veins
Conjunctivitis, keratitis, suddenly cold and suddenly hot, feeling that energy rises to top of body, scapula neuralgia, pain in arm and armpit, asthma, dyspnoea, wailing noise with respiration, pain pulmonary and cardiac region, emphysema, haemoptysis, intercostal neuralgia, brachial neuralgia, claustrophobia, facial paralysis, migraine, insomnia, thirsty, dry mouth, nausea, vomiting, faecal incontinence, oesophageal spasm.

Lung 10
YU JI   FISH BORDER
Fire point
Category II
Throat dry and thirsty, cough, muscular spasm of arm, dyspnoea, heart 'numb', mucus streaked with blood, throat hot and swollen, aphonia, aphasia, upset stomach, cholera, yellow tongue, anorexia, aerophagia, headache, vertigo, insomnia, result of alcoholism, breast abscess.

Lung 11
SHAO SHANG   YOUNG MERCHANT
Wood point
Category I
Last point
Throat and jaws swollen, cerebral congestion, meningitis, intermittent fever, tonsillitis, parotitis, epistaxis, hand and arm numb, swollen chest, lips dry, no mucus or saliva, throat and tongue glistening, nocturnal perspiration, shivering, spasms in frightened children, epilepsy.

Large Intestine

Large Intestine 1

SHANG YANG MERCHANT YANG

Metal point of Yang
metal meridian
Category I
First point

'Dyspnoeic feeling in middle of chest', cough, swollen limbs, fever without perspiration, sudden attacks of fever, tinnitus, deafness, mouth dry, jaws swollen, adenitis of face, neck swollen, throat feels as if it is blocked, stomatitis, laryngitis, toothache, membrane over eye, colour blindness, cerebral congestion.

Large Intestine 2

ER JIAN SECOND INTERVAL

Water point
Category II
Point of sedation (main)

Epistaxis, jaundice, toothache, throat numb, tonsillitis, spasm of oesophagus, 'vision confused', inner canthus of eye diseased, headache, renal pain, pain in shoulder and arm, facial palsy, shivering, tongue tired, intestinal colic or spasm, diarrhoea due to inflammatory causes.

Large Intestine 3

SAN JIAN THIRD INTERVAL

Wood point
Category III
Point of sedation
(secondary)

Throat numb, throat blocked, tonsillitis, pain in eye, palpebral pruritis, dyspnoea, brings up much mucus, mouth dry, tongue swollen, lips cracked, diarrhoea, toothache, brachial neuralgia, likes to stretch himself.

Large Intestine 4

HE GU JOINING OF THE VALLEYS

Category IV
Source
Point of entry
Centre reunion general
point of Yang

Paralysis of limbs, unable to close lips, epistaxis, bleeding from gums, tonsillitis, intermittent fever, sees spots in front of eyes, weak eyesight, headache, migraine, hemiplegia, neuralgia of scapula back and renal area, deafness, tinnitus, aphonia, mute, dyspnoea, insomnia, nervous depression, night sweats, secondary amenorrhoea, pruritis.

Large Intestine 5

YANG XI YANG STREAM

Fire point
Category V

Bleeding from a scab in the nose, incoherent speech, mad laughter, 'sees the devil', fever without perspiration, nervous palpitations, eye red, inner canthus painful, headache, hemiplegia with anaesthesia, deafness, tinnitus, tonsillitis, neuralgia of the teeth, cough with the expectoration of much mucus, pruritis.

Large Intestine 6

PIAN LI INCLINED PASSAGE

Luo point

Dimness of vision, fever, madness, mad speech, throat dry and numb, tonsilitis, epistaxis, deafness, tinnitus, neuralgia of the arm, toothache, retention of urine, constipation.

Large Intestine 7
WEN LIU   WARM CURENT

Accumulation point   Fevers, pain in arm, throat numb, toothache, madness, 'sees devils', swollen tongue, glossitis, sticks tongue out, full of air, good at belching, swollen throat, headache, ulcers o: hand and face, stomatitis, parotitis, tonsillitis.

Large Intestine 8
XIA LIAN   LOWER ANGLE

Anorexia, 'abdomen melancholia', indigestion, abdominal pain, abundant stools, lips dry, headache, hemiplegia, body wastes away, emaciated, tuberculosis, mad speech, urine yellow-red, hernia causing vomiting, breast abscess with discharge, dyspnoea.

Large Intestine 9
SHANG LIAN   UPPER ANGLE

Borborygmi, body yellow, gonorrhoea, knee swollen due to wind and wet, hemiplegia, paralysis of the bladder, loss of sensation in limbs, flatulence, dyspnoea, Wind in the brain with headache, cold feeling in the bones and marrow, this point becomes tender after a lot of brain work.

Large Intestine 10
(SHOU) SAN LI (ARM) THREE MILES

Unable to raise arm, muscular spasm, toothache, pruritis, swelling of neck, adenitis, tonsillitis, indigestion, water brash, hemiplegia, cerebral congestion, pain from loin to navel, pleurisy, poor circulation in extremities.

Large Intestine 11
QU CHI   CROOKED POND

Earth point
Category VI
Point of tonification
Upper meeting point Ho
of large intestine

Eyes red, pain in front of ear, toothache, neck swollen painful and hot, cannot speak, madness, epilepsy, hemiplegia, erythema, anaemia, brachial neuralgia, intercostal neuralgia, torticollis, cervical adenitis, pleurisy, pruritis, amenorrhoea, atonic constipation, depression, dreams of uncultivated fields.

Large Intestine 12
ZHOU LIAO   ELBOW BONE

Elbow joint feels numb, pain in shoulder, unable to raise arm, arm feels wooden and insensitive.

Large Intestine 13
WU LI   FIVE MILES

Feeling of melancholy and pain below the heart, brachial neuralgia, four limbs paralysed, cervical adenitis, cannot see clearly, pneumonia, haemoptysis, peritonitis, very sleepy.

Large Intestine 14
BEI NAO   OUTER BONE OF ARM

? Point of Yang wei mo   Stiff neck, cervical adenitis, brachial neuralgia, unable to raise arm, headache, fever, shivering.

Large Intestine 15

JIAN YU   SHOULDER BONE (YU)

Independent associated
point of shoulder
Point of Yang qiao mo

Brachial neuralgia, hemiplegia, hypertension, muscular spasm in arm and hand, fever of long duration after influenza, spermatorrhoea, dry skin.

Large Intestine 16

JU GU   GREAT BONE

Point of Yang qiao mo

Agitation, epilepsy convulsions in children, brachial neuralgia, haematemesis, toothache.

Large Intestine 17

TIAN DING   HEAVENLY VESSEL

Suddenly dumb, throat numb and painful, tonsillitis, pharyngitis.

Large Intestine 18

FU TU   SUPPORT AND RUSH

Point 'Window of the
sky'

Cough, short of breath, stridor, suddenly dumb, hypersalivation, laryngeal spasm, orbital neuralgia, trembling of upper lip, pain in opposite hip.

Large Intestine 19

HE LIAO   GRAIN BONE

Nose obstructed, nasal catarrh, deviation of mouth, muscular spasm of face, epistaxis, catarrhal deafness, nasal polyp, anosmia, parotitis.

Large Intestine 20

YING XIANG   WELCOME FRAGRANCE

Point of exit
Meeting point sunlight
Yang

Anosmia, coryza, rhinorrhoea, dry mouth, loss of sensitivity of face, nasal polyp, nose blocked, epistaxis, swollen face, dyspnoea.

Stomach

Stomach 1
CHENG QI   RECEIVE TEARS

Reunion S, Cv
Point of Yang qiao mo
Greenish membrane covers eyes, poor vision, eyes twitch and water, dislikes strong light, cannot see well at night, deafness, tinnitus, facial spasm.

Stomach 2
SI BAI   FOUR WHITES

Headache, eyes feel dizzy, membrane over eye, eyes blink, eyes water easily, orbital neuralgia, eyes feel as if they have smoke in them, allergic rhinorrhoea, facial spasm, cannot speak.

Stomach 3
JU LIAO   GREAT BONE

Reunion S, Li
Point of Yang qiao mo
Nose blocked due to wind and cold, rhinorrhoea, abscess of the nose, maxillary sinusitis, weak distant vision, nystagmus, blepharospasm, convulsions, facial paralysis, dental neuralgia, aphonia, swelling of the jaw and lips, swelling and rheumatism of the feet.

Stomach 4
DI CANG   EARTH GRANARY

Reunion S, Li
Point of Yang qiao mo
Suddenly dumb, cannot speak, laryngitis, general catarrhal condition, neuralgia and paralysis of the face, cannot close his eyelids or blink, cannot see clearly at night, nystagmus, swelling of the feet.

Stomach 5
DA YING   BIG WELCOME

Reunion S, G
Neck painful, glandular swelling, stiffness of the tongue, cannot speak, mad fits, fits due to Wind, dry mouth, nystagmus, eyes blink, facial spasm, neuralgia of teeth in lower jaw, parotitis, fever with shivering.

Stomach 6
JIA CHE   JAW CHARIOT

Reunion S, G
Jaw swollen, cannot speak, laryngitis, dental neuralgia, glaucoma, myopia, sees spots in front of eyes, neck rigid, difficult to turn, spasm of facial muscles, trigeminal neuralgia, acne of face.

Stomach 7
XIA GUAN   LOWER GATE

? Reunion S, G
Tinnitus, deafness, otitis externa, orbital neuralgia, feels as if smoke in eyes, poor distant vision, eyes red and painful, foggy distant vision, headache, vertigo, yawning, fainting, facial neuralgia or spasm, maxilla that easily dislocates, pyorrhea, teeth that are loose.

Stomach 8
TOU WEI   HEAD TIED

Point of entry
Headache, head feels as if it is broken, facial paralysis, hemiplegia, loss of sensa-

tion in face, dyspnoea, pain in eye, eye feels as if it has been pulled out, eyes water, dislikes sunlight, conjunctivitis, blinking of eyelids, pain above eyelids.

Stomach 9
REN YING MAN WELCOME

Fullness of the chest, dyspnoea, throat swollen red and painful, cervical adenitis, pharyngitis, tonsillitis, vomiting, feeling as if energy under high tension shoots up and down.

Stomach 10
SHUI TU WATER RUSHING
Dyspnoea, Qi in upper part of body, tonsillitis, pharyngitis, bronchitis, whooping cough, spasmodic cough, pruritis, urticaria.

Stomach 11
QI SHE QI SHELTER
Throat numb and swollen, neck rigid and painful, dyspnoea, pharyngitis, goitre, swelling of glands in neck, 'energy high'.

Stomach 12
QUE PEN BROKEN BOWL

Pain in clavicular fossa, throat numb, cervical adenitis, haemoptysis, incessant cough, middle of chest hot and swollen, dyspnoea, pleurisy, intercostal neuralgia, generalised subcutaneous oedema, excessive loquacity, insomnia due to nervousness.

Stomach 13
QI HU QI COTTAGE
Chest ribs and limbs heavy, dyspnoea, 'energy high', pleurisy, bronchitis, frequent coughing, spasm of diaphragm, loss of taste and smell, loss of appetite, feet perspire too much.

Stomach 14
KU FANG STOREHOUSE
Chest ribs and limbs heavy, dyspnoea, 'energy high', sputum thick and streaked with blood, pulmonary congestion, bronchitis, pleurisy, physical and mental consequences of a shock.

Stomach 15
WU YI ROOM SCREEN
Chest ribs and limbs heavy, little children dyspneic with a swollen belly, whole body itches, dyspneic, asthma, 'energy high', thick phlegm streaked with blood, intercostal neuralgia, melancholic, tumour of the breast.

Stomach 16
YING CHUANG BREAST WINDOW
Ulcers of the breast, breasts too big, 'chest melancholia', short of breath, emphysema, intercostal neuralgia, fever with sensation of cold, insomnia, swelling of the lips, diarrhoea, bitter taste in mouth, heart-burn.

Stomach 17

RU ZHONG   MIDDLE OF BREAST

Most Chinese authors say that this point should not be used. One Chinese author writes that it is recorded in ancient texts that this point cures (or causes?) violent madness.

Chamfrault uses it in all diseases of the nipple.

Stomach 18

RU GEN   BREAST ROOT

Chest pain, hiccough, hacking cough, coughing and panting with much phlegm, breast exhausted, not enough milk, retained placenta, menstruation lasting more than nine days.

Stomach 19

BU RONG   NO ADMITTANCE

Pain in chest, abdomen melancholic and empty with borborygmi, cough, mouth dry, indigestion with much phlegm and painful ribs, eye diseases of little children, cardiac pain.

Stomach 20

CHENG MAN   RECEIVING FULLNESS

Intestinal noises with diarrhoea, lower ribs in the position of full inspiration, dyspnoea, cannot swallow food or drink, jaundice, haemoptysis.

Stomach 21

LIANG MEN   BEAM DOOR

Diarrhoea due to colonic disease, cannot use food or drink, anorexia, acute gastritis, all gastric troubles due to excesses, irritable stomach.

Stomach 22

GUAN MEN   GATE DOOR

Abdomen swollen, aerogastria, gastritis, anorexia, intestinal noises and diarrhoea, feverish, shakes with cold, urinary incontinence, oedema, bad breath.

Stomach 23

TAI YI   BIGGER YI (A CELESTIAL STEM)

Mad, walks about madly, neurasthenia, palpitations, sticks out tongue, bad digestion, cold limbs.

Stomach 24

HUA ROU MEN   SLIPPERY MEAT DOOR

Madness, vomiting, haematemesis, tongue rigid, sticks tongue out, glossitis, pain under tongue, dysmenorrhoea.

Stomach 25

TIAN SHU   HEAVENLY PIVOT

Alarm point of large intestine

Pain round the umbilicus, abdomen bloated, borborygmi, weary, frightened, weak, bowel disease in men, aqueous stools, irregular menstruation, leucorrhoea, sterility in women, dysentery with stabbing pain, retention of urine, ? oedema, ascites — the last two conditions are not altered by food or drink.

Stomach 26
WAI LING   OUTSIDE MOUND
Lower end of heart feels as if it is suspended, pain around umbilicus, intestinal spasm, spasm of rectus abdominus.

Stomach 27
DA JU   BIG GREAT
Shokanten of Sunlight Hernia, lower abdomen swollen and full, premature ejaculation, insomnia,
Yang weakness of limbs, constipation.

Stomach 28
SHUI DAO   WATER PATH
Triple warmer hot and congealed (genito-urinary function of lower triple warmer), retention of urine and faeces, lower abdomen distended, nephritis, cystitis, rectal prolapse, uterine and ovarian disease, inflamation of scrotum, pain going into vagina.

Stomach 29
GUI LAI   THE RETURN
'Hurrying and shuffling' in the lower abdomen, shrunken scrotum, pain in penis, orchitis, uterus cold, amenorrhoea, leucorrhoea, sterility. This point has a special effect on the male and female genitalia.

Stomach 30
QI CHONG   RUSHING QI
Centre reunion parti- Abdominal pain, spasm in foot, unable to use foot, hernia, swelling of penis,
cular point of food pain in penis, impotent, 'uterine cloths' (placenta) retained, amenorrhoea,
Sea of nourishment menorrhagia, energy that rises to top of body, sensation of warmth in
Reunion S, G stomach.
Point of Chong mo

Stomach 31
BI GUAN   THIGH GATE
Pain in loins and knee, lower limbs feel numb — like wood, paralysis of limbs, muscular cramp, inguinal adenitis, gonorrhoea, pain in the lower abdomen radiating to the throat.

Stomach 32
FU TU   PROSTRATE HARE
Reunion of veins Loins thighs and legs painful, knee cold not warm, atrophy of arm, uterine trouble, head heavy, abdomen distended, very mild varicose veins, oedema of legs, asthma in the middle of the night.

Stomach 33
YIN SHI   YIN MARKET
Painful hernia, pain in abdomen, paralysis and numbness of limbs, spasm

and cramp in feet, ascites, very thirsty, uterine spasm, irregular menstruation, trembling hands, no energy.

Stomach 34
LIANG QIU   BEAM MOUND

Accumulation point   Pain in loins knees and feet, limbs cold and numb, stomach pain and cramp, breast swollen and painful.

Stomach 35
DU BI   CALF NOSE

Pain in knee, unable to bend knee, rheumatism of feet, oedema of feet due to humidity.

Stomach 36
(ZU) SAN LI   (LEG) THREE MILES

Earth point of Yang   Globus hystericus, gastritis, anorexia, intestinal noises, abdominal pain,
earth meridian   abdomen swollen, anuria, food does not change abdominal pain, indigestion,
Category VI   constipation, appendicitis — slightly below S36, weak limbs, agitated and
Centre reunion parti-   emaciated, general lack of energy, tinnitus, eye diseases, nervousness, difficulty
cular point of energy   in speaking.
Lower meeting point   Some books mention practically every disease under this point.
Ho of stomach
Sea of nourishment
Reunion of energy

Stomach 37
SHANG JU XU   UPPER GREAT VOID

Lower meeting point   Chest ribs and limbs swollen, arthritis of knee, intestinal noises, diarrhoea,
Ho of large intestine   hemiplegia, unable to raise hand or foot, spleen and stomach empty and weak,
Sea of blood   gastritis, colitis, anorexia, marrow of the bone feels cold.

Stomach 38
TIAO KOU   LINE MOUTH

Weakness of legs, hemiplegia, loss of sensation in limbs and renal area, rheumatism caused by humidity, tonsillitis, gastritis, entero-colitis, diarrhoea.

Stomach 39
XIA JU XU   LOWER GREAT VOID

Lower meeting point Ho   Pain in lower abdomen associated with diarrhoea, pain in loins and legs,
of the small intestine   diseases of the breast, madness, cerebral anaemia, generalised aches and pains
Sea of blood   in body, intercostal neuralgia, tonsillitis, hypersalivation, lips dry, no sweat, loss of hair.

Stomach 40
FENG LONG   ABUNDANT BULGE

Luo point   Throat numb, cannot speak, headache, swollen face, dyspnoea with much phlegm and coughing, asthma hindering sleep, paralysis of leg, constipation, oliguria, madness, sees ghosts, laughs madly.

Stomach 41
JIE XI DISSOLVE STREAM

Fire point
Category V
Point of tonification

Head and face swollen, toothache, gingivitis, vertigo, madness, fits, convulsions in children, stomach hot with incoherent speech, eyes red with headache, muscles numb, rheumatism of feet, frightened and agitated.

Stomach 42
CHONG YANG RUSHING YANG

Category IV
Source
Point of exit

Fever without perspiration, always cold, seeks warmth, wants to undress in public, walks around aimlessly, 'every month madness', wishes to climb on to tables etc. and sing, paralysis of foot, toothache, gingivitis, anorexia, vomiting, yawning.

Stomach 43
XIAN GU SINKING VALLEY

Wood point
Category III

Chest ribs and limbs heavy, face swollen, congestion of eyes, thirsty with indigestion and fever, ascites, abdomen swollen with much belching, coughing that does not stop, very high fever.

Stomach 44
NEI TING INNER COURT YARD

Water point
Category II

Pain around navel, abdomen distended, asthmatic and melancholic, pain with fear and trembling, nightmares, dislikes the human voice, toothache, gingivitis, epistaxis, throat numb, anorexia, diarrhoea — the motion having pus and blood, skin rash and pustules with intermittent fever, dysmenorrhoea.

Stomach 45
LI DUI GENERAL EXCHANGE

Metal point
Category I
Point of sedation
Last point

Fainting, cerebral anaemia, 'like a corpse', deviation of mouth, face swollen, epistaxis, acute rhinitis, cold nose, sinusitis, throat numb, tonsillitis, fever with no perspiration, toothache, epigastrium swollen, eyes twitch, madness awaking and sleeping all the time with many dreams.

Spleen

Spleen 1
YIN BAI   HIDDEN WHITE

Wood point
Category I
Point of entry

Dyspnoea, asthma, abdomen swollen, little children cantankerous, severe vomiting, thirsty, hyperacidity, menorrhagia, epistaxis, haemorrhoids, foot cold and paralysed, madness, cannot remain still in bed.

Spleen 2
DA DU   BIG CAPITAL

Fire point
Category II
Point of tonification

'Humors of the body hot', spermatorrhoea, abdomen distended, agitated, melancholic, indigestion, does not absorb food, epigastric pain, spasm of stomach, general fatigue, body heavy, lumbago, limbs cold, cannot remain still in bed, foggy vision.

Spleen 3
TAI BAI   SUPREME WHITENESS

Earth point of Yin earth
meridian
Category III & IV
Source

Fever, melancholic, agitated, chest ribs and abdomen swollen, intestinal noises with stabbing pain, diarrhoea, intestinal haemorrhage, constipation, diarrhoea with pus and blood, mad, body heavy, lumbago, haemorrhoids cardiac pain, cold feet.

Spleen 4
GONG SUN   GRANDFATHER GRANDSON

Luo point
Master point of Chong
mo
Coupled point of Yin wei
mo

Intestine swollen, stabbing pain in intestines, abdomen swollen, ascites, cardiac pain, pleurisy, vomits foul food, intestinal haemorrhage, fever with yellow ulcers and excessive perspiration, face swollen, very thirsty.

Spleen 5
SHANG QIU   MERCHANT MOUND

Metal point
Category V
Point of sedation
Reunion of veins

Vomits a lot, a gourmand — but cannot digest his food, headache, swollen face, spleen empty, indigestion, pain along inside of thighs, hernia, abdominal pain, agitation in little children, dreams of ghosts, sighs often, haemorrhoids, spasm in feet, yellow ulcer, yellow urine, jaundice, sterility.

Spleen 6
SAN YIN JIAO   THREE YIN CROSSING

Group Luo point of 3
lower Yin
Reunion Sp, K, Liv

All diseases of the genitalia of both sexes, menorrhagia, spermatorrhoea, pain in genitalia, abdomen swollen, diarrhoea, symptoms not changed by food or drink, chest in position of inspiration with phlegm and cough, dysuria, retained foetus, foot paralysed numb or painful, haemorrhoids, insomnia, nervous depression.

Spleen 7
LOU GU   LEAKY VALLEY

Abdomen swollen, borborygmi, indigestion, flatulence, eats much without gaining weight, numbness, not able to walk, very little urine, mad, foot and ankle swollen and painful.

Spleen 8
DI JI   EARTH ORGAN

Accumulation point Abdomen swollen, ascitis, anorexia, spermatorrhoea, irregular menstruation, leucorrhoea, very little urine, haemorrhoids, lumbago, intermittent fever.

Spleen 9
YIN LING QUAN   YIN MOUND SPRING

Water point Water swelling eliminates umbilicus — ascites, spermatorrhoea, very little
Category VI urine, pain in loins and knees, chest ribs and abdomen heavy, intermittent fever, dyspnoea, dysmenorrhoea, weakness of legs, cramps.

Spleen 10
XUE HAI   SEA OF BLOOD

Dysmenorrhoea, menorrhagia, metritis, oligomenorrhoea, orchitis, perineal eczema, indigestion.

Spleen 11
JI MEN   BASKET DOOR

Very little urine, incontinence of urine, gonorrhoea, inguinal adenitis.

Spleen 12
CHONG MEN   RUSHING DOOR

Reunion Sp, Liv Abdomen swollen and painful, gastric spasm, retention of urine, hernia, haemorrhoids, dyspnoea, menorrhagia, dysmenorrhoea, orchitis, epididymitis, insufficient milk, breast abscess, rectal prolapse.

Spleen 13
FU SHE   MANSION COTTAGE

Reunion Sp, Liv Hernia, pain in buttocks, indigestion, intestinal spasm, abdominal pain.
Point of Yin wei mo

Spleen 14
FU JIE   ABDOMEN KNOT

Periumbilical pain, abdominal pain, diarrhoea, heart agitated, cough, dyspnoea, weakness of legs, excessive perspiration.

Spleen 15
DA HENG   BIG HORIZONTAL

Point of Yin wei mo Unable to use limbs, excessive perspiration, influenza, constipated, enterocolitis, always sad.

Spleen 16
FU AI ABDOMEN SORROW

Point of Yin wei mo   Intestinal haemorrhage, blood in stools, pus in stools, periumbilical pain, symptoms not altered by food or drink, peptic ulcer, hypo or hyperacidity.

Spleen 17
SHI DOU FOOD DRAIN

Chest ribs and limbs heavy, diaphragmatic pain, intestines make sound like thunder, intermittent fever of the spleen, paralysis and numbness, ascites, pulmonary congestion.

Spleen 18
TIAN XI HEAVENLY STREAM

Middle of chest full and painful, bronchitis, breast swollen and large, insufficient milk, rebellious cough, throat noises, peptic ulcer.

Spleen 19
XIONG XIANG CHEST VILLAGE

Chest ribs and limbs heavy, bronchitis, loss of appetite, difficulty in lying down or turning.

Spleen 20
ZHOU RONG ENCIRCLING GLORY

Chest ribs and abdomen distended, cough, 'energy high', purulent and blood stained sputum, haemorrhoids, eyelids swollen.

Spleen 21
DA BAO BIG ENVELOPING

Luo point of all Luo   Dyspnoea with chest pain, pain on one side of head and body while other
points   side is relaxed; harmonises right and left, upper and lower, inside and outside
Point of exit   of body.

Heart

Heart 1

JI QUAN   EXTREME SPRING

Point of Entry   Inflammation of the heart, dry throat, cardiac pain, very thirsty, pain in the chest and ribs, feeling of fullness in chest, spasm of the chest, 'frog in throat', nausea, hysteria, moral depression, hypotension, paralysis of all limbs, forearm cold, tip of tongue tender or numb, eyesight weak, excessive perspiration due to weakness, too impulsive.

Heart 2

QING LING   GREEN SPIRIT

Dislike of cold, shivering, fever, frontal headache, generalised headache, neuralgia and spasm of arm, unable to raise arm or shoulder, cannot wear clothes, intercostal neuralgia, congestion and feeling of constriction in middle and lower thorax.

Heart 3

SHAO HAI   LESSER SEA

Water point   Glandular disease, scrofulous swellings, adenitis, hand and fingers cold, *Category VI*   epilepsy, madness, eyes dizzy, diplopia, fainting, bleats like a sheep, toothache, headache due to wind or cold, dizzy, intercostal neuralgia, facial neuralgia, spasm of shoulder or arm, trembling and shaking of hand, pleurisy, torticollis, spasm of elbow, fever with sensation of cold, feels as if energy goes to top part of body, stupidity, forgetfulness, mental depression, coughing up mucus, cannot move limbs, mammary pain, pruritis, trembling in infants, adds stability to nervous exhaustion.

Heart 4

LING DAO   SPIRIT PATH

Metal point   Arthritis of elbow and wrist, spasm and neuralgia of arm, loss of sensation in *Category V*   upper arm, convulsions, hysteria, cardiac pain, fear, anxiety, suddenly mute, unable to speak, paralysis of tongue muscles, nausea, ice cold feeling in bone.

Heart 5

TONG LI   PENETRATING INSIDE

Luo point   Headache, eyes dizzy, dizziness, vertigo, palpitations, tonsillitis, sudden dumbness, throat spasm, pharyngitis, neuralgia and spasm of upper limbs and shoulder blade area, hysteria, not happy, anxiety, fear, fear of people, words fall over one another, dysmenorrhoea, metrorrhagia, incontinence of urine, urinary frequency, clear urine, lack of energy, face warm without sweat, yawning, vomiting, conjunctivitis, abdomen swollen, constipation.

Heart 6

YIN HUNG   YIN ACCUMULATION

Accumulation point   Epistaxis, nose blocked, dizziness, headache, palpitations, tonsillitis, brachial neuralgia, hysteria, startled, frightened, short of breath, pain in chest, fullness of chest, shivering, leucorrhoea, endometritis, night sweats, haematemesis, fainting, suddenly dumb, tongue without strength, sudden diarrhoea, cannot bend elbow.

Heart 7

SHEN MEN   SPIRIT DOOR

Earth point
Category III & IV
Point of sedation
Source

Psychological and physical cardiac diseases, heart big and dilated, warmth and pain in cardiac area, shortness of breath, palpitations, inflammation of the nose, nose blocked, red face, desire for cool drinks, loss of speech, hysteria, shortness of breath with a hot body, face purple and raving, likes to laugh, frightened, laughing and sobbing alternating, hallucinations, loss of taste and appetite, dry throat, tonsillitis, insomnia due to excitement, post-partum haemorrhage, urinary incontinence, cold feet, fear of cold, shivering, palms of hands warm, cardiac and renal energy weak, sighing, forgetfulness, irregular cardiac rhythm, fibrillation, oedematous tongue, cannot stop talking, cardiac oedema, retention of fluid, cold sweat, migraine.

Heart 8

SHAO FU   LESSER MANSION

Fire point of Yin,
Princely, fire meridian
Category II

Diseases and a feeling of calamity in the heart and chest, palpitations, precordial pain, hysteria, fear, frightened of people, trembling, throat dry, sighing, shivering, intermittent fever, neuralgia and numbness of arm and shoulder, hand contracted — cannot be extended, pain and muscular spasm on front of shoulder and armpit, palm of hand warm, difficulty in urination, urinary incontinence, one side of scrotum larger than the other, impotent, general uterine disease, pruritis vulvae, prolapse of the uterus, metrorrhagia.

Heart 9

SHAO CHONG   LESSER RUSHING

Wood point
Category 1
Point of tonification
Point of exit

General cardiac disease, palpitations, heart weak, atonic, steady pulse, mental discouragement, eyes not clear, expressionless voice, neuralgia of arm from palm to armpit, intercostal neuralgia, pleurisy, fullness of chest, bronchial hypersecretion, pharyngitis, dry throat, fever, weakness after fever, fever with sensation of cold, feeling of energy in upper part of body, vaginal odour, white or red vaginal discharge, dreams of fire and smoke.

Small Intestine

Small Intestine 1
SHAO ZE   LESSER MARSH

Metal Point
Category I
Point of Entry

Headache, pharyngitis, cough, tonsillitis, cardiac pain, breathless on exertion, brachial neuralgia, torticollis, pain in chest, agalactia, membrane over eye, diarrhoea, dry mouth, polyuria, epistaxis, convulsions in children.

Small Intestine 2
QIAN GU   FRONT VALLEY

Water point
Category II

Intermittent fever, fever without sweating, cough, haematemesis, tonsillitis, throat and cheeks red and swollen, nose blocked, coryza, agalactia, mastitis, brachial neuralgia, not able to lift arm, epilepsy, tinnitus, weak eye sight.

Small Intestine 3
HOU XI   BACK STREAM

Wood point
Category III
Point of tonification
Master point of Du mo
Coupled point of Yang qiao mo

Madness, epilepsy, epistaxis, deafness, eye red and painful, white membrane over eye, tonsillitis, spasm and pain in arm and forearm, stiff neck, torticollis, pruritis, night sweats, recovers slowly after a shock, bad digestion, greasy stools.

Small Intestine 4
WAN GU   WRIST BONE

Category IV
Source point

Arthritis of arm forearm and fingers, pain and spasm of fingers, not able to bend or stretch fingers, creaking of neck, pharyngitis, white membrane over eye with tears, tinnitus, headache, vomiting, irritated stomach, pleurisy, hemiplegia, convulsions, meningism, apprehension, sense of touch dulled, excessive perspiration, alternately hot and cold.

Small Intestine 5
YANG GU   YANG VALLEY

Fire point of Yang,
Princely, fire meridian
Category V

Dizziness, fainting, tinnitus, deafness, stomatitis, gingivitis, neuralgia of arm and wrist, cannot raise arm, intercostal neuralgia, weakness, fears and spasm of children, epilepsy, stiff tongue, children cannot suckle, talks or laughs excessively, painful haemorrhoids.

Small Intestine 6
YANG LAO   SUPPORTING THE OLD

Accumulation point

Paralysis and neuralgia of the arm, arm feels as if it is broken and uprooted, unable to raise or lower arm, eyes bloodshot, diminished strength of vision.

Small Intestine 7
ZHI ZHENG BRANCH STRAIGHT

Luo point   Forearm and front of shoulder-spasm and not able to bend or stretch, pain in hand, cannot hold objects, face red and feels dizzy, vertigo, throat swollen, headache, intermittent fever, psychopathic apprehension, fear, cyst of eyelids.

Small Intestine 8
XIAO HAI SMALL SEA

Earth point
Category VI
Point of sedation
Upper meeting point Ho
of small intestine

Spasm and neuralgia of the whole upper limb, eyes bloodshot, dizzy Wind? listening and feeling dulled, gingivitis, dancing madly, tics, trembling, insanity, cervical adenitis, lower abdominal pain, pulmonary oedema, swellings, pruritis, shivering.

Small Intestine 9
JIAN ZHEN SHOULDER CHASTITY

Tinnitus, deafness, headache, neuritis, arthritis and pain of upper limbs and scapula, numbness due to wind, unable to raise hand or foot, fever after having been exposed to wind.

Small Intestine 10
NAO YU SHOULDER BLADE YU

Independent associated
point of shoulder blade
Point of Yang wei mo
and Yang qiao mo

Shoulder and scapula region: muscular pain, numbness, arthritis, weakness, hot-cold feeling, swelling, unable to raise arm.

Small Intestine 11
TIAN ZONG HEAVENLY ANCESTOR

Scapula region-neuralgia and numbness, neuralgia of forearm, cannot lift arms, swelling of lower jaw.

Small Intestine 12
BING FENG FACING THE WIND

Reunion Si, Li, T, G   Shoulder and arm neuralgia and numbness, cannot raise arm, pneumonia, pleurisy.

Small Intestine 13
QU YUAN CROOKED WALL

Neuralgia and numbness of the shoulder and arm, shoulder hot, unable to embrace.

Small Intestine 14
JIAN WAI YU OUTSIDE OF THE SHOULDER YU

Independent associated
point of the outside of
the shoulder

Spasm, muscular pain and neuralgia of shoulder and arm, sensation of coldness encircling shoulder and going as far as elbow, spasm of neck muscles, pneumonia, pleurisy.

Small Intestine 15

JIAN ZHONG YU MIDDLE OF THE SHOULDER YU

Bronchitis, shortness of breath, mucus streaked with blood, torticollis, weak eye sight.

Small Intestine 16

TIAN CHANG HEAVENLY WINDOW

Point 'Window of the sky' Half of the body not co-ordinated, aphonia, movements slow and lethargic, not fully under voluntary control, neck slanting to one side, spasm of neck and shoulder, unable to twist neck, intercostal neuralgia, inflammation of jaw, deafness, tinnitus, anal fistula.

Small Intestine 17

TIAN RONG HEAVENLY APPEARANCE

Point 'Window of the sky' Pleurisy, dyspnoea, sternal pain, intercostal neuralgia, difficulty in straightening body, neuralgia, swelling and immobility of neck, tinnitus, deafness, swollen tongue, gingivitis, nausea, vomiting.

Small Intestine 18

QUAN LIAO CHEEK BONE

Reunion Si, T, G Trigeminal neuralgia face red, not able to eat, facial neuralgia and numbness, mouth twisted, eyes blinking, eyes that always move, pharyngitis, toothache.

Small Intestine 19

TING GONG LISTENING PALACE

Point of exit Tinnitus, deafness, otitis externa, hoarseness.
Reunion Si, T, G

493

Bladder

Bladder 1

JING MING   EYES BRIGHT

Point of entry
Meeting point greater
Yang
Reunion B, S, Si, T, G
Point of Yang and Yin
qiao mo

Eye disease, eyes dizzy, inner canthus red and painful, white membrane over eye, conjunctivitis, tears flow in wind, master point for the eyes, dim vision, retinitis, poor night vision, vertigo, headache.

Bladder 2

ZAN ZHU   DRILLING BAMBOO

Brain tired, stiff neck, madness, eyes red, eyes red and painful with headache, eye lazy, eye wanders, excessive blinking, vision foggy, eyes water, convergent strabismus, hay fever, allergic rhinorrhoea, sneezing especially in light and wind, sinusitis, supraorbital neuralgia, nausea, vomiting, nightmares, hallucination, perspiration acid and rancid.

Bladder 3

MEI CHONG   EYEBROW RUSHING

Headache, fainting, epilepsy, nose blocked, catarrh, not able to smell foul smells, maxillary sinusitis.

Bladder 4

QU CHAI   CROOKED SERVANT

Headache, pain on summit of head, facial neuralgia, burning heat in head, stiff neck, rhinophyma, nose blocked, epistaxis, ulcer in nose, nasal polyp, acute dyspnoea, dislikes sunlight in eyes, weak eyesight, no perspiration.

Bladder 5

WU CHU   FIVE PLACES

Spine rigid, spine arched backwards, headache, eyes dizzy, eyes weak, madness, epilepsy, loss of consciousness, does not recognise people, pain in renal area, pain in cervical and upper thoracic vertebrae, neuralgia of canine teeth, heartburn.

Bladder 6

CHENG GUANG   RECEIVE LIGHT

Fever without perspiration, vomiting, vertigo after a shock, palpitations, white membrane covers eye, keratitis, dim vision, foggy vision, cataract, nose blocked, allergic rhinorrhoea, anosmia, cardiac disease, pain over deltoid.

Bladder 7

TONG TIAN   PENETRATE HEAVEN

Headache, head heavy, torticollis, cervical adenitis, nose blocked, epistaxis, rhinitis, anosmia, face swollen, facial neuralgia, dyspnoea, chronic bronchitis, dry mouth, thirsty, convulsions, vertigo, eyesight weak.

Bladder 8

LUO QUE CONNECTING DEFICIENT

Epilepsy, falls down and lies as stiff as a corpse, obsessions, walks around madly, head revolves, tinnitus, eyes see dimly, abdomen swollen, rheumatism of neck and shoulder.

Bladder 9

YU ZHEN JADE PILLOW

Pain in eye and supraorbital region, eyes feel as if they have been torn out, shooting pain in eye on bending or raising head, eyes water in cold wind, dim vision, myopia, vertigo, head and neck heavy and painful, occipital neuralgia, nose blocked, anosmia, grieved, weary, neuralgias, hypertensive encephalopathy.

Bladder 10

TIAN ZHU HEAVENLY PILLAR

Point 'Window of the sky'
Sea of energy
Supposedly vago-sympathetic

Head heavy, spasm of neck muscles, brachial neuralgia, torticollis, writers cramp, light-headedness, limbs and body not co-ordinated, legs collapse under body, throat swollen, difficulty in speaking, nose blocked, weak sense of smell, epistaxis, neurasthenia, nymphomania, seems to have a regularising effect on medullary functions.

Bladder 11

DA ZHU BIG SHUTTLE

Sea of blood
Special point for bone
Reunion B, ? Si, ? T, G

High fever without perspiration, influenza, generalised spasms in the body, generalised muscular rheumatism, headache, vertigo, epilepsy, fainting, nervous agitation, chest full, bronchitis, pain in loins, muscular spasm in back, abdominal distension, arthritis of knee, an important point for all osseous diseases, stiffness of the vertebral column.

Bladder 12

FENG MEN WIND GATE

Reunion B, Gv

Severe muscular spasm of the neck, headache, head feels dizzy, spermatorrhoea, dyspnoeic, cough, asthma, unable to lie down, vomiting, preventative for the after effects of a chill, influenza, fever, tosses about in his bed, delirious with fever, allergic rhinorrhoea, sneezing, epistaxis, acne of the shoulders and back, abscess of the back.

Bladder 13

FEI YU LUNG YU

Associated point of lung

Cough, asthma, dyspnoea, chest feels heavy, pneumonia, bronchitis, agitated, perspiration, pruritis, vomits, haemoptysis, gastritis, water brash, anorexia, mouth and tongue dry, carditis, bored.

Bladder 14
JUE YIN YU   ABSOLUTE YIN YU

Associated point of circulation — sex

Pleurisy, middle of chest feels agitated and depressed, bouts of coughing, cardiac pain, enlarged heart, vomiting, neuralgia of the teeth especially molars, epistaxis, sunstroke, heatstroke, mountain sickness.

Bladder 15
XIN YU   HEART YU

Associated point of heart

Palpitations with shortness of breath, cannot sleep lying down, cardiac pain, easily sad, haemoptysis, vomiting, madness, eyesight poor, body empty and weak, face as red as a beetroot, body below heart feels dead, impotence, perspiration localised over sternum, cannot stop talking, wishes of heart and brain not co-ordinated.

Bladder 16
DU YU   GOVERNING VESSEL YU

Associated point of governing vessel

Cardiac pain, dilatation of heart, hiccough, flatulence, colic, borborygmi, abdominal pain, pain in loins, fever with shivering, nervous breakdown.

Bladder 17
GE YU   DIAPHRAGM YU

Associated point of diaphragm
Centre reunion general point of Yang and Yin and blood

Cardiac pain, throat numb, carditis, body feels empty weary and emaciated, vomiting of food, does not digest food, haemoptysis, gastritis, anorexia, enteritis, chest and abdomen distend 'hot blooded,', night sweats, pleurisy, dyspnoea.

Bladder 18
GAN YU   LIVER YU

Associated point of liver

Haemoptysis, dyspnoea, chest and ribs full and melancholic, enlarged liver, dark rings round eyes, epistaxis, pale stools, bitter taste in mouth, jaundice, duodenal ulcer, bad tempered, haemorrhoids, angio-neurotic oedema, intercostal neuralgia, bronchitis, asthma.

Bladder 19
DAN YU   GALL BLADDER YU

Associated point of gall bladder

Weary, fever, shivering, choleric, dry mouth, bitter taste in mouth, jaundice, pain in lower ribs, epigastrium distended, haemoptysis, vomits food, hypertension, pleurisy, eyebrows tender, eyes yellow, eyes bloodshot.

Bladder 20
PI YU   SPLEEN YU

Associated point of spleen

Chest painful, abdomen protruding, oesophogeal and tracheal pain, colitis, gastritis, indigestion, vomits dark food, eats a lot but remains thin, poor digestion, anorexia, diarrhoea, undigested stools, defective night vision, intermittent fever.

Bladder 21
WEI YU   STOMACH YU

Associated point of the stomach

Stomach ache, borborygmi, gastric haemorrhage, vomiting, diarrhoea, stool mixed with pus and blood, abdomen swollen, gastritis, flatulence, green stools in children, regurgitation of milk, eats a lot but remains thin, anorexia, poor eyesight, does not see well at dusk, dyspnoea, limbs heavy.

Bladder 22
SAN JIAO YU   TRIPLE WARMER YU

Associated point of triple warmer Bowels 'congealed', borborygmi, distended abdomen, enterocolitis, anorexia, melaena, flatulence, cannot digest food, pain in loins, incontinence of urine, feeling of tightening in back and shoulder, stiff vertebral column.

Bladder 23
SHEN YU   KIDNEY YU

Associated point of kidney Weary, empty, emaciated, deafness due to the kidney being empty, sexual and oppressive dreams, nocturnal emissions, premature ejaculation, cramp and paralysis of foot, red or white vaginal discharge, amenorrhoea, dysmenorrhoea, kidney weak, pain in loins, haemorrhoids, haematuria, face yellow-black, asthma.

Bladder 24
QI HAI YU   SEA OF QI YU

Extra associated point of upper lumbar region Pain in loins, periumbilical pain, haemorrhoids, intestinal spasm, hypertension, gonorrhoea.

Bladder 25
DA CHANG YU   LARGE INTESTINE YU

Associated point of large intestine Borborygmi, pain around umbilicus, diarrhoea, dry large intestine?, symptoms not changed by food or drink, pain in small intestine, loins cold and painful, weak legs, little urine, urethritis, dysuria, constipated, spasm of lumbar muscles.

Bladder 26
GUAN YUAN YU   GATE ORIGIN YU

Extra associated point of lower lumbar region Pain in loins, passes little urine, abdomen swollen and tight, generalised disease of bowels, diarrhoea, emaciated, weakness after influenza, uterine spasm, lumbago, sciatica.

Bladder 27
XIAO CHANG YU   SMALL INTESTINE YU

Associated point of small intestine Colitis, enteritis, diarrhoea, blood in stools, metritis, leucorrhoea, gonorrhoea, haemorrhoids, sacral pain, feet swollen.

Bladder 28
PANG GUANG YU   BLADDER YU

Associated point of bladder Dysuria, haematuria, cystitis, urine dark yellow, lumbago, cramp in calves, abdominal pain, pain in lower leg, weakness of lower leg, head cold, metritis, poor circulation in young women.

Bladder 29
ZHONG LÜ YU   MIDDLE OF BACK YU

Extra associated point of sacrum   Kidneys weak, no perspiration, lumbago, back stiff, sciatica, dysentery with red and white flecks in motion, hernia, enterocolitis, abdominal pain.

Bladder 30
BAI HUAN YU   WHITE CIRCLE YU

Extra associated point of anal sphincter   Urine dark yellow or red, spermatorrhoea, amenorrhoea, metritis, incontinence of urine and faeces, spasm of anus, dysuria, lumbago and sacral pain, sciatica, quadriplegia.

Bladder 31
SHANG LIAO   UPPER BONE

Reunion B, G   Anuria, constipation, unable to become pregnant, prolapse of the uterus, red and white vaginal discharge, sciatica, lumbago, impotance, gonorrhoea, orchitis, epistaxis, a general point for genital diseases of both sexes

Bladder 32
CI LIAO   SECOND BONE

Pain and stiffness in loin and knee, swollen epigastrium, vomiting, dysuria, urine red, borborygmi, diarrhoea, red and white vaginal discharge, inflammation of scrotum, sterility, irregular menstruation, uterine prolapse, a general point for genital diseases of both sexes.

Bladder 33
ZHONG LIAO   MIDDLE BONE

Reunion B, G   Anuria, constipation, vomiting, abdominal swelling, diarrhoea, sterility, red and white vaginal discharge, amenorrhoea, pain in middle of lumbar and sacral region, a general point for genital diseases of both sexes.

Bladder 34
XIA LIAO   LOWER BONE

Borborygmi, blood in stools, diarrhoea, acute pain in lower abdomen, constipation, anuria, lumbago, coccydynia, pain and coldness down back and inside of thigh, a general point for genital diseases of both sexes.

Bladder 35
HUI YANG   MEETING OF THE YANG

Diarrhoea, pain in anal region, blood in stools, haemorrhoids, anal discharge, perianal diseases, gonorrhoea, sciatica, impotence, a general point for genital diseases of both sexes.

Bladder 36
FU FEN   SUPPLEMENTARY DIVISION

? Reunion B, Si   Brachial neuralgia, spasm of shoulder, neck painful and stiff, intercostal neuralgia, bronchitis, 'Wind and Cold enters the pores of the skin'.

Bladder 37

PO HU   SOUL SHELTER

Lungs are empty, weary and paralysed, dyspnoea, 'upper Qi', bronchitis, acute pain of the shoulders, vomiting, similar effect to that of the associated point of the lung B13.

Bladder 38

GAO HUANG   THE VITALS DIAPHRAGM

Specialised point for haematopoiesis

Weak, emaciated, five types of weariness, anaemia, spermatorrhoea, 'upper Qi', vomiting, dyspnoea, dry phlegm, madness, night sweats, loss of memory, difficulty in speaking, haemoptysis.

Bladder 39

SHEN TANG   SPIRIT HALL

Dyspnoea, asthma, all types of cardiac disease, 'upper Qi', contracture of back and renal area, shivering.

Bladder 40

YI XI   SIGHING GIGLING

Dyspnoea, epistaxis, pericarditis, brachial neuralgia, intercostal neuralgia, fever without perspiration, slight fever, headache, fainting, cannot see clearly, spasm of back and loins, anorexia, vomiting.

Bladder 41

GE GUAN   DIAPHRAGM GATE

Gastric bleeding, enterocolitis, middle of chest feels full, vomiting, belching, neither food nor drink can be swallowed, back rigid and painful, hypersalivation, nausea, fear of cold, dark yellow urine.

Bladder 42

HUN MEN   SOUL DOOR

Chest feels full and melancholic, pleurisy, neither food nor drink can be swallowed, borborygmi, periumbilical pain, poor digestion, urine red or yellow, rheumatism, syncope.

Bladder 43

YANG GANG   YANG ESSENTIALS

Abdomen distended, flatulence, diarrhoea due to large intestinal disease, urine red, dysuria, body hot with yellow eyes, unable to swallow food or drink, rheumatism.

Bladder 44

YI SHE   THOUGHT SHELTER

Abdominal distension and flatulence, diarrhoea, weary, rheumatism, unable to swallow food or drink, vomiting without stopping, eyes yellow, urine dark yellow, intercostal neuralgia, afraid of cold, very thirsty, the more one drinks the greater is the thirst, localised oedema.

Bladder 45

WEI CANG STOMACH GRANARY

Abdomen distended, ascites, unable to swallow food or drink, vomiting, backache, localised oedema

Bladder 46

HUANG MEN VITALS DOOR

Inflammation of breast, pain below heart, spasm of stomach, constipation.

Bladder 47

ZHI SHI AMBITIOUS ROOM

Pain and swelling in penis, all genital diseases, dysuria, kidney weakness, vomiting, abdominal swelling, back and kidney area rigid and painful, spermatorrhoea.

Bladder 48

BAO HUANG WOMB AND VITALS

Pain in lower abdomen, constipation, retention of urine, heavy feeling pressing downwards, dysuria, pain and stiffness in back and renal area, orchitis, gonorrhoea, metritis, haemorrhoids, urethritis.

Bladder 49

ZHI BIAN FOLDING EDGE

Lumbar and sacral pain, sciatica, pain and heaviness of genitalia, gynaecological diseases, difficult urination, cystitis, haemorrhoids of all types.

Bladder 50

CHENG FU RECEIVE AND SUPPORT

Haemorrhoids, constipated, rectal pain, lumbago, pain in back, sciatica, coccydynia, difficulty in urination, pain in penis, spermatorrhoea, gynaecological diseases.

Bladder 51

YIN MEN PROSPEROUS GATE

Pain in back and loins, sciatica, unable to move foot, unable to look up or down — i.e. bend, bleeding haemorrhoids, circulatory disturbance of the thighs.

Bladder 52

FU XI FLOATING ACCUMULATION

Unable to bend knee, muscular spasm of lateral side of thigh, muscular spasm of calf, lower abdomen hot and hard on pressure, cystitis, constipation, vomiting.

Bladder 53

WEI YANG COMMANDING YANG

Lower meeting point Ho of triple warmer

Abdominal distension, muscular spasm of calf, muscular spasm in general, pain in loins, urinary incontinence, unable to look up or down — i.e. bend, cannot bend knee, chest feels full, pain and swelling of armpit, epilepsy, fever, fainting.

Bladder 54
WEI ZHONG   COMMANDING MIDDLE

Earth point
Category VI
Lower meeting point Ho
of bladder

Lumbago with stiff neck, arthritis of knee, foot swollen, body feels heavy, night sweats due to weakness, epistaxis, diarrhoea with a lot of blood in the motion, bleeding haemorrhoids, madness, spasms in children, nervousness, hemiplegia, abdominal pain, shivering, loss of hair head and eyebrows, skin diseases in general.

Bladder 55
HE YANG   UNITING YANG

Hernia, rheumatism, madness, fits in children, pain in loins and abdomen, heaviness and muscular spasm in knee and calf, orchitis, menorrhagia, leucorrhoea, vaginal spasm.

Bladder 56
CHENG JIN   SUPPORTING MUSCLES

Pain and heaviness in foot and calf, pain of the instep of foot, muscular cramps, haemorrhoids of all types, epistaxis, constipation.

Bladder 57
CHENG SHAN   SUPPORTING MOUNTAIN

Head feels hot, epistaxis, epilepsy, abdominal pain, anorexia, swollen and bleeding haemorrhoids, knee swollen and painful, swelling of feet, lumbago, muscular cramps, gonorrhoea.

Bladder 58
FEI YANG   FLYING HIGH

Luo point

Epilepsy, head and eyes feel dizzy, vertigo, weakness of legs, lumbago, sciatica, supraorbital neuralgia, haemorrhoids, constipation, cystitis, irritable bladder, nocturia, pain in hypochondrium.

Bladder 59
FU YANG   FOOT BONE YANG

Point of Yang qiao mo
Accumulation point
of Yang qiao mo

Rheumatism of ankle, cramp, unable to bend knee or ankle, head heavy and painful, unable to raise arms or legs, thigh swollen.

Bladder 60
KUN LUN   KUN LUN MOUNTAINS (NEAR TIBET)

Fire point
Category V

Convulsions in little children, lumbago, pain in thigh, sciatica, rheumatism of foot, foot swollen, headache, eyes dizzy, vertigo, epistaxis, brachial neuralgia, haemorrhoids, retained placenta, glandular diseases, dyspnoea.

Bladder 61
PU SHEN   OFFICIAL'S AIDE

Point of Yang qiao mo

Foot paralysed, weakness of legs, lumbago, muscular cramp in calf, pain in knee, madness, sees ghosts, faints easily, gonorrhoea.

Bladder 62
SHEN MO   EXTENDED MERIDIAN

Master point of Yang qiao mo
Coupled point of Yin qiao mo
Point of Yang qiao mo

Madness, epilepsy, dizziness, post-concussion symptoms, skin feels as if it is electrified or has too much energy, tinnitus, pain in knee and foot, foot red and swollen, lumbago, sciatica, occipital neuralgia, tension headaches, spastic conditions of uterus.

The symptoms of many diseases of the spinal cord can be helped, though not cured, in the early stages of the disease, by this point.

Bladder 63
JIN MEN   GOLDEN DOOR

Accumulation point
Point of Yang wei mo

Headache, shaking of head with open mouth in children, convulsions in children, tinnitus, pain in knee and lower leg, lower abdominal pain, vomiting.

Bladder 64
JING GU   CAPITAL BONE

Category IV
Source point

Lumbago, sciatica, stiff neck, torticollis, dyspnoea, pneumonitis, headache, epistaxis, epilepsy, madness, cerebral congestion, cardiac disease, inner canthus of eye is red, white membrane covers eye, dim vision, does not eat or drink.

Bladder 65
SHU GU   BIND THE BONE

Wood point
Category III
Point of sedation

Enterocolitis, diarrhoea, fever, dislikes wind and cold, madness, headache, vertigo, inner canthus of eye red and painful, deafness, neck rigid, lumbago, sciatica, all types of haemorrhoids, all types of abscess.

Bladder 66
TONG GU   PENETRATING THE VALLEY

Water point of Yang water meridian
Category II

Headache, vertigo, fear, stiff neck, epistaxis, rhinorrhoea, cannot see clearly, indigestion, gastritis, chest full, symptoms not altered by food or drink.

Bladder 67
ZHI YIN   EXTREMITY OF YIN

Metal point
Category I
Point of tonification
Point of exit

Head heavy, nose blocked, pain in eye, eye covered by membrane, intercostal neuralgia, fever without perspiration, difficulty in urination, effective in early prostatic hypertrophy, spermatorrhoea, 'old man's gait'. Be careful when using this point in a patient who easily gets supraorbital or occipital neuralgia.

Kidney

Kidney 1
YONG QUAN   BUBBLING SPRING

Wood point
Category I
Point of sedation (main)
Point of entry

Fainting with cold limbs, dumbness, prone to fear, madness or epilepsy, disturbed viscera (Zang-solid organs), alarm in children, paralysis (central Feng), pain in head and nape of neck, pain in throat and inability to swallow, throat numb, bleeding from nose, body painful and stiff, throat dry, great thirst, pain in small intestine, loins painful, hot disease spreading from loins around the body causing pain, pain in toes so that patient cannot wear shoes, stomach painful, loss of appetite, 'feet and heart hot', jaundice, chest and ribs full, eyes dizzy, vertigo, coughing, haemoptysis, dyspnoea, constipation, retention of urine, measles, hypertension, hypertensive encephalopathy, head feels congested with red face—looks like a beetroot.

Kidney 2
RAN GU   BLAZING VALLEY

Fire point
Category II
Point of sedation (secondary)

Interior of throat swollen, throat numb, distension of lower abdomen, pain in chest, diarrhoea, dysentery, sharp pains in stomach, coughing blood, pain in legs and feet, oedema of feet, cold-damp feet, spermatorrhoea, impotence, irregular menstruation, pruritis vulvae, menorrhagia, prolapse of uterus, excessive eructation in children, night sweats.

Kidney 3
ZHAO HAI   SHINING SEA

Master point of Yin qiao mo

Coupled point of Ren mo
Point of Yin qiao mo

Throat dry, four limbs weary, sadness, stage fright, madness or epilepsy at night, hemiplegia, lower abdomen painful, irregular menstruation, leucorrhoea, prolapse of uterus, pruritis vulvae, involuntary erections, gonorrhoea, constipation, insomnia, sees stars and spots when he looks into the distance, asthma, neuralgia in arm and hand, headaches, migraine.

Kidney 4
SHUI QUAN   WATER SPRING

Accumulation point

Vision blurred, cannot see in the distance, myopia, periods do not come or when they come patient has much pain in abdomen, a few days before menstruation cries depressed anxious and nervous, abdominal pain, prolapse of uterus, frequent micturition, impotence.

Kidney 5
DA ZHONG   BIG BELL

Luo point

Base of spine stiff and painful, heel swollen and painful, constipation, mouth hot, tongue dry, chest swollen, asthmatic breathing, haemoptysis, throat blocked and unable to swallow, noise in throat, patient fond of lying down, mental stupidity, prone to fear and unhappiness, wishes to remain at home, gonorrhoea, uterine spasm, dislikes the cold, vomits whatever he eats, stage fright, inferiority complex, nocturnal enuresis in children.

Kidney 6

TAI XI BIGGER STREAM

Earth point
Category III & IV
Source

Coughing, coughing glutinous sputum, sharp pains in heart, urine dark yellow, defaecation difficult, fever without perspiration, fond of sleeping, throat swollen, haemoptysis, impotence, irregular periods, toothache, sores on both legs, heel swollen and painful, legs cold after a fever, spasm of diaphragm, anorexia, mammary pain, hand frozen.

Kidney 7

FU LIU RETURNING CURRENT

Metal point
Category V
Point of tonification

Abdomen distended like a drum, four limbs swollen, ascites, oedema, constant sweating, no sweating, hiccough, constipation, flatulence, dysentery, retention of urine, diabetes, spermatorrhoea, extreme fatigue, epistaxis, indigestion, haemorrhoids, pain in loins and back, cannot bear to move, vision dim, prone to anger and ceaseless talking, tongue dry, feet cold, feet paralysed, paralysis in children, myelitis, gonorrhoea, orchitis.

Kidney 8

JIAO XIN EXCHANGE LETTERS

Point of Yin qiao mo
Accumulation point of
Yin qiao mo

Menorrhagia, irregular periods, amenorrhoea, red and white vaginal discharge, prolapse of uterus, loins thighs and legs painful, gonorrhoea, dysuria, orchitis, constipation, dysentery with pus and blood, perspires at night, one sided abdominal pain.

Kidney 9

ZHU BIN BUILDING BANK

Point of Yin wei mo
Accumulation point of
Yin qiao mo

Legs weak, feet painful, insanity, swollen tongue, suddenly sticks out tongue, vomits mucus, muscular spasms in calf of leg, toxaemia of pregnancy with spasm of the lower abdominal muscles, no milk. According to Soulié de Morant, if this point is stimulated at the third and preferably also at the sixth month of pregnancy the infant when born will be healthier than normal, having a greater vitality and resistance to disease.

Kidney 10

YIN GU YIN VALLEY

Water point of Yin
water meridian
Category VI

Pain in thighs, knees painful and cannot be flexed especially inner side, micturition difficult, abdomen and genitalia painful, abdominal pain radiating to umbilicus, abdomen distended like a drum, impotent, scrotum damp and itchy, pain radiating to genitalia on micturition, dysuria, urine dark yellow, incessant vaginal discharge, metrorrhagia, pruritis vulvae, hypersalivation.

Kidney 11

HENG GU TRANSVERSE BONE (PUBIS)

Point of Chong mo

Abdomen swollen, lower abdomen painful, dysuria, five types of urethritis, vaginal prolapse, spermatorrhoea, not enough spermatozoa, penis and scrotum painful, amenorrhoea, eyes red and painful beginning in the inner corner of the eye, keratitis, lack of energy Yin due to abdominal pain, pain in renal area, cannot stand for a long time.

Kidney 12
DA HE   BIG BRIGHTNESS

Shokanten of greater
Yang
Point of Chong mo

Lower abdomen extremely swollen and painful, spermatorrhoea, pain in penis, vaginismus, frigidity, woman unable to conceive, chronic vaginitis, red vaginal discharge, eyes red and painful beginning at the inner corner of the eyes, cystitis, retention of urine, lumbago.

Kidney 13
QI XUE   QI HOLE

Confluence of vital
energy
This point is also called
'the door of infants'
Point of Chong mo

Infertility in women, irregular periods, Qi from upper abdomen attacks ribs and causes pain, Qi rushing madly up and down causing pain in loins, eyes red and painful beginning at the inner corners of the eyes, incessant diarrhoea, spermatorrhoea, impotence, pain in penis, paralysis of bladder.

Kidney 14
SI MAN   FOUR FULL

Point of Chong mo
This point is also called
'the palace of bone
marrow'

Hernia below the navel, abundant stools, indigestion, cutting pain below the navel, shivering with cold, spermatorrhoea, menorrhagia, irregular periods, dysmenorrhoea, urinary incontinence, Qi attacks ribs and causes pain, inner corner of eye red and painful.

Kidney 15
ZHONG ZHU   MIDDLE INJECTION

Point of Chong mo

Heat in upper abdomen, constipation, colitis, urinary incontinence, irregular periods, salpingitis, oophoritis, pain in loins and abdomen, inner corner of eyes red and painful, loss of energy, head clasped in a vice, pain and swelling in the joints of the fingers.

Kidney 16
HUANG YO   VITALS YU

Independent associated
point of intestines
Shokanten of lesser Yin
Point of Chong mo

Abdomen swollen and full, cutting pain in abdomen, constipated, diarrhoea, spasm of stomach, borborygmi, jaundice, eyes red and painful beginning at the inner corner of the eyes, five types of urethritis, spasm of the neck of the bladder, vaginismus.

Kidney 17
SHANG QU   MERCHANT'S TUNE

Point of Chong mo

Abdomen painful, cutting pain when abdomen full, no appetite, constipation or diarrhoea, gastric spasm, hyperacidity, anorexia, jaundice, congestion of eyes, dislikes living, sad, impatient, uterine spasm.

Kidney 18
SHI GUAN   STONE GATE

Point of Chong mo

Asthmatic breathing, hiccoughs, spleen and stomach empty and cold, anorexia, food and drink not digested, vomits food, sialorrhoea, bad blood in organs (Zang-solid organs) of women, unbearable pain in abdomen, constipation, eyes red and painful from inner corner of eyes, gonorrhoea, sterility, congestion and spasm of uterus, urine dark yellow, stiffness of vertebral column, 'upper Qi'.

Kidney 19

YIN DU GHOST'S CAPITAL

Humming noise in adbomen, abdomen distended, abdominal pain, gastritis, duodenal or gastric ulcer, region below the heart distressed and melancholic, borborygmi, vomiting, flatulence, asthmatic breathing, rebellious Qi attacks ribs, eyes red and painful starting from the inner canthus, jaundice, 'upper Qi'.

Kidney 20

TONG GU (FU) PENETRATING VALLEY (ABDOMEN)

Dry mouth, dumbness, yawning, pain in ribs, pulmonary emphysema, dyspnoea, diarrhoea, food and drink not digested, acute and chronic gastritis, duodenal or gastric ulcer, stomach distended, diarrhoea, congestion of the eyes, rhinorrhoea, shaking with fright, stiff neck.

Kidney 21

YOU MEN GATE OF HADES — THE PYLORUS

Whole of chest painful, intercostal neuralgia, bronchitis, region below heart melancholic and full, pain on swallowing, no appetite, vomits mucus, upper abdomen swollen and full, diarrhoea containing blood, gastric or duodenal ulcer, jaundice, vomiting of pregnancy, amnesia, milk from breast does not come out, ulcer in breast, breast abscess, eyes red and painful starting from inner canthus, feeling of energy that rises.

Kidney 22

BU LANG WALKING CORRIDOR

Chest and ribs full, dyspnoea, coughing, asthmatic, cannot raise arms, nose blocked, partial anosmia, vomiting, anorexia, oesophageal spasm, spasm of abdominis rectus, lack of energy, atony of large intestine, inflammation of breast.

Kidney 23

SHEN FENG SPIRIT SEAL

Coughing, chest full, cannot breathe, bronchitis, ulcer of breast, tumour of breast, continually hot and cold, vomiting, anorexia, anosmia, spasm of rectus abdominis, angina pectoris, Judo knock-out point, tinnitus due to congestion, congestion of nose, hot flushes.

Kidney 24

LING XU SPIRIT BURIAL-GROUND

Chest and diaphragm full and painful, incessant coughing, dyspnoea, bronchitis, pleurisy, vomiting, chest melancholia, anorexia, anxious, suspicious, amnesia, angina of effort, neuralgia of forearm, nose blocked, ozena, insomnia.

Kidney 25

SHEN ZANG SPIRIT STORE

Chest and ribs full, coughing and unable to breathe, pulmonary congestion, bronchitis, vomiting, anorexia, stomach distended at midnight, insomia due to worry, does not wish to live, poor hearing.

Kidney 26

YU ZHONG AMIDST ELEGANCE

Coughing, asthmatic breathing, intercostal neuralgia, unable to eat, chest and ribs full, bronchitis, ulcer of breast, excessive perspiration at night, easily becomes bad tempered, quick temperament, cerebral congestion, pruritis of ears, weakness of vocal cords, irritable cough, spits too much, palpitations, weight on chest, cold hands and feet, spasm of oesophagus and stomach, sialorrhea.

Kidney 27

YU FU YU MANSION

Last point Coughing, chest full, cannot breathe, chest painful, chronic asthma, vomiting, anorexia, abdominal distension, oesophageal spasm, painful tongue, sensation that energy rises to top of body, jumps at sudden noises, irritable, headache due to excessive mental strain, pre-menstrual pain and tension, rhinophyma, brachial neuralgia.

507

Pericardium
(Envelope of the Heart or Circulation—Sex)

Circulation—Sex 1
TIAN CHI HEAVENLY POND

Point of entry
Meeting point absolute
Yin
Point 'Window of the
sky'
? Reunion Cx, T

Fever without perspiration but with headache, chest-diaphragm distressed and melancholic, ribs painful, swelling under armpit, adenitis under arm, insufficient milk, mammary pain, cerebral congestion, paralysis of four limbs, foggy vision.

Circulation—Sex 2
TIAN QUAN HEAVENLY SPRING

Cardiac pain, palpitations due to fear, chest-diaphragm full and painful, coughing, pulmonary congestion, bronchitis, chest and back swollen and inside of arm painful, anorexia, vomiting, fear of wind and cold, does not see clearly.

Circulation—Sex 3
QU ZE CROOKED MARSH

Water point
Category VI

Body hot, very thirsty, dry mouth, rebellious Qi, stomach painful, vomiting, diarrhoea, arms trembling and painful, cholera, measles, perspiration of head and neck, chorea, myocarditis, sterility, neuralgia of upper arm, hemiplegia.

Circulation—Sex 4
XI MEN ACCUMULATION DOOR

Accumulation point

Heart and chest painful, myocarditis, haemoptysis, epistaxis, nausea, haemorrhoids, weakness of tissues which bruise easily, spirit (heart) Qi insufficient, lack of energy, fear of surroundings and people, poor memory, neuralgia down middle of forearm and hand.

Circulation—Sex 5
JIAN SHI THE INTERMEDIARY

Metal point
Category V
Group Luo point of
three upper Yin

Cardiac pain, carditis, heart suspended as though hungry, vomiting, cholera, malaria, gastritis, armpits swollen, cramp in elbow, palms of hands warm, insanity, fright in children, irregular periods, vaginal discharge, amenorrhoea, organs (Zang-solid organs) disordered, aphonia, pharyngitis, fear of wind and cold, hypertensive encephalopathy, neurasthenia, as if possessed of a devil.

Circulation—Sex 6
NEI GUAN INNER GATE

Luo point
General Luo point
Master point Yin wei mo

Headache, insomnia, dizziness, palpitation of heart, epilepsy, madness, easily frightened, swelling under armpits, cramp of elbow, cardiac pain, vomiting, middle regions blocked full and swollen, spleen and stomach not harmonised,

| Coupled point of Chong mo | stomach very painful, gastritis, enteritis, swelling of abdomen, diarrhoea, hiccoughs, coughing, depleted and weary, summer-heat diseases, rheumatism of foot, jaundice, irregular periods, post-partum bleeding and dizziness, spermatorrhoea, nearly pulseless. |

Circulation—Sex 7
DA LING   BIG MOUND

| *Earth point*
Category III & IV
Point of sedation
Source | Body hot, head painful, short of breath, chest and ribs painful, fever without perspiration, throat numb, ulcer of breast, arm cramp, armpits swollen, incessant laughter, prone to sadness, weariness and fear, mad speech and unhappiness, summer-heat diseases, ulcers of intestines, eyes red and painful, organs (Zang-solid organs) disordered, insanity, nerves weak. |

Circulation—Sex 8
LAO GONG   LABOUR PALACE

| *Fire point of Ministerial*
Yin fire meridian
Category II
Point of exit | Anger, incessant sadness or laughter, fever without perspiration, stomach painful, indigestion, blood in urine and stools, haemorrhoids, epistaxis, jaundice, very thirsty, pyorrhoea alveolaris, organs (Zang-solid organs) disordered, sensation that energy rises to top of body, writers' cramp, contracture of palmar aponeurosis. |

Circulation—Sex 9
ZHONG CHONG   MIDDLE RUSHING

| *Wood point*
Category I
Point of tonification
Last point | Fainting, delirium, unconsciousness, poor memory, severe fright, fevers with distress and melancholy but no sweating, palms of hands hot, body like fire, tongue rigid, stomach painful, temperature, vomiting and diarrhoea, all Yang diseases with fever, hyper or hypotension, cerebral congestion. |

Triple Warmer

Triple Warmer 1
GUAN CHONG GATE RUSHING

Metal point
Category I
Point of entry

Headache, throat numb, tongue curled up, dry mouth, vomiting, anorexia, pyrexia, cholera, summer-heat diseases, malaria, film over eyes, blurred vision, forearm painful and unable to raise.

Triple Warmer 2
YE MEN FLUID DOOR

Water point
Category II

Hand and arm red and swollen, fingers cramped, forearm painful, all limbs icy cold, dizziness, slight deafness, tinnitus, headaches, eyes red swollen and painful, toothache, gingivitis, pharyngitis, malaria, wandering mind.

Triple Warmer 3
ZHONG ZHU MIDDLE ISLET

Wood point
Category III
Point of tonification

Forearm and elbow painful, fingers cannot grasp objects tightly, fever without sweating, malaria, intermittent fevers, headache, vertigo, dizziness, tinnitus, slight deafness, film over eyes, pharyngitis, pain middle of back.

Triple Warmer 4
YANG CHI YANG POND

Category IV
Source

Wrist painful and weak, wrist red and swollen, cannot be flexed or extended, hand and wrist bent, unable to grasp objects, forearm and elbow painful, brachial neuralgia, unable to raise arm, facial spasm, diabetes, mouth dry, melancholy, intermittent fever, shivering.

Triple Warmer 5
WAI GUAN OUTER GATE

Luo point
General Luo point
Master point of Yang
wei mo
Coupled point of Dai mo

Forearm and elbow cannot be flexed, fingers painful and unable to grasp objects, muscles and bones of upper limb painful, rheumatism in general, slight deafness, epistaxis, toothache, hypertension, headache, pain in chest and ribs, cold, influenza, coughing, fever in general, summer-heat diseases, cholera, intestinal ulcers, infantile paralysis, violent fear, retained placenta.

Triple Warmer 6
ZHI GOU BRANCH DITCH

Fire point of Ministerial
Yang fire meridian
Category V

Fevers without sweating, cholera, shoulder arms loin and back painful, rheumatism in general, ribs painful, pneumonia, pleurisy, chest-diaphragm troubled and melancholic, chest knotted, vomiting, difficulty in defaecation, limbs swollen and puffy, bleeding and fainting after childbirth, amenorrhoea, dumbness, lockjaw, eczema, cardiac pain.

Triple Warmer 7

HUI ZONG   MEETING ORIGIN

Accumulation point   Qi blocked up, epilepsy, nervous trembling, agitation, involuntary movement of fingers and arm, partial deafness, skin and flesh painful, dyspnoea.

Triple Warmer 8

SAN YANG LUO   THREE YANG LUO

Group Luo point of the   Forearm and elbow painful and unable to raise, sleepiness, body does not
three upper Yang   wish to move, deafness, eye diseases, toothache, painful loins.

Triple Warmer 9

SI DU   FOUR GUTTERS

Forearm and elbow-joint painful, deafness, tinnitus, pharyngitis, toothache.

Triple Warmer 10

TIAN JING   HEAVENLY WELL

Earth point   Elbow and shoulder painful, unable to grasp objects, lumbago, cannot lie
Category VI   down, pain behind ear, tonsillitis, cervical adenitis, throat numb, cannot
Point of sedation   speak, jaw swollen and painful, outer corners of eyes red and swollen, one
Upper meeting point Ho   sided headache, tinnitus, partial deafness, heart and chest painful, coughing,
of triple warmer   bronchitis, dislikes food, insanity, excessive perspiration.

Triple Warmer 11

QING LENG YUAN   PURE COLD ABYSS

Elbow arm shoulder and back painful, cannot bend or stretch arm, cannot bear to wear clothes, headache, tinnitus, eyes yellow, ribs painful.

Triple Warmer 12

XIAO LUO   THAWING LUO RIVER

Arms and back swollen and painful, neck stiff, cervical adenitis, ulcers on arms, head dizzy, vertigo, occipital neuralgia.

Triple Warmer 13

NAO HUI   SHOULDER MEETING

Reunion T, Li   Arms painful and cannot be raised, elbow and forearm painful, difficult to
? Point of Yang wei mo   flex or extend arm, shoulders and back painful, arm-pits very painful, goitre.

Triple Warmer 14

JIAN LIAO   SHOULDER BONE

Shoulder and arm painful and cannot move.

Triple Warmer 15

TIAN LIAO   HEAVENLY BONE

? Reunion T, G   Shoulder and back painful, arm and elbow painful and cannot be raised, neck

stiff, pain in centre of clavicle, chest troubled and melancholic, absence of perspiration.

Triple Warmer 16
TIAN YOU   WINDOW OF HEAVEN

Point 'Window of the sky' Shoulder back and arms painful, neck stiff, cannot turn neck, hyperacusis, suddenly becomes deaf, headache due to Wind, lively dreams, face swollen, eyes painful, vision confused.

Triple Warmer 17
YI FENG   WIND SCREEN

Reunion T, G Tinnitus, partial deafness, pain in ears, dumb, inside of ear damp and itchy, facial paralysis, facial spasm, trigeminal neuralgia, mouth tightly clenched, jaw swollen, lower jaw painful, toothache, both sides of throat swollen, cervical adenitis, mumps.

Triple Warmer 18
QI MAI   FEEDING MERIDIANS

Headache, tinnitus, partial deafness, blurred vision, fits in children, epilepsy, convulsions, fear, vomiting, diarrhoea.

Triple Warmer 19
LU XI   SKULL REST

Body hot, head heavy, fits in small children, vomiting in children, convulsions, partial deafness, tinnitus, retinal haemorrhage, vomiting mucus and saliva, dyspnoea, ribs painful at sides, cannot turn body.

Triple Warmer 20
JIAO SUN   ANGLE OF THE EAR

Reunion T, G, ? Si, Lobe of ear red and swollen, lips rigid, difficulty in chewing, gums swollen, optic nerve inflamed, film over eyes, exophthalmos, retinal haemorrhage.

Triple Warmer 21
ER MEN   EAR DOOR

Partial deafness, dumb, tinnitus, inside of ear painful, otitis media, otorrhoea, sores in ear, toothache, gingivitis, lips stiff, epistaxis.

Triple Warmer 22
(ER) HE LIAO   (EAR) HARMONY BONE

Point of exit Headache, facial paralysis, facial spasm, tinnitus, otitis externa, convulsions, *? Reunion T, Si, G* neck and jaw swollen, rhinitis, nasal polyp.

Triple Warmer 23
SI ZHU KONG   SILK BAMBOO HOLLOW

Headache, eyes red and swollen and painful, eyes twitch or blink separately, optic atrophy, vision blurred, tears flow in bright light, inflammation of eyes due to electric light, vomits mucus and saliva, madness.

Gall Bladder

Gall Bladder 1
ZHONG ZI LIAO   EYE BONE

Point of entry
Meeting point lesser
Yang
Reunion G, Si, T

Headache, colour blindness, night blindness, optic atrophy, outer corners of eyes red and painful, myopia, retinal haemorrhage, conjunctivitis, keratitis, weak eye sight, trigeminal neuralgia, mouth and eyes awry, pharyngitis.

Gall Bladder 2
TING HUI   HEARING MEETING

Deafness and dumbness, pain inside ears, tinnitus, otorrhoea, mouth awry, jaw swollen, dislocation of jaw, toothache, gingivitis, dislikes cold food and drink, hemiplegia, convulsions, sad.

Gall Bladder 3
SHANG GUAN   UPPER GATE

Reunion G, S

Dislikes cold and wind, mouth and eyes awry, trismus, tinnitus, deafness, vertigo, pain one side of head, toothache, glaucoma, dislikes bright light.

Gall Bladder 4
HAN YAN   JAW DETESTED

Reunion G, S, T

Feng in the head, pain one side of head, mouth and eyes awry, foggy vision, tinnitus, deafness, vertigo, toothache, frequent sneezing, convulsions in children, hemiplegia, epilepsy, rheumatism, pain in neck.

Gall Bladder 5
XUAN LU   SUSPENDED SKULL

Reunion G, S, T

Pain on one side of head, toothache, epistaxis, purulent nasal discharge, face red and painful, outer corners of eyes red and painful, body hot, no sweating, melancholy.

Gall Bladder 6
XUAN LI   SUSPENDED BALANCE

Reunion G, S, ? T

Fevers without perspiration, headache on one side, trigeminal neuralgia, face red and swollen, outer corner of eyes red swollen and painful, melancholy of heart, anorexia.

Gall Bladder 7
QU BIN   TWISTED HAIR ON THE TEMPLES

? Reunion G, B

Mouth and eyes awry, cheeks and jaws swollen and painful, trismus, neck stiff and painful and unable to turn, headache on one side, retinal haemorrhage, eye diseases in general.

Gall Bladder 8
SHUAI GU   LEADING VALLEY

Reunion G, B

Headache, top of head painful, headache due to Wind on one or both sides, vomiting, eye diseases, melancholy, inability to eat or drink, drunkenness.

Gall Bladder 9
TIAN CHONG HEAVEN RUSHING

Reunion G, B Headache, insanity, epilepsy, muscular contractures, toothache, gums swollen and painful.

Gall Bladder 10
FU BAI FLOATING WHITE

Reunion G, B Throat numb, coughing, chest melancholy, dyspnoea, tinnitus, deafness, toothache, neck swollen and painful, tonsillitis, unable to move shoulders and back.

Gall Bladder 11
(TOU) QIAO YIN (HEAD) EXTREME YIN

Reunion G, B, T Headache, neck and jaws painful, throat numb, bitter taste in mouth, tongue stiff, tinnitus, dizziness, eyes painful, stiffness of limbs, no perspiration.

Gall Bladder 12
WAN GU FINAL BONE

Reunion G, B Headache, Wind affecting the head, face and head swollen, insanity, epilepsy, legs without strength, mouth and eyes awry, facial paralysis, otitis media, deafness, neck painful, torticollis, gingivitis, insomnia, urine dark yellow or red.

Gall Bladder 13
BEN SHEN ROOT SPIRIT

Point of Yang wei mo Penetrating Wind, unconsciousness, eyes dizzy, vertigo, neck stiff and painful, cannot turn neck, insanity, epilepsy, spitting saliva, fear, madness.

Gall Bladder 14
YANG BAI YANG WHITE

Reunion G, Li, T Eyes red and swollen and painful, eyes twitch, dislikes bright light, headache,
Point of Yang wei mo facial spasm, trigeminal neuralgia, nausea.

Gall Bladder 15
(TOU) LIN QI (HEAD) ABOVE THE TEARS

Point of Yang wei mo Outer corners of eyes painful, film over eyes, excessive formation of tears, nose blocked, fear of wind and cold, occipital headache, syncope, cerebral haemorrhage, cerebral congestion.

Gall Bladder 16
MU CHUANG EYE WINDOW

Point of Yang wei mo Colour blindness, eyes suddenly red swollen and painful, face and eyes swollen and puffy, weak eyesight, hazy vision, headache, dizziness, vertigo, fever without perspiration.

Gall Bladder 17
ZHENG YING UPRIGHT YING

Point of Yang wei mo Head and neck painful, toothache, lips stiff, gingivitis, vomiting, dizziness, dislikes hearing men's voices, weak eyesight.

Gall Bladder 18

CHENG LING RECEIVING SPIRIT

Point of Yang wei mo Headache, dislikes wind and cold, dyspnoea, epistaxis, nose blocked.

Gall Bladder 19

NAO KONG BRAIN HOLLOW

Point of Yang wei mo Headache, dizziness, unable to open eyes because of headache, photophobia, palpitations, dyspnoea, body hot, general weakness, neck stiff and cannot turn.

Gall Bladder 20

FENG CHI WIND POND

Reunion G, T Alternately hot and cold, sweatless fevers, colds, summer-heat diseases,
Supposedly vaso- migraine, headache, nervous debility, hemiplegia, cerebral haemorrhage,
sympathetic eyes dizzy, foggy vision, excessive formation of tears, eyes both dull, wind
Point of Yang wei mo causes eyes to water, inner canthus red and painful, night blindness? retinal
and probably Yang haemorrhage, optic atrophy, epistaxis, nose blocked, rhinorrhoea, inflam-
qiao mo mation of eye due to electric light, tinnitus, partial deafness, spine painful, rheumatism, stiff neck, painful shoulder, urticaria, poisoning.

Gall Bladder 21

JIAN JING SHOULDER WELL

Reunion G, T Rheumatism, neck stiff, unable to turn neck, shoulder and back painful, arm
Point of Yang wei mo painful, unable to raise hands to head, hemiplegia, cerebral congestion, vertigo, Qi blocked, phlegm rises, cannot speak, cervical adenitis, ulcers, boils, sores, retained placenta, post-partum haemorrhage, premature labour or miscarriage with cold limbs, breast abscess.

Gall Bladder 22

YUAN YE ARMPIT ABYSS

Chest full, feeling of weakness in chest, pleurisy, intercostal neuralgia, cannot raise arms, goitre.

Gall Bladder 23

CHE JIN FLANK MUSCLE

Alarm point Chest very full preventing sleep, asthmatic respiration, cannot sleep well
(secondary) due to respiratory trouble, nervous depression, cannot speak clearly, vomiting stale fluid, swallowing stale saliva, warmth in the lower abdomen.

Gall Bladder 24

RI YUE SUN AND MOON

Alarm point (main) Ribs painful, kidney Qi rushes against heart, vomiting, swallowing stale
Reunion G, Sp saliva, pain on swallowing, hiccoughs, frequent sighing, does not speak
Point of Yang wei mo clearly, liver diseases, warmth in lower abdomen, spasms in limbs.

Gall Bladder 25

JING MEN CAPITAL DOOR

Alarm point of kidney Loins painful, cannot bend down, pain in hip joint, lumbago, pain back and shoulder, cannot remain standing a long time, abdomen distended, diarrhoea especially in a frightened person, borborygmi, asthma, dysuria, urine dark yellow.

Gall Bladder 26
DAI MO   DAI MO   (WAISTBAND EXTRA MERIDIAN)

Special for gynaeco-
logical diseases
Point of Dai mo

Lower abdomen painful, interior of body feels anxious, posterior part of body feels heavy, irregular menstruation, dysmenorrhoea, red or white vaginal discharge, vaginal prolapse, lower abdominal pain, false urge to go to stool in women due to pelvic pressure, loins as though 'seated in water'.

Gall Bladder 27
WU SHU   FIVE PIVOTS

Point of Dai mo

Loins and back painful, uterine spasm, red or white vaginal discharge, constipation, intestinal tumour? false call to stool in a woman, orchitis.

Gall Bladder 28
WEI DAO   BINDING PATH

Point of Dai mo

Loins and legs painful, lumbago, oedema, ascites, vomiting, anorexia, inflammation of intestines, nephritis, orchitis.

Gall Bladder 29
JU LIAO   DWELLING BONE

Point of Yang qiao mo

Paralysis, loins and lower abdomen painful, dysmenorrhoea, irregular periods, leucorrhoea, cystitis, nephritis, orchitis, diseases of upper limbs, pain radiating from shoulder to chest.

Gall Bladder 30
HUAN TIAO   JUMPING CIRCLE

Reunion G, B.

Half of body uncoordinated, paralysis, epilepsy, loins and spine painful, loins and thighs painful, buttocks over ischium painful, sciatica, unable to turn, rheumatism in general, pain in knee, influenza, nervous exhaustion.

Gall Bladder 31
FENG SHI   WIND MARKET

Paralysis, paralysis of lower limbs, paralysis in children, weakness of the legs in general, sciatica, generalised pruritis, sores.

Gall Bladder 32
ZHONG DU   MIDDLE DITCH

Half of body uncoordinated, sciatica, lumbago, loins and legs painful, weakness in general of the legs, muscular spasms in legs, passage point with three lower Yang.

Gall Bladder 33
(XI) YANG GUAN   (KNEE) YANG GATE

Knees red, swollen and painful, knee cannot be flexed or extended, loss of sensation in knee.

Gall Bladder 34

YANG LING QUAN   YANG MOUND SPRING

Earth point
Category VI
Lower meeting point Ho
of gall bladder
Specialised point for
muscles

Half body uncoordinated, lower limbs cold and numb, legs cold as though without blood, lumbago, sciatica, knees red swollen and painful, special point for the knee, neurasthenia, ribs painful, face swollen, pharyngitis, extreme fright, insanity, madness, constipation.

Gall Bladder 35

YANG JIAO   YANG CROSSING

Point of Yang wei mo
Accumulation point
Yang wei mo

Throat numb, chest full, dyspnoea, pleurisy, face swollen, and puffy, sciatica, weakness and neuralgia of peroneal muscles, weakness of legs, cold feet.

Gall Bladder 36

WAI QIU   OUTER MOUND

Accumulation point

Paralysis, muscular spasm in calves, beri-beri, neck painful, chest and ribs swollen and painful, dislikes wind and cold, insanity, madness.

Gall Bladder 37

GUANG MING   LIGHT BRIGHT

Luo point

Muscular pain in legs, cannot stand for long periods, paralysis of lower limbs, muscular spasm or neuralgia in calves, sweatless fevers, all eye diseases, becomes suddenly mad.

Gall Bladder 38

YANG FU   YANG SUPPORT

Fire point
Category V
Point of sedation

Paralysis, muscular spasm, vascular spasm, generalised arthralgia, generalised aches and pains, pain in chest and buttocks and knees extending to ankles, sciatica, loins as though sitting in water, corners of eyes painful, bitter taste in mouth, throat numb, cervical adenitis, goitre, likes to sigh, pasty skin, axillary and clavicular swellings.

Gall Bladder 39

XUAN ZHONG   SUSPENDED BELL

Group Luo point of
three lower yang
Specialised point for
bone marrow,
leucocytosis

Penetrating wind, cerebral haemorrhage, hands and feet uncoordinated, stomach and abdomen swollen and full, no appetite, acute appendicitis, diarrhoea, haemorrhoids, rheumatism, loins painful, beri-beri, lower part of leg painful, cannot rise after sitting down, Shang han with high fever which does not subside, throat numb, epistaxis, inside of nose dry, chorea, neurasthenia, madness, fear, bad temper.

Gall Bladder 40

QIU XU   GRAVE MOUND

Category IV
Source point

Chest and ribs painful, cannot breathe, swelling under arms, paralysis, cannot rise after sitting, pain in buttocks, lower limbs painful, muscular spasm, sciatica, heels red, heels swollen and painful, neck swollen, pain in lower abdomen, conjunctivitis.

Gall Bladder 41

(ZU) LIN QI (FOOT) ABOVE TEARS

Wood point of Yang
wood meridian
Category III
Point of exit
Master point of Dai mo
Coupled point of Yang
wei mo

Lower part of legs and feet damp and swollen, rheumatic pains that move around, ribs full and painful, irregular menstruation, dysmenorrhoea, ulcers of the breast, axillary adenitis, vertigo, mastoid pain, intermittent fever, excessive perspiration.

Gall Bladder 42

DI WU HUI EARTH FIVE MEETINGS

Extensor surface of foot red and swollen, ulcers of the breast, pain and swelling of axilla, eyes red and painful.

Gall Bladder 43

XIA XI CHIVALROUS STREAM

Water point
Category II
Point of tonification

Extensor surface of foot red and swollen, spasm of the five toes, space between toes damp and rotten, four limbs swollen and puffy, ribs painful, pleurisy, jaw swollen, tinnitus, partial deafness, vertigo, sweatless fever, outer canthus red and swollen, cerebral congestion.

Gall Bladder 44

(ZU) QIAO YIN (FOOT) EXTREME YIN

Metal point
Category I
Last point

Headache, dreams of ghosts, heart troubled, eyes painful, ribs painful, cannot breathe, coughing, excessive sleep, insomnia, cannot raise arm, hands and feet hot, no perspiration, throat numb, tongue stiff, mouth dry, deafness.

Liver

Liver 1
DA DUN   BIG HEAP

Wood point of Yin wood meridian
Category I
Point of entry

Frequency of micturition, incontinence of urine, one side of scrotum enlarged, pain in penis, gonorrhoea, vaginal prolapse, pruritis vulvae, menorrhagia, polymenorrhoea, abdominal pain, abdominal swelling, pain in stomach, 'penetrating Wind', unconsciousness, fainting, appearance as though dead, likes to sleep, headaches, excessive perspiration, lumbago.

Liver 2
XING JIAN   COLUMN INBETWEEN

Fire point
Category II
Point of sedation

Headache, head dizzy, insomnia, angry easily, eyes red swollen and weepy, throat dry and irritated, chest and ribs painful, coughing due to emptyness and weariness, gastric pain, haematemesis, whole abdomen swollen, lower abdomen swollen, retention of urine, excessive and ceaseless menstrual bleeding, loins painful, cannot bend, knees swollen and painful, dry and wet beriberi, inter-digital swelling, hysteria, madness, insanity, epilepsy, fits, convulsions in children, neurasthenia, carbuncle, ulcer or abscess of breast.

Liver 3
TAI CHONG   BIGGER RUSHING

Earth point
Category III & IV
Source
Independent associated point for spasms

Stomach painful, throat dry, nausea, vomiting, dry lips, chest and ribs full and painful, cervical or axillary swelling, lower abdomen swollen, diarrhoea, constipation, loins and lower abdomen painful, incontinence of urine, urethritis, retracted scrotum, haematuria, constant uterine bleeding, pain in front of internal malleolus, difficulty in walking, feet weak, spasms or cramp of toes, face and eyes pale, does not see clearly.

Liver 4
ZHONG FENG   MIDDLE SEAL

Metal point
Category V

Swelling of abdomen, lower abdomen distended, eyes yellow with slight fever, jaundice, anorexia, feels ill after food, pain around body at level of navel, loins painful, feet and legs cold, muscular atony, spermatorrhoea, impotence, urethritis, pain in vagina.

Liver 5
LI GOU   INSECT DITCH

Luo point

Violent pain in abdomen, lower abdomen swollen, retention of urine, sudden pain in scrotum, menorrhagia, irregular periods, vaginal discharge, belching, throat feels obstructed, fear and nervousness, depression, dejection, cramp in back, cannot bend back, skin cold and aching, difficult to flex knee.

Liver 6
ZHONG DU   MIDDLE CAPITAL

Accumulation point

Lower abdominal pain, diarrhoea, large stools, feet weak withered and emaciated, cannot walk or stand, pain in knee, skin cold numb and painful, menorrhagia, pharyngitis.

Liver 7
XI GUAN   KNEE GATE
'Wind' rheumatism, pain in throat, inside of knee and patella painful, cannot bend knee.

Liver 8
QU QUAN   CROOKED SPRING

Water point
Category VI
Point of tonification

Fibroids, abdomen swollen, abdominal colic, irregular periods, vaginal prolapse, pruritis vulvae, pain in vagina and thighs, pain in penis, spermatorrhoea, dysuria, retention of urine, rectal discharge of thick blood, dysentery, knees painful with cramped muscles and inability to flex, knees and shins cold and painful, lower abdominal pain extending to throat, epistaxis, madness, paraplegia.

Liver 9
YIN BAO   YIN WRAPPING
Loins and base of spine painful extending to lower abdomen, muscular spasm of loins and buttocks, dysuria, incontinence of urine, irregular periods, boils on both buttocks, fullness of chest.

Liver 10
(ZU) WU LI   (FOOT) FIVE MILE
Abdomen full, retention of urine, spermatorrhoea, scrotum damp and itching, helps perspiration and sleep.

Liver 11
YIN LIAN   YIN SCREEN
Women cease to bear children, irregular periods, leucorrhoea, pruritis vulvae.

Liver 12
JI MAI   QUICK PULSE
Penis painful, inside of buttocks or thighs painful.

Liver 13
ZHANG MEN   CHAPTER DOOR

Alarm point of spleen
Centre reunion particu-
lar point of five Zang
(solid) organs
Shokanten of greater
Yin
Reunion Liv, G
Point of Dai mo

Oedema, ascites, borborygmi, abdominal swelling, abdomen distended like a drum, food not digested, diarrhoea, stomach painful, flatulence, mouth dry, anorexia, over-eating, chest and ribs painful, ribs painful — cannot lie down, body hot — heart troubled, hypertension, stertorous respiration, loins painful — cannot turn over, jaundice, loss of weight with slightly yellow skin.

Liver 14

QI MEN   PERIOD DOOR

Point of alarm
Point of exit
Shokanten of absolute
Yin
Reunion Liv, Sp, ? G
Point of Yin wei mo

Chest-diaphragm distended, coughing, stertorous respiration, belching, vomiting sour fluid, food and drink do not descend, mouth dry, very thirsty, diarrhoea, abdomen hard, peritonitis, both sides of body painful, sharp pain in wrist, hypertension, difficult delivery, post partum troubles.

Conception Vessel

Conception Vessel 1
HUI YIN   MEETING OF YIN

General Luo point
Reunion Cv, Gv
Point of Chong mo

All diseases of perineal area, pruritis vulvae, excessive perspiration in perineal area, pain in vagina, outer part of vagina swollen and painful, prolapse of vagina, irregular periods, dysmenorrhoea, amenorrhoea in young women, spermatorrhoea, scrotum cold, penis painful and cold, pruritis ani, haemorrhoids, constipation with infrequent micturition, nocturnal perspiration that is not salty.

Conception Vessel 2
QU GU   CROOKED BONE

Reunion Cv, Liv

Lower abdomen swollen and full or extremely painful, retention of urine with overflow, incontinence of urine, cystitis, red or white vaginal discharge, gonorrhoea, vaginismus, metrorrhagia, menorrhagia, uterus does not reduce in size within normal period after delivery, spermatorrhoea, impotance, scrotum wet and itchy, lack of virility.

Conception Vessel 3
ZHONG JI   MIDDLE EXTREMITY

Alarm point of bladder
Reunion Cv, Sp, K, Liv

Lump below navel like upturned cup, fibroids, irregular periods, dysmenorrhoea, menorrhagia, excessive white vaginal discharge, pruritis vulvae, vaginal orifice swollen and painful, pain in vagina, prolapse of vagina, retained placenta, incessant discharge after confinement, impotence, spermatorrhoea, dysuria, haematuria, urinary incontinence, frequent micturition, fainting, general fatigue, ascites.

Conception Vessel 4
GUAN YUAN   GATE ORIGIN

Alarm point of small
intestine
Reunion Cv, Sp, K, Liv

Abdomen painful, dysentery, cholera, diarrhoea, prolapse of rectum, lines of pain around navel, abdomen swollen like a drum, fibroids below navel like upturned cup, dysuria, haematuria, urinary incontinence, spermatorrhoea, impotence, vaginal discharge, irregular menstruation, light periods of long duration, dysmenorrhoea, prolapse of vagina, pruritis vulvae, abdomen painful after confinement, incessant discharge after confinement, retained placenta, jaundice, hypertension, neurasthenia.

Conception Vessel 5
SHI MEN   STONE DOOR

Alarm point of triple
warmer — main
Centre of energy

Abdomen swollen painful and hard, colitis, incessant diarrhoea, pain in lower abdomen, haematemesis, periumbilical pain, ascites, food not digested, micturition infrequent, urinary diseases, menorrhagia, vaginal discharge. Original Qi of lower triple warmer in males and females of all ages empty and cold.

Conception Vessel 6
QI HAI SEA OF QI

Centre of energy Stomach painful, abdomen painful, periumbilical pain, cold and pain below navel, ascites, abdomen swollen like drum, fibroids and tumours in abdomen, swelling in abdomen which does not descend when pressed, hiccoughing, vomiting, constipated, haematuria, dysuria, Zang Qi empty and melancholy, true Qi deficient, chronic Qi diseases, body emaciated, emptyness, weariness, limbs weak, patient wishes to die, Yin diseases, limbs cold, menorrhagia, red and white vaginal discharge, amenorrhoea, irregular periods, dysmenorrhoea, incessant discharge after confinement, abdomen swollen after confinement, retained placenta, prolapse of vagina, spermatorrhoea, impotence, enuresis in children, hypertension, insomnia.

Conception Vessel 7
YIN JIAO YIN CROSSING

Alarm point of triple warmer — lower Reunion Cv, Cx, T Point of Chong mo Pain below navel, cold and pain around navel, abdomen full, abdomen hard and painful, sweating and pruritis of genitalia, urethritis, cannot urinate, sterility, menorrhagia, irregular periods, vaginal discharge, incessant discharge after confinement, fainting, post-partum madness, acute tonsillitis, epistaxis.

Conception Vessel 8
SHEN QUE SPIRIT SHRINE

Incessant diarrhoea, ascites, abdomen swollen like drum, abdominal pain, periumbilical pain, abdomen empty, intestinal noises like sound of flowing water, rectal prolapse, penetrating Wind, fainting, unconsciousness, cerebral haemorrhage, incessant lactation.

Conception Vessel 9
SHUI FEN WATER DIVISIONS

Reunion Cv, L Water diseases, ascites, oedema, abdomen swollen like drum, stomach empty and swollen, anorexia, pain round body at level of navel, borborygmi, flatulence, a rushing up into the chest which causes inability to breathe, pain in renal area, fontanelles weak, epistaxis.

Conception Vessel 10
XIA WAN LOWER CHANNEL

Reunion Cv, Sp Abdomen painful, abdomen distended, vomiting, anorexia, tumour in abdomen (?), food not digested, gradual emaciation, abdomen swollen like a drum, stomach ache, gastritis, gastric spasm, dilation of stomach, haematuria.

Conception Vessel 11
JIAN LI ESTABLISHED MILE

Abdomen swollen, abdomen painful, body swollen, stomach painful, spasms of lower abdomen, vomiting, anorexia, poor digestion, cardiac pain with sensation of energy that moves to upper part of body.

Conception Vessel 12

ZHONG WAN MIDDLE CHANNEL

Alarm point of stomach and triple warmer — middle
Centre reunion particular point of five Fu (hollow) organs
Reunion Cv, Si, S, T, L, Cx, ? Liv

Abdomen painful, abdomen swollen, all gastric diseases, cholera, vomiting, swallowing sour saliva, vomiting sour matter, stomach pain, acute gastro-enteritis, food difficult to digest, abdomen swollen like drum, diarrhoea, constipation, intestinal abscess, prolapse of vagina, jaundice, insomnia, headache, palpitations of heart, chronic spleen Wind, ribs painful, hiccoughing, dyspnoea, hypertension, insanity, madness, paralysis, penetrating Wind, face numb and yellow.

Conception Vessel 13

SHANG WAN UPPER CHANNEL

Reunion S, Si, L

Vomiting, food does not descend, abdomen swollen, abdomen painful, diarrhoea, Qi full, peritonitis, food not digested, pain in stomach, hard mass in abdomen like a dish, haematemesis, jaundice, hiccoughing, pleurisy, bronchitis, insanity, madness, fear, epilepsy, body hot and sweaty, cardiac pain with sensation of warmth.

Conception Vessel 14

JU QUE GREAT SHRINE

Alarm point of heart

Coughing, Qi rises, chest full, dyspnoea, chest painful, cardiac pain, sour taste in mouth, vomits sour matter, vomiting, diarrhoea, abdomen swollen and very painful, jaundice, hiccoughs, acute gastro-enteritis, fainting, confusion and melancholy, insanity, madness, fear, forgetfulness, beri-beri.

Conception Vessel 15

JIU WEI DOVE TAIL

Luo point
Centre reunion particular point of vital centres

Chest full, coughing, haemoptysis, throat numb, throat swollen — fluid does not descend, dyspnoea, hiccoughing, vomiting, gastric pain, palpitations, cardiac diseases, anti-smoking, insanity, hysteria, walks around wildly, cannot choose correct words, unilateral headache, loss of virility.

Conception Vessel 16

ZHONG TING MIDDLE COURTYARD

Chest and ribs swollen and painful, dyspnoea, throat blocked — appears like a plum stone — tonsillitis, food does not descend, nausea, vomiting, vomiting milk by children.

Conception Vessel 17

SHAN ZHONG PLATFORM MIDDLE

Alarm point of Cx
Alarm point of triple warmer — upper and ? of Cx
Centre reunion particular of breath energy
Sea of energy

Dyspnoea, lung abscess, coughing, all lung diseases, haematemesis, haemoptysis, heart and chest painful, anti-smoking, insufficient lactation, abdomen swollen like a drum.

Conception Vessel 18
YU TANG   JADE HALL
Chest painful, coughing, Qi rises, pleurisy, bronchitis, vomiting cold phlegm, chest full, cannot breathe, dyspnoea, cardiac pain, haemoptysis.

Conception Vessel 19
ZI GONG   PURPLE PALACE
Chest painful, coughing, dyspnoea, bronchitis, vomiting cold phlegm, both breasts swollen and painful cardiac pain, food and drink do not descend, vomiting food.

Conception Vessel 20
HUA GAI   SPLENDOUR COVERING
Sides of chest full and painful, coughing, Qi rises, dyspnoea, throat numb, glosillitis, throat swollen, unable to swallow liquids, anti-smoking, spasm of notttis, asthma.

Conception Vessel 21
XUAN JI   PEARL JADE
Sides of chest full and painful, coughing, dyspnoea, throat numb, throat swollen, tonsillitis, aerogastria, unable to swallow liquids.

Conception Vessel 22
TIAN TU   HEAVEN RUSHING
Point 'Window of the Dyspnoea, dry cough, noise in throat like sound of a crane (bird), cardiac pain,
sky' Qi rebellious in chest, lung abscess, bronchitis, asthma, haemoptysis, throat
Point of Yin wei mo swollen, sores in throat which prevent eating, dumbness, aphonia, oesophageal spasm, glottic spasm, stiff tongue, veins on underside of tongue congested, partial deafness, goitre, cervical adenitis, jaundice, vomiting, acute gastroenteritis, falls asleep too easily, face red with sensation that energy rises to the upper part of body.

Conception Vessel 23
LIAN QUAN   SCREEN SPRING
Point of Yin wei mo Tongue stiff, tongue loose, dribbles saliva, sores in mouth, veins under tongue swollen, difficulty in speaking, throat constricted, hacking cough, dyspnoea, bronchitis, deafness and dumbness, excessive thirst.

Conception Vessel 24
CHENG JIANG   RECEIVING FLUID
Reunion Cv, Li, S Head and back of neck stiff and painful, half body uncoordinated, hemiplegia, mouth and eyes awry, trismus, face swollen, toothache, gingivitis, dental caries, excessive thirst, complete dumbness, insanity, fear.

Governing Vessel

Governing Vessel 1
CHANG QIANG LONG STRENGTH

Luo point
General Luo point
Reunion Gv, G, K

Lower back painful, haemorrhoids, intestinal haemorrhage, haematemesis, rectal prolapse, wind in large intestine, extreme nervousness, convulsions, madness, micturition and defaecation difficult, diarrhoea, impotence, spermatorrhoea, pruritis vulvae.

Governing Vessel 2
YAO YU LOINS YU POINT

Independent associated
point of renal area

Loins and back stiff and painful, feet paralysed, haemorrhoids, irregular periods, malaria and other fevers, urine dark red.

Governing Vessel 3
(YAO) YANG GUAN (LOINS) YANG GATE

Lumbago, knees painful, cannot bend knees, spermatorrhoea, leucorrhoea, abdominal distension, diarrhoea, colitis.

Governing Vessel 4
MING MEN GATE OF LIFE

Headache, body extremely hot, no perspiration, intermittent fevers, pain in lumbar region and abdomen together, lumbar pain, nervousness in children, convulsions, tinnitus, red or white vaginal discharge, impotence, spermatorrhoea, haemorrhoids, rectal prolapse, neurasthenia, insomnia, oedema, incontinence of urine.

Governing Vessel 5
XUAN SHU SUSPENDED PIVOT

Loins and back stiff and painful, food not digested, epigastric discomfort, stools loose, frequency of micturition.

Governing Vessel 6
JI ZHONG MIDDLE OF SPINE

Insanity, epilepsy, abdomen distended and full, anorexia, jaundice, stomach turns over, haematemesis, haemorrhoids, blood in stools, diarrhoea, prolapse of rectum.

Governing Vessel 7
ZHONG SHU MIDDLE PIVOT

Pain in lower thoracic and lumbar region, stomach ache, deterioration in eyesight.

Governing Vessel 8
JIN SUO CONTRACTED MUSCLE
Insanity, epilepsy, walking around madly, rolling of eyes, eyes fixed in an upward direction, cardiac pain, lower back extremely stiff, stomach ache.

Governing Vessel 9
ZHI YANG EXTREME YANG
Loins and back painful, chest and back painful, shins aching, limbs weary and heavy, chest distended, dyspnoea, difficulty in speaking, stomach feels cold, cannot eat, jaundice, borborygmi, intermittent fevers.

Governing Vessel 10
LING TAI SUPERNATURAL TOWER
Dyspnoea, asthma, bronchitis, pneumonia, insomnia—especially if caused by dyspnoea, loins and back painful.

Governing Vessel 11
SHEN DAO SPIRIT PATH
Cardiac diseases in general, fever, dislikes cold, headache, intermittent fever, forgetfulness, nervousness, nervousness and insanity in children, convulsions, back rigid and painful.

Governing Vessel 12
SHEN ZHU BODY PILLAR
Epilepsy, convulsions, extreme nervousness in children, body hot, suicidal, incoherent speech, madly walking around, loins and spine rigid and painful, rheumatic diseases, epistaxis.

Governing Vessel 13
TAO DAO KILN PATH

Reunion Gv, B Head heavy, eyes dizzy, vertigo, convulsions, depression, spine rigid, neck, shoulders and back painful, fever with dislike of cold, intermittent fevers, no sweating, inflammatory diseases of bones, numbness in children, amenorrhoea, urticaria.

Governing Vessel 14
DA ZHUI BIG HAMMER — VERTEBRA

Centre reunion general Headache, neck stiff and cannot turn, hysteria, wind diseases, rheumatic
point of Yang (Numb) diseases, paralysis, numbness in children, St. Vitus' Dance, neuras-
Reunion of all Yang thenia, retinal haemorrhage, epistaxis, gingivitis, chest distended, hacking
meridians including cough, loins and spine painful, intermittent fever, fever with dislike of cold,
Gv summer-heat diseases, vomiting, cholera, jaundice, urticaria.

Governing Vessel 15
YA MEN DOOR OF DUMBNESS

Reunion Gv, B Headache, neck stiff, spine rigid, epilepsy, convulsions, tongue moves slowly,
Point of Yang wei mo cannot speak, swelling of sublingual area, complete or partial loss of voice, deafness and dumbness, epistaxis.

Governing Vessel 16

FENG FU   WIND MANSION

Point 'Window of sky'
Sea of bone marrow
Reunion Gv, B
Point of Yang wei mo

Headache, vertigo, epistaxis, nose blocked, throat swollen and painful, deafness and dumbness, neck stiff, cannot turn neck, toothache, hemiplegia, cerebral haemorrhage, tongue slow — cannot speak, walks around madly, eyes move wildly, suicidal, fear, colds, influenza.

Governing Vessel 17

NAO HU   BRAIN SHELTER

Reunion Gv, B

Eyes painful, cannot see long distances, head heavy, neck stiff and painful.

Governing Vessel 18

QIANG JIAN   STRENGTH INBETWEEN

Unbearable headaches, vertigo, vomiting, epilepsy, insomnia, depression, neck stiff — cannot turn, cardiac discomfort.

Governing Vessel 19

HOU DING   POSTERIOR SUMMIT

Headache, migraine, fear of wind and cold, head and neck stiff, vertigo, epilepsy, walks around madly, insomnia.

Governing Vessel 20

BAI HUI   HUNDRED MEETINGS

Centre reunion general point of Yang
Reunion Gv, B, ? Liv
Sea of bone marrow

Headache, penetrating Wind, vertigo, hemiplegia, cerebral haemorrhage, fainting with trismus, delirium, extreme nervousness, forgetfulness, frequent weeping, unable to choose words, madness, insanity, severe fright, hysteria, neurasthenia, eclampsia, menorrhagia, cardiac discomfort, tinnitus, partial deafness, nose blocked, anosmia, rectal prolapse, haemorrhoids, retention of urine, sterility in women, convulsions in children, stiff spine, heavy head.

Governing Vessel 21

QIAN DING   ANTERIOR SUMMIT

Headache, vertigo, extreme nervousness in children, convulsions, epilepsy, rhinorrhoea, nasal polyp, face red and swollen.

Governing Vessel 22

XIN HUI   SKULL MEETING

Vertigo, nervousness, eyes stare upwards, cannot recognise people, face swollen, face too red or pale, epistaxis, nose blocked, anosmia.

Governing Vessel 23

SHANG XING   UPPER STAR

Headache, eyes painful, cannot see far, nose blocked, nasal polyp, purulent rhinorrhoea, epistaxis, face red and swollen, fever without perspiration.

Governing Vessel 24

SHEN TING SPIRIT COURTYARD

Reunion Gv, S, B Violent headache, eyes weepy, eyes red swollen and painful, rhinorrhoea, eyes stare upwards and cannot recognise people, climbing to high place and singing, taking off clothes and walking, suddenly sticks tongue out, dyspnoea with thirst, vomiting.

Governing Vessel 24.5

YIN TANG SEAL PALACE

Nervousness in children, headache, vertigo, eye diseases in general, nasal catarrh, nose blocked, trigeminal neuralgia, uterine bleeding after confinement, eclampsia, vomiting, diarrhoea.

Governing Vessel 25

SU LIAO ELEMENT BONE

Nose blocked, nasal polyp, sores inside nose, bulbous nose from drinking excessive alcohol, epistaxis.

Governing Vessel 26

REN ZHONG MIDDLE OF THE MAN

Reunion Gv, Li, S Fainting, delirium, epilepsy, madness, hysteria, severe fright, Penetrating Wind, eclampsia, menorrhagia, bleeding and dizziness after confinement, oedema, excessive thirst, summer-heat diseases, lumbago, pain along vertebral column.

Governing Vessel 27

DUI DUAN EXTREME EXCHANGE

Fainting, delirium, epilepsy, hysteria, incessant epistaxis, lips stiff, toothache, gingivitis, tongue dry, excessive thirst, swelling of chin, urine yellow.

Governing Vessel 28

YIN JIAO GUM CROSSING

Reunion Gv, Cv Sores on face in children, gingivitis, excessive weeping, inner corners of eyes red itching and painful, white film over eyes, nose blocked, nasal polypus, cardiac pain, melancholic feeling in cardiac area.

Non Meridian Points

Head

SI SHEN CONG   FOUR SPIRIT ABILITY

XH1   Headache, dizziness, epilepsy.
(One Chinese inch in front, behind, to left and right of Gv 20.)

YIN TANG   SEAL PALACE

XH2   See Gv 24.5

TAI YANG   SUPREME YANG

XH3   Headache, head dizzy, neurasthenia, trigeminal neuralgia, optic nerve atrophy, retinal haemorrhage, eyes red swollen and painful, toothache.

NEI JING MING   INNER BRIGHT EYES

XH4   Conjunctivitis, optic nerve atrophy, retinal haemorrhage, various eye diseases.
(Medial corner of eye — middle of caruncle.)

Nose

NEI YING XIANG   INNER WELCOME FRAGRANCE

XN1   Severe headaches, severe pain in eyes, fevers.
(Inside ala of nose.)

SHANG YING XIANG   UPPER WELCOME FRAGRANCE

XN2   Headaches, nose blocked.

Mouth

JU QUAN   COLLECTED SPRING

XM1   Rigid tongue, dyspnoea, coughing.

XM2 left   JIN JIN   GOLDEN FLUID

YU YE   JADE FLUID

XM2 right   Tongue swollen and painful, throat obstructed, sores in mouth, excessive thirst, vomiting, diarrhoea.

HAI QUAN   SEA SPRING

XM3   Excessive thirst, throat obstructed, tongue swollen and painful, vomiting, diarrhoea.

Ear

ER JIAN   EAR POINT

XE1   Film over eyes.

Back

HUA TUO   FLOWERY HUMP

XB1   Coughing, dyspnoea, asthma, pain in back and loins, all mild complaints.
(These points are about half an inch on either side of the spines of the thoracic and lumbar vertebrae. A total of 34 points.)

*XB*2   Indigestion, feeling as if food does not pass through.

SI HUA   THE FOUR FLOWERS
*XB*3   Exhaustion, Qi weak, blood weak, bones weak, coughing phlegm, dyspnoea, emaciation.
(Another name for the two diaphragm and two gall bladder associated points: B17 and B19.)

Arm
SHI XUAN   TEN PROCLAMATIONS
*XA*1   Delirium, fainting, hysteria, epilepsy.
(Beneath the middle of the nail at the tips of the ten fingers.)

SI FENG   FOUR CRACKS
*XA*2   Pyloric stenosis ? throat, larynx.
(Middle of the palmar crease of the proximal-phalangeal joint. None for the thumb.)

ZHOU JIAN   ELBOW POINT
*XA*3   Adenitis.

Leg
HE DING   CRANE SUMMIT (BIRD)
*XL*1   Pain in knee, weakness of legs.

NEI XI YAN   INNER KNEE EYE
*XL*2   Pain and numbness in knee, difficulty in bending or flexing knee, knee swollen and painful.

LAN WEI   INTESTINE TAIL (APPENDIX)
*XL*3   Appendicitis.

NEI HUAI JIAN   INNER ANKLE POINT
*XL*4   Toothache in lower jaw, muscular cramp medial side of leg.

WAI HUAI JIAN   OUTER ANKLE POINT
*XL*5   Muscular cramp lateral side of leg, beri-beri.

A General Survey of Common Diseases and their Treatment by Acupuncture

(CHANGJIAN JIBING SHENJIU ZHILIAO BIANLAN)

COMPILED BY: THE PEKING SCHOOL OF CHINESE MEDICINE
PUBLISHED BY: THE PEOPLE'S HYGIENE PUBLISHING
HOUSE, PEKING, 1960

SECTION 2

Acupuncture Points used in the Treatment of Specific Diseases or Symptoms

TAKEN FROM THE CASE HISTORIES OF DR. FELIX MANN
AND OTHER EUROPEAN DOCTORS
PRACTISING ACUPUNCTURE

Section 2 is envisaged as an extension to Section 1, mainly from the point of view of enlarging the variety of acupuncture points that may be used in a certain disease. For this reason only combinations of acupuncture points not mentioned in Section 1 have been included. The symptomatology of the individual point should determine which acupuncture point to use.

General Diseases

1. INFLUENZA, COLDS and related conditions   *GAN MAO*

Section 1

CAUSE OF DISEASE	SYMPTOMS	DIAGNOSTIC FEATURES	MAIN POINTS	SECONDARY POINTS
1. Affected by Wind Evil.	Dislikes the cold; fever; headache; clear mucus flows from nose; sneezing; nose blocked.	Pulse Floating; tongue slightly furred white.	Gv14 B12 T5 G20 Li4 B11	S8 Gv23 Li20
2. Affected by Wind and Cold.	Head and body painful; fever; dislikes cold.	Pulse Floating and Tight; tongue slightly furred white.	as above	Gv16 S36 XH3
3. Affected by Wind and Heat.	Headache; fever; mouth parched; eyes red.	Pulse Floating and Over-flowing; tongue slightly furred yellow.	as above	Li11 XH3 (let blood)
4. Affected by Seasonal Evil.	Sudden high fever; head and nape of neck painful; body painful; breathing harsh; coughs up thick sputum; throat painful; eyes red; face flushed.	Pulse Floating and Over-flowing; tongue furred yellow; chest melancholy.	as above	L7 L9 L11 L10 B13 Gv13
5. Affected by Wind and Damp	Headache; neck stiff; joints swollen and painful; no thirst.	Pulse Floating, Slow but Weak-floating; tongue white; no thirst; joints swollen and painful.	as above	Gv16 Li11 G34
6. Dormant Evil.	Headache; heart troubled; Shen weary; troubled sleep; urine red; mouth dry; no wish to drink; delirious speech.	Pulse Rapid; tongue red.	as above	Li11 B54
7. Summer-heat and Wind on exterior of body.	Headache; no sweating; heart distressed.	Pulse Floating but Weak-floating; tongue slightly red and yellow.	as above	Cx6

Section 2

INFLUENZA	SHIVERING
Cx6 Li4 L7 Li20 S16 G20 B11 B12 B13 The Yu points	T5 K1 Cv12 B54 L10 Liv2 S36 Gv16 G25 Si14 S12 Sp9

2. PAROTITIS   *ZHA SAI*

Section 1

CAUSE OF DISEASE	SYMPTOMS	DIAGNOSTIC FEATURES	MAIN POINTS	SECONDARY POINTS
Warm Poison erupts on jaws and neck.	Swelling from behind ears to nape of neck and from in front of ears to the jaw; body hot; spontaneous sweating.	Pulse Rapid; tongue red.	G20 Li4 L7	T17 T5

Section 2

MUMPS	INSUFFICIENT SALIVA
T5 Li4 Si3	Liv4

535

3. COUGH   KE SOU
Section 1

CAUSE OF DISEASE	SYMPTOMS	DIAGNOSTIC FEATURES	MAIN POINTS	SECONDARY POINTS
1. Wind and Cold invade lungs.	Coughing; nose blocked; sneezing; dislikes cold; fever.	Pulse Floating; tongue slightly furred white.	G20 B12 B13	T5 L8
2. Wind and Heat injure lungs.	Coughing; mouth parched; body hot; sweating.	Both Inch Pulses Large; tongue furred white and slightly yellow.	B13 B12 Li4 L7	T5
3. Lung meridian Dry and hot.	Sputum difficult to cough up; sputum yellow; slight fever; palms of hands hot.	Right Inch Pulse Overflowing and Large; tongue furred yellow and white but dry.	B13 B12 Li4 L7	Cv22
4. Phlegm hot, obstructed and Full.	Coughing; chest melancholy; thick sputum causes obstruction and is difficult to cough up.	Pulse Slippery and Full; tongue yellow and greasy; stools hard; urine red.	Li4 L7 L5	S36 Sp9 T6
5. Cough due to Empty lung. (Note 1)	Continuous coughing; short of breath; Shen weary; movement causes dyspnoea; mouth parched; throat dry.	Pulse Empty.	B37 B38 Cv6	Cv12 S36
6. Cough due to Exhausted lung. (Note 2)	Continuous cough; blood in sputum; cheeks red; body emaciated; hot and flushed after midday.	Six Pulses Empty and Rapid; appearance haggard.	B37 B38 Gv12	S25 Cv6 S36

NOTES

1. *'Empty Lung: the Empty Lung is caused by a slight weakness in the lung Qi. Its symptoms are: light breathing, voice low and weak, skin dry and withered, frequent sweating, face dry and white, body fears the cold.' (Jianshi)*

2. *'Exhausted Lung: one of the Five Exhaustions (i.e. exhaustion of the Five Zang Organs: see Glossary). It is caused by damage to the Qi by Grief and Worry. The Symptoms are: gathering of the skin, loss of hair on body, appearance haggard, shivering and dislike of cold, coughing.' (Jianshi)*

Note that both Empty Lung and Exhausted Lung are diseases in themselves and have other symptoms apart from the coughing discussed here.

Section 2

LARYNGITIS
K7 K3
Cv23 Cv22 Cv18
G20 B10
B11 B12 B13

TRACHEITIS
Li4 L2
Gv12 G12 Cx3

COUGH
Yu points as indicated by the pulse
L8 L10 B13
K19 S41 Si2
B18 Liv8 H5 Cx8

COUGH—cont.
Gv12 Cv17 L11
S14 S15 S12 S36 Li10
K1 Sp14 L4
G21 K26 K27
Cv23 S19 K22 Cx2

COUGH WITH EXCESSIVE EXPECTORATION OR MUCUS THAT CANNOT BE EXPECTORATED
K2 B60 K5
T16 B13
Si1 H9
Cv12 S40 Cv17
B38 Sp9 Cx6
G10 Cv28

4. APHONIA   BAO YIN
Section 1

CAUSE OF DISEASE	SYMPTOMS	DIAGNOSTIC FEATURES	MAIN POINTS	SECONDARY POINTS
Cool Wind restrained outside the body; lung Qi does not circulate.	Sudden loss of speech.	Onset of disease sudden, not gradual	Gv16 Cv23 Li4	T5 Cx5

Section 2

HYSTERICAL APHONIA
K1 Liv1 L11 Li10
Li13 B10 Cv23 T17 Si15
Gv15 G12 Li17
Li4 K4 H5

5. DYSPNOEA, Asthma, Pneumonia, Bronchitis and similar conditions (Note 1)   *CHUAN*

Section 1

CAUSE OF DISEASE	SYMPTOMS	DIAGNOSTIC FEATURES	MAIN POINTS	SECONDARY POINTS
1. Wind and Cold restrict lungs.	Fever; dislikes the cold; no sweating; coughing; sputum rattles in bronchi; dyspnoea.	Pulse Floating and Wiry; tongue furred white.	B13 B12 Li4 K7 L7 L10	T5 Cv12
2. Fire depressed in lungs.	Dyspnoea; body hot; sputum difficult to cough up; mouth dry; face red; disease at its worst after midday.	Inch Pulse Rapid; tongue thinly furred and slightly yellow.	B13 B15 L5 L9 L10	Cx6 Si4 L1
3. Phlegm obstructed.	Dyspnoea; sputum rattles; chest-diaphragm blocked and melancholy.	Pulse Large and Slippery; tongue furred yellow and greasy.	Cv22 L5 Cx6	Cv12 S40
4. Phlegm in bronchi attacks upwards.	Inability to sleep due to coughing and difficult breathing; thin saliva causes blockage.	Inch and Connecting Pulses Deep and Wiry; tongue furred white but not parched.	Cv12 Liv13 L5	Cx6 S36 B20
5. Qi rebels and attacks upwards.	Dyspnoea; no sputum; chest-ribs swollen and melancholy.	Inch Pulse Large; Foot Pulse Deep.	Cv17 B13 Gv10 S36	Cv22 L1
6. Lungs Empty and Qi weak.	Breathing short and difficult; unable to rest; night sweats; face white.	Pulse Empty; tongue substance pale.	B37 B38 Cv17 Cv6	S36 (moxa)
7. Kidney does not transmit Qi.	Qi does not return to its source; appearance haggard and emaciated; mouth dry; no wish to drink.	Both Foot Pulses have no source; tongue substance pale; urine clear and frequent.	B23 Cv4 K6	S36
8. Wind and Heat dyspnoea: Wind and Heat enter lungs.	Fever; dislikes the cold; face red; lips red; dyspnoea.	Tongue slightly furred white; Pulse Floating and Rapid.	Cv17 (moxa) B12 B13	Cv22 L7 S40
9. Wind and Cold dyspnoea: Wind and Cold injure lungs.	Dislikes the cold; dyspnoea; coughing; sputum watery; mouth not parched.	Pulse Floating and Slow; tongue furred white.	B12 B13 Cv6	Cv12 S36
10. Hot Interior dyspnoea: rich foods and intemperate eating lead to excess Heat inside body and cause dyspnoea.	Coughing; sputum glutinous; lips red; mouth parched; heart troubled; face red.	Pulse Slippery but does not show disease, which is indicated only by dyspnoea.	Cv12 Liv3	Cx6 S40
11. Empty dyspnoea: good constitution but Empty lungs; after prolonged illness may be prone to excessive colds and diarrhoea.	Breathing short and rapid; dyspnoea only intermittently; low-pitched voice; face white; Qi of spleen and stomach not connected.	Pulse Minute; tongue not furred.	B37 B38 Cv6	Li10
12. Phlegm-fluid dyspnoea: Phlegm-fluid remains in lungs (see Notes for No. 6 Gastritis).	Sputum rattles in throat; dyspnoea; unable to rest.	Pulse Slippery; tongue furred white and thick.	B13 Cv12 S40	Cv22
13. Chronic dyspnoea: Phlegm floating in lungs.	Unseasonal weather causes attacks which are intermittent and cease spontaneously; sputum rattles; dyspnoea; breathing difficult if	Pulse Wiry and Slippery or Wiry and Weak.	Cv22 B13 B38	S36 L5

537

CAUSE OF DISEASE	SYMPTOMS	DIAGNOSTIC FEATURES	MAIN POINTS	SECONDARY POINTS
	attack is heavy; face white; lips colourless; all types of food may cause attack.			
14. Lung Qi does not accumulate.	Slight dyspnoea at all times but deteriorates with exertion; face white; breathing light; voice weak.	Pulse Minute and Weak.	Gv12 B13 B38	Cv6 S36
15. Horse-spleen Wind (Note 2): Cold Evil Visitor inside lungs; Cold changes to Heat.	Dyspnoea; chest withered; ribs on both sides collapse and become concave; Shen Qi melancholy and confused; appearance haggard and fierce.	Pulse Floating and Rapid.	Gv12 Cv17	T2 L10
16. Chronic dyspnoea brought on by external influences (e.g. other diseases).	Dyspnoea; sputum rattles; nose blocked; small amount of clear mucus from nose; nostrils sometimes red.	(no observations)	B38 (moxa) Gv16 B12 B13	S36 (moxa) T5 L7

NOTES

1. *The heading Chuan, normally means 'asthma' 'dyspnoea' 'difficult breathing' etc., though most commonly, 'asthma'. However, this sub-division clearly deals with pulmonary diseases other than asthma alone; consequently the Chinese word Chuan has been translated throughout as 'dyspnoea' to avoid giving the impression that we are here concerned with asthma alone.*

2. *'Horse-spleen Wind: popular name "severe dyspnoea" (Bao Chuan); symptoms: chest withered, breathing hurried, lungs swollen and full, ribs and nose agitated, Shen Qi (see Introduction) melancholy and distressed. Caused by Heat restrained in lungs.' (Jianshi)*

Section 2

ASTHMA
Often allergic—Liv8
Associated with fear, rigidity and gastric symptoms—K5
Anguish, a staring hollow look—L9
Local points—Cv17 K27 B11
  Cv12 G25
Si14 B10 S36 G20
Cv17 H9 T3 L1
Cv13 L3
B51 Cv3 K1
Li8 Sp9 Gv10

BRONCHITIS
L7 Liv13 Li10 Li4
B11 B12 B13 B14 B36 B38
S12 Cv20
H3 Cv14

PNEUMONIA
L7 K3
Cv17
K24 K25 K26 K27 S16 S15
  S14 S13

PNEUMONIA—cont.
B42 B43 B44 B36 B37
Li4 Li13
Sp21 Liv14 Sp17 Sp18

EMPHYSEMA
L11 Li1
L1 L2
Cv13 Cv16 Cv20 Cv21
K3 H3 L7
B17 B18 B22

PNEUMOCONIOSIS
K5 Cx6

PLEURISY
G37 G34 S40 Sp4
Liv3 Liv13
B43 Si9 Sp21 K23 S16
Li7 H3 Si4
B17 G35
S13 S15 S16
T5 K27 B11 B12 B13

6. GASTRITIS (Note 1)   *TAN YIN*

Section 1

CAUSE OF DISEASE	SYMPTOMS	DIAGNOSTIC FEATURE	MAIN POINTS	SECONDARY POINTS
1. Phlegm-fluid: spleen loses its strength and movement.	Previously robust, now emaciated; chest-diaphragm swollen.	Pulse Wiry and Slippery.	B20 B21 Cv12 Liv13 S36	Cx6 L5

CAUSE OF DISEASE	SYMPTOMS	DIAGNOSTIC FEATURES	MAIN POINTS	SECONDARY POINTS
2. Suspended-fluid (Note 2): water stopped below ribs.	Ribs on both sides painful; water stops between ribs and is audible; excessive coughing and vomiting.	Pulse Deep and Wiry.	Liv13 Cv12 L5	S24 S28
3. Overflowing-fluid (Note 3): water and Damp leak into the four limbs.	Body painful and heavy; four limbs swollen and puffy.	Pulse Floating and Wiry.	B20 B23 Liv13 K7	T5 S36
4. Branch-fluid (Note 4): fluid stops between chest and diaphragm.	Coughing prevents rest; vomits mucus; body swollen and puffy.	Inch and Connecting Pulses Wiry and Full.	B17 Cv21 Liv13 Cv12	S28 Sp9

NOTES

1. *Gastritis is a somewhat fortuitous translation of the Chinese heading Tanyin, which literally means Phlegm-drink or Phlegm-fluid. No direct English equivalent exists. The Cihai gives: 'Chronic gastritis (normal Chinese medical term); fluid blocks the stomach and cannot be absorbed; it is audible. Ancient doctors called it Tanyin and it is also known as Tingyin (Stopped-fluid).' Under Tingyin is also given:*
'One of the symptoms of gastric inflammation or gastric catarrh. The function of the digestive juices is impaired so that fluid remains in the stomach. It also causes distress of the heart and vomiting of yellow or acid fluid. If acute, the noise of water can be heard when the body is shaken. Inflammation of the stomach must be cured before this complaint will cease.'
Under Tanyin, Jianshi gives:
'Thick and turbid fluids are called Tan, thin and clear fluids are called Yin; the two characters together are used as a short name for Tanyin Disease.'
Nos. 2, 3 and 4 are also given by Jianshi as variations of Tanyin, as below:
2. *Suspended-fluid: 'The Yang Qi of the Middle Warmer (see Glossary) is deficient, the blocked fluid cannot move to the bladder but is suspended beneath the ribs; this leads to coughing and vomiting and pain beneath the ribs.' (Jianshi)*
3. *Overflowing-fluid: The blocked fluid leaks into the skin of the limbs and cannot move down to the bladder as urine; it also cannot pass out of the body as sweat but remains in the body, causing swelling and pain.' (Jianshi)*
4. *Branch-fluid: 'One of the Tanyin Diseases, characterised by coughing, inability to sleep, dyspnoea, face and eyes swollen and puffy.*
Note also that Tanyin is given under item 12 of No. 5 Dyspnoea, as a cause of one of the pulmonary conditions listed there.

Section 2

GLOBUS HYSTERICUS
L3 Cv14
Sp17 Cv12 H5

EPIGASTRIC PAIN
S45 Sp4 S25 Sp13
S36 K21 S21 L11
Cv12 Liv1

POOR DIGESTION
Liv13 Liv14
Sp15 S36 G25

POOR DIGESTION—cont.
B17

GASTRIC PTOSIS
Cv8 (S de Morant from Jap.)

ANOREXIA
S39 S45
Liv4
B17 B18 B19
Cv6

7. INTERMITTENT FEVERS, REMITTENT FEVERS, MALARIA and related conditions NUE JI

Section 1

CAUSE OF DISEASE	SYMPTOMS	DIAGNOSTIC FEATURES	MAIN POINTS	SECONDARY POINTS
1. Affected by Wind and Cold.	Dislikes the cold; fever at regular intervals; desires to vomit; head dizzy.	Pulse Wiry; tongue furred white; side of tongue purple.	Gv14 Gv13 Cx5 T6 Si3	Gv16 Li4 Li11
2. Affected by Damp and Heat.	During attacks patient alternates rapidly between extremes of heat and cold; sweating relieves attack; great thirst; patient hot more than cold.	Left Pulse Wiry; tongue purple and slightly furred.	as above	Li4 Li11 S36

539

CAUSE OF DISEASE	SYMPTOMS	DIAGNOSTIC FEATURES	MAIN POINTS	SECONDARY POINTS
3. Attack caused if Dormant Qi exposed to Summer-heat.	Bones and joints painful; occasional vomiting; continually hot, never cold; muscles and flesh waste away.	Pulse normal; mouth parched; tongue furred yellow and greasy.	as above	B11 K6
4. Fever due to tiredness; Yin Qi ceases to function, only Yang Qi in operation.	Patient continually hot, never cold; mouth dry and hot.	Pulse Overflowing.	as above	XH2 Li4
5. Starvation or immoderate eating and drinking.	Patient feels hot and cold simultaneously; bouts of fever at regular intervals; stomach obstructed and full; dislikes food; breath putrid.	Pulse Wiry, Slippery and Full; tongue thickly furred and greasy.	as above	Cv12 S44 Sp4
6. Recurrent fever brought on by exhaustion; fever all day long; spleen and stomach Qi Empty.	Hot and cold simultaneously and at regular intervals; bout lasts whole day; limbs weary; fluctuation in temperature slight; sweating; dyspnoea.	Pulse Empty; tongue pale.	as above	B20 Liv13 L8 XB2

Section 2

PYREXIA OF UNKNOWN ORIGIN
K3 B62

8. DYSENTERY   *LI JI*

Section 1

CAUSE OF DISEASE	SYMPTOMS	DIAGNOSTIC FEATURES	MAIN POINTS	SECONDARY POINTS
1. Cold dysentery: Zang organs Cold and Empty; this also causes cold in rest of body.	Face and lips blue-green and white; likes warm fluids; abdomen painful; intestinal noises; diarrhoea; if severe, feet and hands become cold; eyes prominent and red; stools like those of a duck.	Pulse Deep; tongue not furred.	S25 Cv6	B25 B29
2. Heat dysentery: Warmth congealed.	Fever; tongue red; lips burning; likes cold fluids; abdomen painful; incessant diarrhoea; small quantities of red urine; bowel painful and heavy.	Pulse Rapid; tongue thickly furred yellow.	Cv12 S25 Li4	Sp2 S44
3. Periodic dysentery: affected by Wind Evil from outside and injured by cold from within.	Fever; no sweating; whole body painful; diarrhoea and vomiting; abdomen painful; bowel heavy.	Pulse Floating and Slippery	B12 Cv12 T5	Li4 S36
4. Dysentery with trismus: Great Poison rushes into stomach; diarrhoea injures Yin.	Body hot; tongue red; lips red; diarrhoea without having eaten; likes cold fluids.	Pulse Rapid.	B20 B21 Cv12 S25	K7 Sp4
5. Nourishment dysentery: caused by food and water.	Diarrhoea; abdomen painful; bowel heavy.	Pulse Slowed-down.	B20 B21 Cv11	B25 B29
6. Chronic dysentery.	Intermittent dysentery may continue for 6–12 months; face yellowish-white; eats and drinks normally.	Pulse Fine and Rapid.	B20 B23 Cv4	K2 Sp4
7. Five-colour dysentery: due to use of purgative medicine or incomplete coagulation of food in bowel.	Stools of various colours, purulent and bloody.	Both Foot Pulses Fine.	B25 B27	S36 S25

Section 2

DYSENTERY
Liv6 Sp6
Cv12 S36 S28 S39 K21 Cv6
T5 Cx6
S11 Gv1 K7
B62 Li4 G26 Liv2

9. DIARRHOEA *XIE XIE*

Section 1

CAUSE OF DISEASE	SYMPTOMS	DIAGNOSTIC FEATURES	MAIN POINTS	SECONDARY POINTS
1. Damp diarrhoea: cold produced by food and drink, sitting on damp surface, or excessive drinking of alcohol.	Limbs weary; stools watery; dysuria; insipid taste in mouth; inability to taste; chest-diaphragm suffering and melancholy; abdomen painful.	Pulse Weak-floating and Blocked; tongue furred, dirty and greasy.	Cv12 S25 B20 B25	Cv9 S36 Sp6
2. Fire diarrhoea: caused by overflowing of Heat, or by eating bitter, hot foods and excessive drinking of alcohol; Fire in body depressed and congealed.	Precipitous diarrhoea; abdomen painful; stools hot and foul-smelling; rectum burning and painful; burning pain in bowel during passing of stools; mouth parched; dreads the heat.	Tongue purple and furred yellow; small quantities of red urine; Pulse Deep and Rapid.	Cv12 S25 S36 S44	Li11 Li4 Sp9 S39
3. Food diarrhoea: excessive eating and drinking; food accumulates and congeals and is not broken down.	Belching; abdomen full; stools putrid and glutinous.	Pulse Full and Large; tongue furred, rough and yellow.	Cv13 Cv12 S25 Liv13	Cx6 S36 S37 S39
4. Water diarrhoea: food and water produce cold; water accumulates and is not digested.	Intestinal noises; lower abdomen painful; diarrhoea frequent and completely liquid; mouth parched despite drinking; dislikes cold.	Pulse Slow; tongue furred white and greasy.	Cv12 S25 B20 B23	Cv9 S28 S36 Sp6
5. Summer-heat diarrhoea: Summer-heat Qi damp, remains in intestines and stomach.	Face dirty; sweating; mouth parched; heart anxious; abdomen rumbles like thunder; stools watery.	Pulse Weak-floating; tongue furred and greasy.	Cv12 S25 B20 B25	Cx7 S36 Sp6
6. Phlegm diarrhoea: Damp and Phlegm flowing; large intestine not strong, allowing food to slip out as diarrhoea.	Intermittent diarrhoea; chest melancholy; food only slightly digested; patient may wish to vomit phlegm.	(no observations)	Cv12 S25 B25	Cx6 S36 S40
7. Cold diarrhoea: spleen Yang Empty and Cold.	Intestinal noises; severe pain in intestines; stools like those of a duck; dislikes the cold.	Pulse Slow; urine white.	Cv12 Cv6 Liv13 B20 B21	S25 B25 S36 Sp6
8. Spleen diarrhoea: spleen Empty; Pure Yang cannot ascend, thus producing diarrhoea.	Abdomen Empty and Full(?); diarrhoea after meals; patient appears emaciated; no strength; Jing Shen failing; stomach transmits Qi inadequately.	Pulse Empty and Pliable; no variations in colour of tongue (i.e. whole tongue of uniform colour).	Gv20 Cv12 Liv13 B21 B20	S25 Cv4 S36 Sp6
9. Kidney diarrhoea: kidney Empty and Cold; Yang Qi deficient.	Diarrhoea on rising in the morning (the so-called 'Fifth watch of the night diarrhoea'); limbs weary and cold; dislikes the cold; abdomen rumbles.	Pulse Empty and Weak; no variations in colour of tongue.	Cv12 Liv13 Cv8 B20 B23	Gv20 Cv4 S36 K6
10. Slippery diarrhoea: disease persists for long time; intestines slippery and weak.	No control of bowel action when passing stools.	Pulse Empty and Pliable; no variations in colour of tongue.	Gv20 Cv12 Cv6 B20 B23	B44 Gv4 Gv1 Cv8 S36

Section 2

COLITIS	COLITIS—cont.
K5 B23	L9 B54 Li11 S36
Liv11 Liv2 Liv8	Sp1 Sp3 S44
S25 S27 Cv12 Cv4	Sp4 G41 Sp14 K14
Sp9 K2 B65	K7 Cv9 B35

541

10. CHOLERA *HUO LUAN*

Section 1

CAUSE OF DISEASE	SYMPTOMS	DIAGNOSTIC FEATURES	MAIN POINTS	SECONDARY POINTS
1. Affected by Wind and Cold from outside the body; inside the body food and drink are obstructed; the Pure and Impure Qi contest; stomach and intestines are not in accord.	Vomiting; diarrhoea; vomitus like dirty water; dislikes the cold; fever; muscular spasms in severe cases.	Pulse Deep and Wiry; tongue furred white and slippery.	Cv12 S25 S36 S44 T5	B57 Sp4
2. Affected by Summer-heat Evil.	Fever; no sweating; excessive vomiting; muscular spasms in severe cases; fingers cracked and shrivelled.	Pulse Floating and Wiry; tongue furred white.	XA1 S25 Li4 S36	B57 Cv12
3. Summer-heat attacks inside the body.	Mouth parched; heart troubled; body hot; sweating; vomiting; diarrhoea; limbs cold; spasms of limbs; eyes sunken.	Pulse Empty and Large or Weak-floating; face red; small quantities of urine.	L5 B54 (let blood) Li4 Cv12 S36	S44 S25 B57
4. Cold and Damp injure spleen.	Abdomen painful; vomiting; diarrhoea; hands and feet cold; muscular spasms in severe cases.	Pulse Deep and Fine; tongue furred greyish-white and not parched.	Cv8 Cv4 B20 B25	Cv6 S25 S36 B57

11. CHOLERA SICCA *GAN HUO LUAN*

Section 1

CAUSE OF DISEASE	SYMPTOMS	DIAGNOSTIC FEATURES	MAIN POINTS	SECONDARY POINTS
1. Sudden attack of Cold and Damp; impurities in the body are obstructed and do not descend.	Abdomen extremely painful; heart troubled, agitated and melancholy; patient wishes to vomit and defaecate but cannot.	Pulse Deep and Wiry but Slow; Pulse Buried in severe cases; limbs cold; tongue furred, greasy and moist.	XA1 (let blood) Cv12 Cv6 Cv4 Cv8	Li4 S36
2. Summer-heat is impure and attacks within the body, preventing ascent or descent of Qi.	Lines of pain running through the abdomen; patient wishes to vomit and defaecate but cannot.	Pulse Deep and Slippery; Pulse Buried in severe cases; tongue red and furred yellow.	XA1 L5 B54 (let blood) Cv12 Cx6	S36 S44 Sp4

12. VOMITING *OU TU*

Section 1

CAUSE OF DISEASE	SYMPTOMS	DIAGNOSTIC FEATURES	MAIN POINTS	SECONDARY POINTS
1. Stomach hot: savoury foods collect and become hot; stomach loses control and causes vomiting.	Vomiting immediately after meals; vomitus hot and foul-smelling; likes the cold and dislikes the heat; mouth parched and thirsty.	Pulse Overflowing and Large; tongue furred yellow and parched.	Cx6 Cv12 S36	Cv22 S44 XM2 (let blood)
2. Spleen cold: spleen and stomach Empty and Cold; Yang Qi does not circulate; food not digested; Yin Qi turbid, does not descend.	Vomits large amounts of gastric secretions mixed with saliva, which is clear and cold; violent vomiting after food in morning; vomitus not hot or foul-smelling; no thirst; likes heat and dislikes cold; limbs cold.	Pulse Slowed-down and Fine; tongue furred white.	Cv12 Liv13 Cv17 B20 B21 B23	Cx6 Cv13 S36 Sp6
3. Qi obstructed: heart anxious; Qi uneasy and rebels upwards against the stomach.	Vomiting immediately after eating; chest and abdomen bloated and melancholy; obstruction below ribs; mouth bitter and hot; head and nape of neck may be painful, or not painful but swollen.	If hot: Pulse Wiry and Slippery; tongue furred yellow and burning.	Hot: Cx6 Cv12 S36	Hot: G34 Li4 Liv2 S41 XM2

542

CAUSE OF DISEASE	SYMPTOMS	DIAGNOSTIC FEATURES	MAIN POINTS	SECONDARY POINTS
	Patient may be either hot or cold: If hot: vomitus hot and foul-smelling; dislikes the heat; thirsty. If cold: vomits large amounts of clear fluid; no thirst; dislikes cold, likes heat.	If cold: Pulse Fine; tongue furred white.	Cold: Cx6 Cv12 S36 B17 Liv13 (moxa)	Cold: B18 B20 B21 Liv2 S44
4. Phlegm-fluid: (see Note to No. 6 Gastritis): previously body contained much Phlegm; spleen Yang may be immobile.	Vomiting if cold; vomits phlegm and saliva; no appetite; chest-diaphragm full and melancholy.	Pulse Slow and Slippery; tongue furred white.	Cx6 Cv12 S36 S40	Cv6 B17 B20 B21
5. Food accumulation: excessive eating causes accumulation and failure to digest.	Chest-diaphragm bloated and melancholy; dislikes smell of food; stools usually hot and foul-smelling; lines of pain in more severe cases; vomitus putrid.	Pulse Full and Rough; tongue thickly furred and greasy.	Cx6 Cv12 Liv13 S36	Li4 Cv21 G34 Sp4
6. Middle Empty: spleen and stomach Empty and Weak; the Transforming Action of Qi is not effective (see Introduction).	Food cannot pass beyond the stomach which rebels and causes vomiting; limbs and body weary; body emaciated.	Pulse Empty and Fine; tongue thickly furred and greasy.	Cv12 Liv13 B20 B21	S25 S36 Sp6

Section 2

AT CERTAIN TIMES AFTER S. DE MORANT
Acid vomiting at night—G23 G24
Vomiting with pyloric spasm—K21
Food vomited several hours after eating—G30
Vomiting after meals—Liv13
Vomiting, shoulder pain, food undigested—B22
Water brash—B13 Liv14 Liv2 Sp6

HAEMATEMESIS
B17 B18
Spl T5

13. HICCOUGH *E NI*

Section 1

CAUSE OF DISEASE	SYMPTOMS	DIAGNOSTIC FEATURES	MAIN POINTS	SECONDARY POINTS
1. Food produces cold; stomach may be Empty, and Cold.	Breath travels downwards then immediately upwards producing a short, sharp noise on leaving the mouth. Special symptoms: gullet swollen and full; hiccough may be cured by drinking hot water.	Pulse Slow and Fine; tongue thinly furred white.	B20 B21 Cv12	S25 S36
2. Liver Fire rises.	As above. Special symptoms: thirst.	Pulse Wiry and Rapid; tongue furred yellow.	B18 Liv2 Cx6	S36 G34
3. Spleen and stomach Qi Empty and weak.	As above. Special symptoms: noise slight; breathing light.	Pulse Minute or Fine.	B38 B17 Cv17 Cv6	S36
4. Stomach Hot, Dry and Full.	As above. Special symptoms: noise loud; breathing heavy; constipation.	Pulse Slippery and Full.	Cv12 S25 Cx6	L7 S36 S44

HICCOUGH
B38
Cv12 Li9 K17
Liv13 Liv14 B17

HICCOUGH—cont.
Cx8 Li5 Cv17
Sp3 B19

14. NAUSEA AND VOMITING *FAN WEI*

Section 1

CAUSE OF DISEASE	SYMPTOMS	DIAGNOSTIC FEATURES	MAIN POINTS	SECONDARY POINTS
1. Middle Warmer Empty and Cold.	Food rejected on entering stomach.	Pulse Slow and Weak; tongue pale.	Cv12 Liv13 B20 B21	S36 Sp6
2. Middle Warmer Cold and Empty; much Phlegm; Qi obstructed.	Vomits phlegm and saliva.	Pulse Weak; tongue furred and greasy.	G21 Cv17 Cv6 Cv12	Cx6 S36 S40
3. Stomach Empty; Qi obstructed.	Vomiting and hiccough; chest full.	Pulse Weak; tongue pale.	Cv12 B21 K16	Cx6 S36
4. Cold Phlegm Visitor in Upper Warmer.	Coughing and vomiting.	Pulse Slippery; tongue furred and greasy.	G21 Cv17 B17 Cv12	S36 Sp4
5. Lower Warmer Empty and Cold; Fire weak; Earth sinking.	Food eaten in morning vomited in in evening.	Pulse Slow and Weak; tongue pale.	Cv6 Cv4 B20 B23	S36 Sp6
6. Spleen and stomach Qi Empty; True Yin dried up.	Chronic nausea; constipation.	Pulse Rough.	Cv12 Liv13	S36
7. Alcohol injures spleen.	Vomiting.	Pulse Slow and Weak; tongue furred white and greasy.	Cv12 Liv13 B20	Cx6 S36
8. Damp depressed, becomes Heat; stomach Fire rushes upwards.	Vomiting immediately after eating.	Pulse Rapid; tongue purple.	G21 Cv12 Liv13	Cx6 S36 S44

Section 2

NAUSEA, VOMITING
Liv8 Liv14
B62 Gv12
Cx6, S36
B17
Cx5 Li11 Sp5
Si3 L7 Li4
Cx8 Si1
L9 Cx7

AEROGASTRIA
L8 L10 Cx6
Liv14 G25 Liv13 Sp16
Cv12 Gv6 Cv12
Sp2 Sp4

OESOPHAGEAL SPASM
B38 Cv17
Sp6 B17
K21 B45 Cx8
G20 B18 Cv22 Li11 Sp5

15. GASTRALGIA *WEI TONG*

Section 1

CAUSE OF DISEASE	SYMPTOMS	DIAGNOSTIC FEATURES	MAIN POINTS	SECONDARY POINTS
1. Affected by Cold Evil from outside and by cold matter from within; Cold Visitor in stomach.	Stomach suddenly painful.	Pulse Deep and Tight.	Cv13 Cv12 Cv10 Cx6 S36 S25 Cv6	S34 S21
2. Stomach depressed and Hot.	Pain in stomach; feels extremely hot.	Pulse Slippery and Rapid; thirsty; tongue red; likes cool drinks.	as above	S44

CAUSE OF DISEASE	SYMPTOMS	DIAGNOSTIC FEATURES	MAIN POINTS	SECONDARY POINTS
3. Qi obstructed.	Stomach painful, swollen, full and uncomfortable.	Pulse Deep and Rough.	as above	B18 Liv13
4. Dead blood.	Pain in stomach at particular points which feel as though being pierced.	Pulse Rough; tongue black.	as above	B20 B21 B18 B19 B17
5. Stomach Empty.	Continuous pain in stomach; likes to press stomach to relieve pain.	Pulse Empty, Slowed-down and without strength; face white; small appetite.	as above	B20 B21 B18
6. Stomach Full and obstructed.	Stomach painful, obstructed and swollen; constipated.	Pulse Deep and Full; right Connecting Pulse has strength; tongue thickly furred yellow.	as above	S44

Section 2

PEPTIC ULCER

Acid-base imbalance: the kidneys and to some extent the lungs, keep the pH of the blood normal — K5 L9
Purely gastric type — S45
Really a hepatic disturbance, but has nearly indistinguishable symptoms — Liv8 G40
Abdominal type — Cx6 Cv12 Cv13 Cv10 S25 S36
A large proportion of patients with peptic ulcer respond to one of the above four combinations. There are of course in addition an infinite number of different combinations or variations:
B17 B18 B19 B20 B21 B22
B41 B42 B43 B44 B45
Gv6 Gv7 Gv8 Gv9
Any point on the upper abdomen may be used, according to its symptomatology. If the abdominal point is excessively tender or large, it should not be used, as it might easily cause an aggravation.

16. ABDOMINAL PAIN   *FU TONG*

Section 1

CAUSE OF DISEASE	SYMPTOMS	DIAGNOSTIC FEATURES	MAIN POINTS	SECONDARY POINTS
1. Affected by Cold.	Lines of pain in abdomen; stools may be loose.	Pulse Deep and Slow; tongue furred white; likes heat and not thirsty.	Sp4 Cx6 S36 Cv12 Cv4 S25	
2. Qi of the Seven Emotions depressed.	Abdomen painful, obstructed and swollen; no appetite or thirst.	Pulse Deep; face haggard.	as above	
3. Empty and Cold.	Pain not severe.	Pulse Deep and Wiry; tongue pale; no thirst; urine clear; likes warmth; presses abdomen to relieve pain.	as above	
4. Food stopped up.	Abdomen painful, swollen and full; dislikes food; halitosis; saliva sour.	Pulse Deep and Slippery; tongue thickly furred and greasy; presses abdomen.	as above	S44
5. Inside Hot; Fire depressed.	Abdomen painful; vomiting; thirsty and likes cold drinks.	Pulse Rapid; tongue red; small quantities of red urine.	as above	Li4

Section 2

'TUMMY ACHE'	ABDOMINAL DISTENSION
Sp4 Liv4	L9 Li11
S37 Cv9 S22	Cv3 Cv5 Cv10 Cv12
B57 Cx6 Li8	Liv13
S25 Sp6 Cv12 Liv13	
	AEROCOLON
	K8 S19 S29 Sp6
	S36 Cv8 Li3 Liv3

17. INTESTINAL INFLAMMATION *CHANG YONG*
Section 1

CAUSE OF DISEASE	SYMPTOMS	DIAGNOSTIC FEATURES	MAIN POINTS	SECONDARY POINTS
Damp and Hot Qi obstructed and congealed.	Abdomen extremely painful when pressed; bowel action heavy.	Pulse Slow or Tight.	XL3	Li11 S36

Section 2

INTESTINAL SPASM
B62 Li4

18. CONSTIPATION *BIAN MI*
Section 1

CAUSE OF DISEASE	SYMPTOMS	DIAGNOSTIC FEATURES	MAIN POINTS	SECONDARY POINTS
1. Hot and Dry Yang congealed.	Faeces in bowels dry and congealed, and not passed.	Pulse Deep and Rapid and has strength; tongue furred yellow; abdomen swollen, obstructed and full.	T6 S25 B25 G34	Cv12 S36 Li4 S44
2. Cold and Dry Yin congealed.	Stools dense and congealed.	Pulse Deep and Slow and has strength; tongue thickly furred white; no appetite.	Cv12 Cv4 S25 B25	T6 S36 Sp6
3. Qi dense.	Qi penetrates and obstructs the frame of the body; stools dense and congealed.	Pulse Deep; chest-diaphragm obstructed and full; abdomen swollen.	Cv12 Cv6 T6 G34	Cx6 S36 Gv1 Liv1 S44
4. Blood dense.	Stools dense and congealed.	Pulse Empty and Large; tongue substance purple; mouth dry; heart troubled; sleep restless.	B17 B18 B15 T6	Cx7 Sp6
5. Wind dense.	Stools dense and congealed.	Pulse Floating and Wiry.	B12 B14 B25	T6 G34 S36 K3

Section 2

CONSTIPATION
Yin — T6 S36
Yang — Gv1 Liv1 G34
   (A. Chamfrault)
Weak abdominal muscles — Sp13
Distended abdomen — B28
Habitual constipation — T7 G34
K17 K16 B46 (S. de Morant).

CONSTIPATION—Cont.
Unable to pass motion — Sp6 B57 Cv6 B31
   (S. de Morant)
Liv13 Liv3 Sp3 Cv12
B57 K6
B23 B24 K15 K16

19. JAUNDICE *HUANG DAN*
Section 1

CAUSE OF DISEASE	SYMPTOMS	DIAGNOSTIC FEATURES	MAIN POINTS	SECONDARY POINTS
1. Damp and Heat jaundice: spleen and stomach Damp and Hot.	Eyes and body yellow; urine yellow; abdomen full; constipation.	Pulse Deep, Slippery and Full; tongue furred yellow and greasy.	Cv12 S36 Gv9 B19	Gv14 G34 S44 Sp4
2. Damp and Heat depressed inside the body; bladder Qi does not Transform.	Body and face completely yellow; dysuria.	(no observations)	B19 Gv9 B27 B28 Cv3	Cv12 S36 S28 Sp9
3. Yin yellow: spleen and kidney Empty and Cold; Damp is stored up and is not transformed.	Body and face yellow and of dark complexion; arms and legs cold from extremities to elbows and knees.	Pulse Deep and Fine; tongue pale and furred white; intestines melancholy; no appetite; no constipation.	Cv12 Gv9 B20 B23	Si4 S36 Sp9 Sp6

546

CAUSE OF DISEASE	SYMPTOMS	DIAGNOSTIC FEATURES	MAIN POINTS	SECONDARY POINTS
4. Nourishment jaundice: Damp, Heat and stale foods attack each other.	Stomach bitter and melancholy; head dizzy after eating; body and face hot.	Pulse Slippery; tongue furred, slippery and greasy.	Cv12 B19 B20 B21	Cx6 S36 L7 Li4 S44
5. Alcohol jaundice: excess of alcohol; Damp and Heat steaming	Heart melancholy and disordered; sometimes painful and hot and unable to eat, or having eaten wishes to vomit; soles of feet hot; dysuria; body and face yellow.	Pulse Wiry and Slippery; tongue furred, slippery and greasy.	Sp4 B19 Gv9 B54	Si4 B27 B28 Cv12 S36 Sp9
6. Woman-weary jaundice (Note 1): Heat Evil injures kidney.	Body yellow; forehead black; lower abdomen full; soles of feet hot; stools black and loose.	Pulse Deep, Fine and Rapid; tongue furred black and insipid.	B23 B67 Sp4	K6 K2

NOTES

1. *Mathews gives 'Woman-weary jaundice' as 'chlorosis' while Jianshi says simply 'a type of jaundice'. Although from the symptoms given here it seems unlikely that 'chlorosis' is correct, it is interesting to note that the modern Chinese term for that condition is 'withering yellow disease' whereas in English it is known as 'green sickness', (chlorosis).*

Section 2	JAUNDICE Liv8 K5 G21 Si14 B44 S44 Li4 Cv12 Cx7 K7 Liv4	JAUNDICE—Cont. Li2 Li13 Si8 G38 G40 Sp5 Liv8 B38 Sp10 B54 (S. de Morant)

20. SWELLING OF ABDOMEN ONLY (Note 1)   *DAN FU TONG*

Section 1

CAUSE OF DISEASE	SYMPTOMS	DIAGNOSTIC FEATURES	MAIN POINTS	SECONDARY POINTS
1. Abdomen swelling: the Swelling Disease has its roots in the spleen where the Yin is injured. Although the stomach transmits Nourishment, the spleen does not transform it (i.e. into Qi, Blood, Ying, Wei etc. see Introduction); Anger may injure the liver and gradually encroach upon the spleen, the spleen is extremely Empty so Yin and Yang do not meet; Pure and Impure Qi are mixed together, so the Way cannot be penetrated, and this causes Heat; Damp and Heat are both generated, so the abdomen becomes swollen.	Abdomen swollen and Empty; skin taut; if the patient eats in the morning he cannot do so in the evening. (If the navel protrudes (Note 2) dark veins appear on the abdomen and the skin is like oil, then the disease is severe and cannot be cured).	Pulse Floating and Large in mild cases, Empty and Small in severe cases.	Cv12 B20 B23 B22 Liv13 Cv9 Cv6	Cx6 K7 Sp4 S36 Sp6
2. Qi depressed: great anger or frustration cause liver Fire to	Either right or left or both sides of body painful.	Qi painful; pain intermittent; abdomen swollen; slight relief from pain if	Cv12 Cv6 B18	Liv14 Sp4 Cx6

CAUSE OF DISEASE	SYMPTOMS	DIAGNOSTIC FEATURES	MAIN POINTS	SECONDARY POINTS
move vigorously and make the sides of the body painful. Dead blood: bad blood remains below the ribs and makes the sides of the body painful; extreme pain when pressed.		warm; pain circulates; Inch Pulse Wiry. Blood painful: painful whether pressed or not; pain continuous; no swelling; dead blood causes obstruction; disease mild during day, severe at night; fever after midday; Pulse Short and Rough.	Liv13 B17 B18 Liv13	S36 Liv14 B54 G40 Cx6
3. Swelling in abdomen only: violent anger injures liver; anxiety injures spleen. (This disease is popularly called the 'spider drum' disease.)	Only abdomen, not limbs, swollen. The Yi Zhi (Purpose of Healing) says: 'There is a disease called 'Spider poison swelling' in which only the abdomen is swollen and the four limbs are very emaciated.'	Abdomen visibly swollen: ribs on both sides must be examined in order to make sure there is no swelling and pain; and the abdomen should be examined to make sure there is no accumulation of fluid. The ribs should also be examined for symptoms of other diseases which may be caused by the liver and spleen.	Cv12 Cv6 Liv13 B20 B18 B22 Cv9	S36 Sp6 Sp9

NOTES

1. *In this case the English title is a direct translation of the Chinese. The condition should be contrasted with Nos. 21 and 22.*

2. *The 'protruding navel' is also found as a condition in itself, occurring in children. The protrusion may apparently vary greatly in size. In fact the same term, Qi Tu Chu, is now used for 'umbilical hernia': in this case the modern and the traditional use of a Chinese term are virtually identical, but this is uncommon. The older usage is rarely as precise as the modern one, and not infrequently has a completely different meaning.*

Section 2

ASCITES
Cv9 S28 Sp6 G28
K7

21. QI-ACCUMULATION DISEASES (Mainly gastric) (Note 1) *JI JU*

Section 1

CAUSE OF DISEASE	SYMPTOMS	DIAGNOSTIC FEATURES	MAIN POINTS	SECONDARY POINTS
1. Immoderate eating and drinking gradually cause blockage and accumulation of Qi.	Hard obstruction in abdomen which is swollen, painful and melancholy.	Pulse Rough; tongue thickly furred.	Cv12 Liv13 XB2 B20 B21	S36 Sp4
2. Phlegm-fluid, blood and Qi accumulated.	Chest and abdomen obstructed.	Pulse Deep, Full and Fine.	Cv12 Liv13 B20 B18 XB2	Cx6 S36 S40 S44
3. The Five Exhaustions and the Seven Injuries; dried blood within the body.	Body emaciated; abdomen full; cannot eat and drink; skin dry and scaly; both eyes black.	Pulse Rough.	Cv12 Liv13 B17 B18 XB2	Sp10 K6 B54 S36 Sp6
4. Affected by the Seven Emotions.	Acute dyspnoea; chest-diaphragm listless; heart distressed; no appetite.	Pulse Rough; no indication of accumulated Qi; Qi sometimes scattered, sometimes accumulated.	Cv13 Liv13 Cv6 B13 B17	Cx6 S36 S44
5. Qi Cold and accumulated.	Limbs obstructed; bowel cold and constipated.	Pulse Rough.	Cv12 Cv6 S25 B25	S36 Sp6

CAUSE OF DISEASE	SYMPTOMS	DIAGNOSTIC FEATURES	MAIN POINTS	SECONDARY POINTS
6. Spleen weak and loses its movement; Empty Evil becomes accumulated.	Obstruction in bowel; emaciated, weak and weary.	Pulse Fine and Rough.	Cv12 Liv13 B20 B21 B23 XB2	S36 S40 Sp4
7. A prolonged accumulation causes Gan (see No. 90 GAN JI) and activates the liver Fire.	Cheeks swollen; mouth wasted away; teeth and gums rotten; constipated.	Pulse Wiry and Rapid; mouth hot, thirsty and painful.	Cv12 Liv13 S25 B20 B19 B22	Li4 S36 G34 Liv2

NOTES
1. *Separately Ji, and Ju, have a more precise meaning than is evident here. According to Jianshi: 'An accumulation of Qi is called Ji; it occurs in a definite place and its pain is not far from that place. A gathering together of Qi is called Ju; it does not occur in any definite place and its pain has no fixed location. The combination of Ji and Ju means that a Qi disease of accumulating, obstructing, gathering and congealing affects the Zang and Fu organs.'*

22. OEDEMA *SHUI ZHONG*

Section 1

CAUSE OF DISEASE	SYMPTOMS	DIAGNOSTIC FEATURES	MAIN POINTS	SECONDARY POINTS
Fluid causes obstruction inside the body; Wind and Cold restrained outside the body; the Triple Warmer transforms but does not activate; the skin becomes swollen.	Eyes, limbs, abdomen and genitals all swollen; if the disease attacks upwards it causes difficult breathing, coughing and vomiting; if it collects below, retention of urine occurs.	1. Empty Swelling: disease usually protracted; fatigue; appearance dejected; voice weak and hesitant; Pulse Empty. 1a. Lung Qi Empty and unable to circulate; region below the heart rebellious and full; Qi attacks chest. 1b. Spleen Qi Empty and unable to vaporize; water saturates the middle of the body. 1c. Kidney Qi Empty and unable to activate the water; oliguria.	B13 B23 B20 B28 Cv9 S28 Cv8	Cv6 Cv4 Cv3 S36 Sp6 Sp9 K7
		2. Full Swelling: usually severe; Pulse always Abundant; oliguria and constipation.	Li4 L7 Sp9 K7 S28 Cv9	S43 S36 Sp6 B27 Gv26

Section 2

OEDEMA OF FEET
G31 Sp4 Sp9 G30
B54 B57 B58 B62

CARDIAC OEDEMA
H7 B15 B23
H9 K8
S36 S43 G30 Li4

CARDIAC OEDEMA—cont.
Sp6 T7 Cv5

VARICOSE VEINS
Only slight effect
Gv14 Gv12 G21 Gv4
Plus local points on legs (A. Chamfrault)

23. PENETRATING WIND (Cerebral Haemorrhage: see Note 1.) *ZHONG FENG*

Section 1

CAUSE OF DISEASE	SYMPTOMS	DIAGNOSTIC FEATURES	MAIN POINTS	SECONDARY POINTS
1. Penetrating the Luo: Wind Evil penetrates the Luo.	Mouth and eyes awry; flesh and skin numb; movement causes pain.	Pulse Floating, Wiry and Anxious.	S6 S4 T17 Li4 L7 S36	Gv26 Cv24 G14 S2 G20 Si18 S42 Li20
2. Penetrating the meridians: Wind penetrates the meridians.	Hands and feet paralysed; tongue feeble.	Pulse Deep and Wiry.	Gv20 Gv16 Li15 Li11 Li4 G30 G34 G39	G20 T5 Si3 G21 Li10 S36 G31 B60
3. Penetrating the Zang and Fu organs.	Patient suddenly collapses and becomes unconscious; mouth tightly closed and unable to open; face red; hands tightly clenched; breathing harsh.	Pulse Slippery and Unyielding.	all or any of Category 1 points. XA1 (let blood) Gv20 Gv26	Li4 S6 K1
4. (no observations)	Special symptoms: eyes and mouth wide open; no control of body; urinary incontinence: heavy sweating.	Pulse Minute and Weak.	Cv8 Cv6 Cv4	Gv26 Cx9 Gv20

NOTES

1. *Although this subdivision seems in fact to be concerned with various results of cerebral haemorrhage, in order to make use of the material supplied here, it is more profitable to retain the Chinese terminology and seek to understand the traditional Chinese interpretation of the cause of the symptoms listed. It is unlikely that the Chinese knew of the existence of cerebral haemorrhage until fairly recent times, but this in no way effects the validity of the argument: cerebral haemorrhage, or any other 'cause' of this condition, would simply be regarded as a result of the primary cause, in this case Wind Evil.*

Moreover 'cerebral haemorrhage' does not cover all that is implied in the term Penetrating Wind; for instance the Cihai says:

'Chinese medicine says the cause of the disease is Wind (see Introduction); Western medicine says it is caused by cerebral haemorrhage. There are also conditions (embraced by the term Penetrating Wind) due to bleeding in the stomach and intestines, and in the pericardium.'

24. SECONDARY PENETRATING WIND (Note 1) *LEI ZHONG FENG*

Section 1

CAUSE OF DISEASE	SYMPTOMS	DIAGNOSTIC FEATURES	MAIN POINTS	SECONDARY POINTS
1. Fire penetrating: the Fire of the Five Desires erupts inside the body.	Sudden collapse and loss of consciousness; body hot; constipation.	Face red; tongue red; Pulse Overflowing and Rapid.	XA1 (let blood) Gv26 Gv20	Li4 K1 Cx9
2. Cold penetrating: Yin Cold penetrates the Zang organs.	Sudden lockjaw; hands and feet trembling; face sad and colourless.	Pulse Deep and Slow or Buried.	Cv4 Cv6 Cv12	Li4 Liv3 Gv26 Gv20
3. Food penetrating: excessive eating or drinking.	After eating patient suddenly becomes delirious; cannot speak; cannot raise limbs; chest and abdomen hard and full.	Pulse Deep and Full or Buried.	XA1 (let blood) Li4 Gv20 Gv26	Cx6 Cv12 S36

CAUSE OF DISEASE	SYMPTOMS	DIAGNOSTIC FEATURES	MAIN POINTS	SECONDARY POINTS
4. Emptiness penetrating: Qi Empty and extremely weary.	Sudden collapse and delirium; face pale and yellow.	Pulse Empty; tongue pale.	Cv6 Cv4 Cv12 Cv8	S36 Cx6
5. Qi penetrating: Qi of the Seven Emotions rebels.	Sudden delirium; Tide of Phlegm confined and obstructed; teeth tightly clenched; body cold.	Inch Pulse Deep.	Gv26 Gv20 XA1 Li4	S6 Cv22 S40
6. Summer-heat penetrating: Summer-heat Evil invades the interior of the body.	Shen Jing confused; severe sweating; dyspnoea; thirst.	Face dirty or red; Pulse Hollow and without strength.	XA1 Gv26 Li4	B54 (let blood) L5 S36

NOTES

1. The term 'secondary' is a purely arbitrary one to make a distinction with No. 23 Penetrating Wind; the Chinese word Lei means something like 'in the same category as', 'similar to'. In fact the physiological causes of the symptoms of Secondary Penetrating Wind may have no connection whatsoever with cerebral haemorrhage (see Notes to No. 23); but to the Chinese mind are intimately bound up with Penetrating Wind. Jianshi says: 'This disease is similar to Penetrating Wind, but does not have the symptoms of hemiplegia and contortion of the eyes and mouth.'

25. TRISMUS KOU JIN
Section 1

CAUSE OF DISEASE	SYMPTOMS	DIAGNOSTIC FEATURES	MAIN POINTS	SECONDARY POINTS
1. Wind and Cold stopped outside the body.	Teeth tightly clenched.	Unable to open mouth.	S6 Li4	T17 T5
2. Heat blazing and convulsed.	As above.	Unable to open mouth; mouth may be twisted.	S6 S7 T17	Li1 (let blood) T1 S36

Section 2

FACIAL SPASM
L7 S40 T5
S6 Li4
Li20 S5

26. CONVULSIONS (allied to Insanity) (see Note 1) DIAN, KUANG, XIAN

Section 1

CAUSE OF DISEASE	SYMPTOMS	DIAGNOSTIC FEATURES	MAIN POINTS	SECONDARY POINTS
Dian: (Note 2) Principal causes: Heart Qi Empty; Phlegm Hot and abundant. Secondary causes: Fright; Anger; Qi and blood deficient; Phlegm remains surrounding the Luo; Excessive worry; Heart meridian stores Heat; Yin Empty; Shen Empty.	At first unhappy; head heavy and painful; eyes red; weeping; Shen foolish; speech incoherent; severe loss of balance and patient collapses; muscular spasms and rigidity.	Heavy Yin Dian: (Note 3) 1. Bone Dian: teeth and jaws diseases; space between skin and flesh full (Note 4); sweating; depression. 2. Sinew Dian: severe muscular spasms. 3. Blood-vessel Dian: severe loss of balance; blood-vessels in limbs swollen and full; patient may vomit phlegm. In cases where Qi descends and leaks away the disease is incurable. Pulse Large and Slippery, eventually returning to normal; in this case there is Qi in the stomach. If Pulse Small, Strong and Anxious, there is no cure and patient dies; in this case there is no Qi in stomach.	Gv12 Gv26 Cv12 H7	Cx6 Si3 S40

CAUSE OF DISEASE	SYMPTOMS	DIAGNOSTIC FEATURES	MAIN POINTS	SECONDARY POINTS
Kuang: (Note 5) Principal causes: Heat Evil in heart; Phlegm accumulates in the holes of the heart. Secondary causes: Upper Warmer Full; Large intestine and stomach meridians hot; Heat enters the Chong Mo; Fire excessive, mad and reckless; Frightened, sorrowful Phlegm accumulates; Animal Soul lost; Sorrow and pity move in the middle of the body and injure the Spiritual Soul. Excessive pleasure injures the Animal Soul.	Forgetful; prone to rage and fear; sleeps little; no appetite; previously a reputable person capable of rational thought and possessing knowledge and sound moral values; prone to use abusive language; does not rest day or night; fond of singing and music; moves about wildly and without pause; eats much; prone to see ghosts.	Wild speech; does not avoid vulgarity; if case is severe may remove clothes and walk about naked; may also climb to high places and sing.	Gv16 B15 Gv26 Cv12	Cx5 S40 Sp6
Xian: (Note 6) Principal causes: kidney meridian ceases to function; the two Yin are agitated and become Xian and Cold. The kidney Dragon Fire ascends and the liver Lightening follows in order to assist. Although all the forms of Xian have their origin in the kidney, their manifestations are according to the Five Zang: 1. Horse Xian (heart) 2. Ox Xian (spleen) 3. Pig Xian (kidney) 4. Chicken Xian (liver) 5. Sheep Xian (lung)	Spits saliva; Shen confused; suddenly does not know or recognise anything; trismus; convulsions lasting any length of time; after attacks behaves normally. 1. Patient opens mouth wide and shakes head; neighs like a horse; this corresponds to the heart. 2. Stares straight ahead; abdomen swollen; makes noise like an ox; corresponds to spleen. 3. Spits saliva; grunts like a pig; corresponds to kidney. 4. Shakes head to and fro; clucks like chicken; corresponds to liver. 5. Raises eyes and ejects tongue; bleats like a sheep; corresponds to lung.	Yang Xian: Phlegm hot, lodges in heart and stomach. Attack occurs when startled. Yin Xian also basically due to hot Phlegm. If doctor uses too much medicine (i.e. herbs, drugs, etc.) the spleen and stomach become Yin. When attack occurs in early morning, disease is in liver. When attack occurs in early evening, disease is in spleen. When attack occurs at dawn, disease is in gall-bladder. When attack occurs in middle of day, disease is in bladder. When attack occurs in late evening, disease is in stomach. When attack occurs in middle of night, disease is in kidney.	G20 Gv14 B15 H7	Cx5 Si3 S40 Liv2

NOTES

1. *As in the previous two diseases, we are here chiefly concerned with conditions of the brain. There are no exact equivalents for Dian, Kuang and Xian in European languages. From the symptoms it seems clear that both symptomatic and idiopathic fits are included — Blood-vessel Dian might possibly be hypertensive encephalopathy, whereas Xian seems more likely to be epilepsy. To the Chinese this is of no consequence, since primarily their classification of diseases is according to observed symptoms rather than etiology as recognised in the West.*

2. *Dian is defined as 'a type of nervous condition' by the Cihai. Note however that a modern Chinese medical word compounded of Dian and Xian is the normal term for epilepsy.*

3. *Heavy Yin Dian: i.e. Dian occurring in a person with an excess of Yin.*

4. *The 'space between the skin and flesh' is a common Chinese 'anatomical' term. (See Introduction under Wei.)*

5. *Kuang is the common Chinese word for 'mad' 'insane' in a general sense. More precise terms such as schizophrenia, paranoia etc. may well be included in Kuang, but are probably of less use here than the more vague 'insanity' — though conversely 'insanity' in English may embrace more than Kuang.*

6. *Xian is vaguely defined as 'fits' 'convulsions' 'epilepsy' etc.*

Section 2

MENTAL DISEASES
Depression — treat liver and gall bladder
Fears — treat kidney and bladder
Obsessions — treat spleen and stomach
Anguish — treat lung and large intestine
Emotional states — treat heart and small intestine
　　See pages 106–107 in my other book.

27. ZANG ORGANS AGITATED *ZANG ZAO*

Section 1

CAUSE OF DISEASE	SYMPTOMS	DIAGNOSTIC FEATURES	MAIN POINTS	SECONDARY POINTS
1. Liver Qi depressed and congealed; Ying and blood deficient.	Patient prone to grief and weeping; often stretches the body (as when tired).	Pulse Wiry; tongue red and not furred.	Gv26 H7 Gv20 Cv12 Cx7 K1 Gv14 B15	Li4 Liv3 Si3 S40

Section 2

EXCESSIVE NERVOUS TENSION
Si3 B62
Yu points.

28. INSOMNIA *SHI MIAN*

Section 1

CAUSE OF DISEASE	SYMPTOMS	DIAGNOSTIC FEATURES	MAIN POINTS	SECONDARY POINTS
1. Mental anxiety and weariness injure heart and spleen.	Patient startled and agitated; night-sweats; cannot sleep having woken; tired and lethargic; eats little; forgetful.	Pulse Weak; tongue pale.	H7 Sp6 B15 B20	H6 Si3 Cv4 S36
2. Heart blood deficient; Fluid dried up.	Shen Zhi ill at ease; palpitations of the heart; forgetful; constipated; sores in mouth and on tongue.	Pulse Fine and Rapid; tongue deep red; urine red; mouth dry.	B15 B23 H7 B42	Li4 S36 Sp6
3. Kidney water deficient; heart Fire burning.	Heart troubled; cannot sleep.	Pulse Rapid; tongue deep red.	B15 B23 Cx7 Sp6	H7 K6 S36
4. Weariness injures lungs; extreme weariness damages liver.	Empty exhaustion, Empty irritation (Note 1); cannot sleep.	Pulse Rapid; tongue deep red; slight fever.	H7 L9 Sp6 B13 B18	Cx6 S36 K6
5. Fright and fear.	Restless sleep; patient jumps up in alarm during dreams.	Pulse Wiry and Fine or Empty and Floating.	H7 L9 Sp6 B13 B19 B23	Li4 Liv3 B39 B42
6. Damp and Phlegm obstructed.	Cannot sleep peacefully at night; vomitus foul; Qi melancholy; chest-diaphragm not in order.	Pulse Slippery; tongue greasy; mouth acrid.	Cv12 B17 B20	Cx6 S36 S40 Sp6
7. Stomach not in harmony and has accumulation of food	Restless sleep; stomach swollen, melancholy and painful.	Pulse Full; tongue thickly furred.	Cv12 B20 B21 Cx6 S36	H7 Sp6 Sp1 S45

NOTES

1. *'Empty exhaustion, Empty irritation': as usual what is here a symptom is given by Jianshi also as a 'disease' in itself.*
'Empty exhaustion' (Xu Lao) is an Exhaustion Disease (see Glossary) characterised by an Emptiness in the Qi, Blood, Fluid and Marrow. It is caused by irregular eating habits, emotional repression, excessive sexual intercourse.
'Empty irritation' is a condition which applies to the heart and is associated with Heat in the stomach. It is characterised by an unfulfilled desire to vomit, dizziness and anxiety. Jianshi stresses that the 'Empty' is 'hollow' rather than 'weak'. Nervous dyspepsia?

INSOMNIA
H7 Sp6 Sp9 Sp1 Cx6 (A. Chamfrault)
B62 G41 L9
S36 T19 S27
B13 B30 G17
L1

29. PALPITATION OF THE HEART   *ZHENG CHONG*
Section 1

CAUSE OF DISEASE	SYMPTOMS	DIAGNOSTIC FEATURES	MAIN POINTS	SECONDARY POINTS
1. Yin Empty and has little blood.	Heart agitated and palpitating.	Pulse Empty and Rapid.	Cv4 B15 H5 Cx7 S36	H7 Cv7 Cx6
2. Kidney water dried up and exhausted; heart Fire burns upwards.	Heart and Shen confused and disordered; heart agitated and palpitating; continuous discomfort waking and sleeping.	Pulse Rapid; tongue deep red.	H7 Cx6 H5 B15 B23	Cx7 S36 G35 S41

Section 2

PALPITATIONS
H7 H3 B15
Cx6
K24 K25
Cv12 Liv13
B10 G20

TACHYCARDIA
H5 Gv11 Gv14
G20 B10
Liv2
B38 B39 B13

ANGINA PECTORIS
K5 T7 Cv3
S36 B17 K2 Cv12 S19

ANGINA PECTORIS—cont.
Sp6 H8 Cx8 H3 G41
Cx1 Cx7 Si1 B60 B42

HYPERCHOLESTEROLAEMIA
Liv2

CARDIAC ASTHMA
H9 H4
Si14 Si15
L1 L2
Gv17 Cv18

ANAEMIA
B38 S36
L9 Sp5

30. AMNESIA   *JIAN WANG*
Section 1

CAUSE OF DISEASE	SYMPTOMS	DIAGNOSTIC FEATURES	MAIN POINTS	SECONDARY POINTS
1. Kidney Empty; Knowledge deficient; heart Empty; Shen not filled up; heart and kidney both Empty; Fire and Water have not passed into their respective organs.	Shen and Si scattered; patient forgets what has happened.	Foot and Inch Pulses Empty.	B15 B23 Cv4 S36	H7 H3
2. Phlegm set in motion by Fire and covers the pericardium.	Shen Zhi confused.	Pulse Slippery; tongue greasy.	Cv12 S40 B15 S36	L7 H7 Cx6 K1

Section 2

AMNESIA
H9 H7 H3 Gv11 B15 B38 B39
Cx9 L3 Li11
Gv20
K1

31. LIVER WIND *GAN FENG*

Section 1

CAUSE OF DISEASE	SYMPTOMS	DIAGNOSTIC FEATURES	MAIN POINTS	SECONDARY POINTS
1. Yin deficient and has little blood; extreme Heat generates Wind.	Head and eyes dizzy; may have headache and tinnitus; muscular spasms.	Tongue deep red and not furred; Pulse Wiry, Fine and Rapid.	G20 B18 Cx6	G34 Liv2 Liv3
2. Violent anger; Qi anxious.	Patient suddenly collapses and becomes unconscious; teeth tightly clenched; face blue-green.	Pulse Wiry and has strength.	Gv20 Gv26 Cv12 XA1 (let blood)	Li4 Liv3 B54

32. HEADACHE *TOU TONG*

Section 1

CAUSE OF DISEASE	SYMPTOMS	DIAGNOSTIC FEATURES	MAIN POINTS	SECONDARY POINTS
1. Affected by Wind Evil.	Headache; dislikes the wind; nose blocked.	Pulse Floating; tongue thinly furred white.	Gv16 B12 Gv23 S8	Li4 T5 Li20
2. Affected by Cold Evil.	Headache; dislikes the cold; no sweating.	Pulse Floating and Tight.	as above	Li4 T5
3. Phlegm obstructs the Pure Yang.	Head dizzy and painful; vomiting and dizziness.	Pulse Wiry and Slowed-down; tongue furred and slippery.	G20 S8 Gv20	S40 Cx6 S36
4. Fire depressed and attacks upwards.	Head extremely painful; teeth also painful.	Pulse Wiry and Rapid; sides of tongue deep red.	XH3 (let blood) G20 Li4	Liv2
5. Weariness injures Qi	Headache; body weary; dyspnoea; little appetite.	Pulse Empty and Large; tongue pale.	Gv20 XH2 (or Gv24.5) B10	S36 Cv6
6. Yin blood deficient and damaged.	Continuous headache.	Pulse Hollow; pain in Fish Tail (?).	T23 B17 B18	XH3 S36
7. Side of head painful; Qi and blood Empty; liver Wind rebels.	Lateral headache; pain inter-mittent; headache continues inter-mittently all day.	Pulse Deep and Wiry.	G20 S8 T23 T3 G41	XH3 G14 S2 Li20 S7 Gv26
8. Phlegm and Heat attack upwards.	Left or right lateral headache (but consistently on one side, in con-trast with 9).	Pulse Rapid or Slippery; tongue red, furred and greasy.	G20 S8 XH3 Cv12	L7 S40
9. Wind Evil invades the Luo.	Pain alternately severe and mild; may occur on either side of head.	Pulse Floating.	G20 G5 G4 B54	T5 G34

Section 2

HEADACHE, MIGRAINE
Hepatic type migraine — Liv8 G40
Fear and tension type — K5 L6
Feeling of heat — Sp2 Liv2 K2 S44
Many headaches or migraines respond to the first two of the above three groups.
Other points, including localised points are often also needed:
G20 B10 Gv16
B2 G1 T17 T18 G12 G11 G10
L7 Si3 Si5
Pain in the temporal area is often due to liver and gall bladder.
Pain on the vertex is often due to kidney or bladder.
Supraorbital pain is often due to stomach or bladder.

Head heavy, tension: triple warmer.
Congestive headache: B62
Alcoholic hangover: G8 (S. de Morant).
S36 T12 Si1 B60 B57 G3 G4 G5 G6 Gv4 B22 Gv10
S41 G18 Cv4 Gv23 H3 B9 S1 S2 S3 S4 B12
B63 Gv18 Gv28 Li11 Si11 Li1
Li4 H7 Cv5 Gv20 S36 K1 B54 S8 G20

33. VERTIGO *XUAN YUN*

Section 1

CAUSE OF DISEASE	SYMPTOMS	DIAGNOSTIC FEATURES	MAIN POINTS	SECONDARY POINTS
1. Phlegm and Fire depressed in Upper Warmer; Wind Evil ascends into the Qiao Luo.	Head and eyes dizzy.	Both Inch Pulses Empty and Large; sides of tongue deep red.	Gv20 G20 S8 Li4	XH3 CX7 Liv3
2. Yin Empty; Fire brilliant; Water dried up; Fire ascends.	Dizziness; heart troubled.	Both Foot Pulses Empty and Rapid; mouth dry.	Cv4 B23	S36 K6
3. Phlegm-fluid rebels upwards.	Dizziness; desire to vomit.	Pulse Wiry and Slippery; tongue furred, slippery and greasy; mouth glutinous; no thirst.	Gv20 Cv12 G20 Li4 Gv23	G34 S40 S36 S41
4. Liver Fire rushes upwards.	Dizziness; quick tempered and prone to anger.	Left Connecting Pulse Wiry and Full.	Gv20 G20 B18 H7 K1	Li4 Liv3 G34 K6

Section 2

VERTIGO
Li4 S40 G20
B16 Gv20 B62 B67 B8
Gv23 G20 Cx1 Gv19
Si3 B62 Si7
B66

SYNCOPE
Li10 Gv26
L9 T2 Liv1
H9 Cx9

SYNCOPE—cont.
Sp6 G43 S45
B57

CEREBRAL CONGESTION
K1 B62
Li1 L11
S36 Cx7

MENINGISM
B62 S13

34. INTERCOSTAL NEURALGIA *XIE TONG*

Section 1

CAUSE OF DISEASE	SYMPTOMS	DIAGNOSTIC FEATURES	MAIN POINTS	SECONDARY POINTS
1. Left ribs painful: dead blood in ribs.	Left ribs painful; pain does not move.	Pulse Wiry and Rough; tongue substance dark purple.	Liv14 Liv13 B17 B18	Cx6 Liv4
2. Right ribs painful: Phlegm stopped up; Qi obstructed.	Right ribs swollen and painful; pleuritic rub.	Pulse Wiry and Slippery; tongue furred, slippery and white.	Liv14 (rt.h.side) B18 Cv12 Cv17	Cx6 (rt.h.side) S40 (lt.h.side) G40 (lt.h.side) Sp17 (rt.h.side)
3. Liver Full: liver brilliant; Qi rebels.	Ribs on both sides painful; difficult to turn the body.	Pulse Deep, Wiry and has strength; face blue-green.	Liv14 B18 Liv13	T6 G34 Cx6 Liv3

CAUSE OF DISEASE	SYMPTOMS	DIAGNOSTIC FEATURES	MAIN POINTS	SECONDARY POINTS
4. Liver Empty: liver Empty and depressed, rebels.	Slight pain in ribs on both sides; pain extends to shoulders and chest.	Pulse Wiry and Empty.	Cv14 Liv13 Liv14 B18	Cx6 G40 K6
5. Liver Hot: liver meridian Full and Hot.	Ribs on both sides painful; heart troubled, anxious and prone to anger; constipation; urine yellow.	Pulse Full and Rapid; tongue yellow and greasy; tinnitus.	Liv14 Liv13 B18 Cv3	T6 G34 S36
6. Food stopped up: food and drink obstructed.	Taste in mouth foul and sour; stomach obstructed and full; dislikes food.	Pulse Deep and Slippery; tongue thickly furred.	Liv14 Liv13 Cv12 S25	Cx6 Sp4 G34 S36

Section 2

INTERCOSTAL NEURALGIA
L9 Li4 B13
B17 Liv13 Cv17
G41 S36 Si5
T6 B62 K1

35. NUMBNESS including Rheumatism and similar conditions *BI ZHENG*

Section 1

CAUSE OF DISEASE	SYMPTOMS	DIAGNOSTIC FEATURES	MAIN POINTS	SECONDARY POINTS
1. Moving numbness: Wind, Cold and Damp Qi lodge in meridians; Wind exceeds Cold and Damp.	Wind Evil flows up and down, fighting with the Good Qi in places where it is Empty; muscles flaccid; pain does not occur in any fixed place.	1. Wind Evil attacks Damp and moves into the four limbs and shoulders; Pulse Floating, Rough and Tight.	Gv14 Li15 Li11 G31 G34	T5 B58 Li4 B54
		2. Limb joints swollen and painful; pain never ceases.	G39	
2. Painful numbness: Cold exceeds Wind and Damp.	Limbs cramped and painful; severe if cold, relieved if warm.	1. Occurs only at night; pain like the bite of a tiger (this is called the 'White Tiger passing through the joints Wind); Pulse Rough and Tight. 2. If associated with Damp it occurs in dull (i.e. Yin) weather; body feels heavy.	Li15 Li11 Li4 G31 G34 B19 B20	T5 G38 Sp6
3. Summer-heat numbness: Damp exceeds Wind and Cold.	Painful and does not shift; heavy sweating; limbs slow and weak; Jing Shen confused and obstructed; skin numb.	1. Numb as though Insect moving in the flesh, unlike itching or pain. Empty Qi is the Root, Wind and Phlegm are the Signs (Note 1). 2. Does not itch, is not painful; not sensitive when pressed or pinched; it is like the solidity of wood; dead blood congeals and forms blockage; Wind and Cold attack outside.	Cv12 Cv6 S36 B17 B20 B23 Li11 G34	B12 T5 B53 Sp6

NOTES
1. *Empty Qi is the principal cause of the condition, Wind and Phlegm are the 'external manifestations', the secondary contributary factors.*

RHEUMATIC DISEASES
Muscular or early arthritic.
Often the Luo point on the opposite side is useful i.e.: Very early osteo-arthritis of the right hip, with pain going down lateral side of leg (gall bladder meridian) and inside groin (kidney meridian). Use K6 left and G37 left. Brachial neuralgia on right, with pain along course of small intestine meridian. Use Si7 left and possibly local points such as G20 G21 T15.
Pain base of thumb. Use L7 and Li6 on opposite side, with possibly L9 and Li5 on same side. Sprained knee, with pain behind knee, and on either side of patella. Use B58 Sp4 G40 on opposite side.
Damaged ring finger or early rheumatism. T5 on opposite side.
Category III points may be used.
The above, and other, basic principles may be used in any part of the body.

LUMBAGO, SCIATICA	NUMBNESS
K5 B62 B54	Cx8 H3
B23 K5 Cx9	
Gv4 B28 B48 B49	
B31 to 35	

36. NUMBNESS OF THE CHEST   *XIONG BI*

Section 1

CAUSE OF DISEASE	SYMPTOMS	DIAGNOSTIC FEATURES	MAIN POINTS	SECONDARY POINTS
1. Yang Qi in chest does not move; Yin Evil ascends.	Dyspnoea; coughing; chest and back painful; chest blocked and melancholy.	Inch Pulse Deep and Slow; superficial Connecting Pulse Small, Tight and Rapid; tongue furred white.	Gv12 Gv10 B13 Cv17 Cx6	L5 Cv12 S36
2. Yang Qi in chest does not move; Phlegm-fluid rebels upwards.	Chest numb; cannot sleep; whole of chest and back painful; noise in chest.	Pulse Deep, Wiry, Minute and Slippery, or Deep and Slippery.	Cv12 Liv13 Cx6 B17 B13	
3. Cold and rebellious Qi in chest attacks upwards.	Chest blocked and full; region below the heart rebels against the heart.	Pulse Deep and Full.	B16 B17 Liv13 Cx6 Cv17	

Section 2

See other pulmonary and cardiac diseases:
Nos. 3, 5, 22, 29.

37. PARALYSIS   *WEI*

Section 1

CAUSE OF DISEASE	SYMPTOMS	DIAGNOSTIC FEATURES	MAIN POINTS	SECONDARY POINTS
1. Damp and Heat: affected by Seasonal Damp and Heat.	Both legs paralysed and weak; limbs extremely weary.	Pulse Weak-floating and Rapid; face pale and yellow; tongue furred white and slippery; head heavy.	S30 S36 G30 G39 G34	B20 G20
2. Damp and Heat flow downwards; Damp in Lower Warmer overflowing.	Both feet paralysed and weak; fever; urine red; polyuria.	Pulse Deep and Slippery; tongue furred and greasy; mouth glutinous.	as above	Sp6 K6 Gv16
3. Yin Empty and associated with Damp and Heat.	Legs have no strength to move; feet hot.	Pulse Fine and Rapid; tongue dry; heart troubled.	as above	K6 Sp10 Gv16
4. Chronic disease in which Qi and blood are Empty and weak.	Both legs paralysed and weak; dyspnoea; spontaneous sweating.	Six Pulses Empty and Pliable; tongue pale; face paralysed and yellow.	as above	B20 B21
5. Liver and kidney Empty and damaged.	Muscles and bones paralysed and weak; cannot walk.	Pulses in both feet Fine and Weak; tongue pale; no Shen; flesh wasted away.	as above	B23 B18 B11

WEAKNESS OF LEGS
S35 XL2
G30 G41
K2 K10

38. DIABETES (see Note 1)   *XIAO KE*

Section 1

CAUSE OF DISEASE	SYMPTOMS	DIAGNOSTIC FEATURES	MAIN POINTS	SECONDARY POINTS
1. Upper Wasting: lung meridian Dry and Hot.	Excessive drinking, micturition normal.	Right Inch Pulse Large; face red; tongue furred yellow.	B13 B15	Cx6 L10
2. Middle Wasting: stomach Dry and Hot.	Thirsty; good appetite; emaciated.	Right Connecting Pulse Overflowing and Rapid; tongue red and furred yellow; constipated.	B21 Cv12	K3 S44
3. Lower Wasting: kidney Yin Empty and dried up.	Thirsty; micturition immediately after drinking; limbs emaciated.	Both Foot Pulses without strength; feet and shins painful and weak.	B15 B23 Cv4 Cv3	K7 B60

NOTES
1. *The heading of the disease is literally 'wasting and thirst' which the Cihai gives as an old term for the Chinese word now used for 'diabetes'.*

39. GOITRE   *YING QI*

Section 1

CAUSE OF DISEASE	SYMPTOMS	DIAGNOSTIC FEATURES	MAIN POINTS	SECONDARY POINTS
Qi obstructed, blood congealed; Phlegm and Heat may be congealed.	Large hard swelling on neck.	Does not move when pressed; no pain when touched.	appropriate local points.	G21 T10 Toxic Goitre: 1. With palpitations of the heart Cx6 H7 2. With heavy sweating Li4 3. With swollen eyes B1 B2 S2 G20 4. With high blood-pressure Gv20

40. SPONTANEOUS SWEATING   *ZI HAN*

Section 1

CAUSE OF DISEASE	SYMPTOMS	DIAGNOSTIC FEATURES	MAIN POINTS	SECONDARY POINTS
1. Exterior Yin Empty.	Sweating not due to natural causes such as wearing thick clothes in hot weather, or strenuous movement.	Sweating for no reason.	Gv14 Cv4 B38 B23	Li4 K7 S36
2. Wei Yang not strong, Wind Evil affects the	Fluid moves wildly and pours out of the body.	For no reason sweat pours out of the body.	Gv14 Cv4	Li4 S44

559

CAUSE OF DISEASE	SYMPTOMS	DIAGNOSTIC FEATURES	MAIN POINTS	SECONDARY POINTS
Wei, Wei Qi cannot keep it out, so the skin becomes slow and the pores flaccid; as a result of this, Fluid pours wildly out of the skin.				
3. Body fat; pores dilated; Sunlight Yang Hot.	Sweating for no reason.	Intermittent spontaneous sweating.	Cv12 S36	Li4 S44

Section 2

EXCESSIVE PERSPIRATION	LACK OF PERSPIRATION
L11 Sp15 B17 T10 Gv16	L8 Sp2 Li4
B13 H7	G11 G44
B62	Cx9 S43 S45
	Li1 Li4 Si2 L8

41. NOCTURNAL SWEATING   *DAO HAN*

Section 1

CAUSE OF DISEASE	SYMPTOMS	DIAGNOSTIC FEATURES	MAIN POINTS	SECONDARY POINTS
Yin is Empty and cannot stimulate its Mai Qi outside the body (Note 1); Fluid cannot be restrained; during sleep the Wei Qi activates the Yin, blood and Qi have nothing on which to rely for support, so the pores open and sweat is emitted.	Sweating when asleep; sweating ceases on waking.	Sweating when asleep.	Gv14 H6 Si3 B13 Cv6 Cv4	Cv7 Sp6

NOTES
1. *Mai Qi: the Qi which pertains to the Mai or blood-vessels.*

Section 2

NOCTURNAL SWEATING
L1
Cv6 B15 H7
K2
Si3 K7 T5 (S. de Morant)

42. RECTAL BLEEDING   *BIAN XUE*
Section 1

CAUSE OF DISEASE	SYMPTOMS	DIAGNOSTIC FEATURES	MAIN POINTS	SECONDARY POINTS
1. Near blood: large intestine Damp and Hot.	Blood passed through rectum; blood visible before stools.	Pulse Deep and Rapid; urine red.	B25 Gv1 B57	B35
2. Distant blood: small intestine Cold and Damp.	Blood passed through rectum; stools visible before blood.	Pulse Deep and Slowed-down; urine white.	Sp1 S36	B27 (moxa) Sp6
3. Intestine Wind: blood in large intestine Hot and affected by Wind.	Blood passed through rectum; blood thin and bright.	Both Foot Pulses Floating.	B25 Gv1 B57	B17
4. Damp and Heat collect poison.	Blood passed through rectum; blood thick and dark.	Both Foot Pulses Slippery.	Gv1 B57 B20 B23	Sp10 B17

HAEMORRHOIDS
B58 B57 B54
Gv1 B35 B47 B48 B49
Liv8 Cx7
Sp5 G39
K5 K8 K10 B50
Gv20 B60

43. EPISTAXIS *NU XUE*

Section 1

CAUSE OF DISEASE	SYMPTOMS	DIAGNOSTIC FEATURES	MAIN POINTS	SECONDARY POINTS
1. Fire pursues, blood rebels.	Sudden bleeding from nose with great force.	Pulse Overflowing and Slippery; blood purple; face red.	Li4 Gv23 Gv14 Gv16	Li20 Gv26 XH2 B64
2. Qi Empty, blood not strong.	Bleeding from nose continues intermittently for whole day.	Pulse Hollow and without strength; blood light red; face hoary-white.	B20 Sp1 Cv13	Gv23 B17 S36
3. Wind and Cold obstructed and overflow into meridians; blood moves wildly.	Dislikes the cold; fever; headache; no sweating.	Pulse Floating and Tight; tongue furred white.	Gv23 Gv16 Gv14 B12	Li4 G20
4. Interior of body Empty and Cold; upper part of body False and Hot.	Nose bleeds all day long; not stopped by Cool Medicine.	Pulse Hollow and Sloweddown or Empty and Fine; tongue pale; mouth dry but no wish to drink.	Gv14 B20 (moxa)	Cv4 (moxa) S36

Section 2

EPISTAXIS	EPISTAXIS—cont.
Liv5 Si1 B18	Li11 Li10 Li4 S44
Gv24 Gv20 Gv15 Li19	Cv4 B54 S36
G21 Si15 G20 B10	Si2 L3 G39 B64 Liv1

44. INTERNAL WEAKNESS *LONG BI*

Section 1

CAUSE OF DISEASE	SYMPTOMS	DIAGNOSTIC FEATURES	MAIN POINTS	SECONDARY POINTS
1. Heat congealed below.	Hot feeling in abdomen; stools hard.	Pulse Deep and Full; tongue furred yellow.	Cv4 Cv3 B23 B28 B22	Liv8 Sp9 Sp6 K1
2. Yang Empty.	Dislikes the cold.	Pulse Empty and Fine; tongue furred pale and white.	Cv4 Cv3 B20 B23	S36 Sp6
3. Yin Empty.	Fever after midday; mouth parched; tongue burning.	Pulse Empty and Wiry.	Cv4 Sp6 Cv3	Cx7 Sp9 Li4
4. Middle Qi deficient.	Abdomen not anxious or full; extremely weary; dyspnoea; no Strength in speech.	Pulse Empty and Weak.	Cv6 Cv4 B38 B20	S36 Sp6

Section 2

RETENTION OF URINE	PROSTATIC HYPERTROPHY
Cv6 Cv4 K2 K11	B67 K3
Sp9 Sp10	Cv2 Cv3 Cv4
Li9 S37 B54	Sp9 Sp10

45. INTERMITTENT SWELLINGS (Note 1) *SHAN QI*

Section 1

CAUSE OF DISEASE	SYMPTOMS	DIAGNOSTIC FEATURES	MAIN POINTS	SECONDARY POINTS
1. Rushing Swelling: liver Evil rebels upwards.	Lower abdomen painful; Qi rushes upwards to the heart; constipation and dysuria.	Pulse Deep, Wiry and Tight; face blue-green.	B23 Cv4 Liv3	Sp6 K6
2. Lonely Swelling: Cold and Damp invade testicles.	When lying down the testicles retract, when standing up they descend.	Pulse Deep and Wiry.	Cv3 Liv1 B23	S29 Sp6
3. Tui Swelling: Cold and Damp congealed in scrotum.	Scrotum swollen and large.	Pulse Hard.	B23 Cv6 Cv4	Sp9 Liv1
4. Cold Swelling: spleen receives liver Evil.	Lower abdomen painful; desire to vomit.	Pulse Deep and Tight.	B23 Cv4	Liv2 S36
5. Gui Swelling: dead blood congeals and forms abscess.	Lower abdomen swollen on both sides like a cucumber.	Pulse Deep and Slippery.	Cv4 Cv3 Sp10	Liv1 T5
6. Swelling of small intestine: Wind and Cold invade small intestine.	Pain in lower abdomen extending to testicles.	Foot Pulse Wiry and Tight.	Cv4 B23	K6 Liv3
7. Bladder Qi: Cold congeals in bladder.	Lower abdomen swollen and painful; unable to micturate.	Pulse Deep and Slow.	B23 Cv3	Liv8 Sp6

NOTES

1. *The heading is a combination of what is now a common term for 'hernia', Shan, plus the ubiquitous Qi. But although hernia is probably represented here, it is difficult to reconcile all the above symptoms with herniae alone. Moreover none of the Chinese definitions of Shan specifically refer to any 'protrusion' (Tu Chu). Jianshi gives: 'Acute pain in testicles and lower abdomen; may be greater on one side than the other. Scrotum swollen, pain generally over whole area; if severe, abdomen is gathered like a cup or a bowl.' Cihai gives: 'The Su Wen says: "Pain in lower abdomen, inability to micturate or defaecate". Yin Qi accumulates inside the body, Cold Qi in the abdomen causes Ying and Wei to be out of harmony (see Introduction), blood and Qi to be Empty and Weak; thus Cold Wind enters the abdomen and causes Shan. There are many varieties of Shan.' The scant definitions of these 'many varieties' provide no more information than is given above as symptoms. Nos. 3 and 4, Tui, and Gui, have no meanings other than types of Shan.*

46. INCONTINENCE OF URINE *YI NIAO*
Section 1

CAUSE OF DISEASE	SYMPTOMS	DIAGNOSTIC FEATURES	MAIN POINTS	SECONDARY POINTS
1. Bladder Empty and Cold.	Incontinence of urine which is passed without cause.	Both Foot Pulses Deep and Fine; face withered and dark.	B23 B28 Cv6 Cv4 Cv3	Sp9 Sp6 Liv1
2. Bladder Empty and Hot.	Incontinence of urine which is passed without cause.	Both Foot Pulses Fine and Rapid; urine red.	Cv6 Cv4 Cv3 B23 B28	B24 Sp9 Sp6

Section 2	INCONTINENCE OF URINE B67 Cv1 Sp9 B27 B28 S36 L7 L9 Gv4 T4	NOCTURNAL ENURESIS K10

47. URETHRAL DISCHARGE (Note 1) *CHI BAI ZHUO*

Section 1

CAUSE OF DISEASE	SYMPTOMS	DIAGNOSTIC FEATURES	MAIN POINTS	SECONDARY POINTS
1. White discharge: Lower Warmer Damp and Hot.	Thick purulent discharge; sometimes purulent matter remains in urethra.	Pulse Deep and Slippery; mouth glutinous and greasy.	B23 Cv6 Cv4 Liv13	Liv8 Sp6 K6 Sp4
2. Red discharge: Damp and Heat injure the blood.	Sometimes red purulent matter in urethra.	Pulse Deep and Rapid; mouth parched; heart troubled; restless sleep.	B15 B23 B28 H8 Cv4	Sp9 Sp6

NOTES

1. *The Chinese heading literally means 'red and white turbid-fluid'. Confusion arises since 'white turbid-fluid' is a modern word for 'gonorrhoea', but so too is Lin, the heading of the next section, No. 48. This problem is not really solved by omitting 'gonorrhoea' from both headings, as has been done; but it is certainly far safer to rely on the symptoms given, rather than on a possibly inaccurate modern equivalent for an old Chinese term.*

Section 2

URETHRITIS
B31 B32 B33 B34 B35
Cv1 K11
K9 K10 Sp6
S25 S28 Cv4 Cv12 Liv1

48. URINARY DISEASES (see Notes to No. 47) *LIN*

Section 1

CAUSE OF DISEASE	SYMPTOMS	DIAGNOSTIC FEATURES	MAIN POINTS	SECONDARY POINTS
1. Qi leakage: Transforming action of Qi not effective.	Retention of urine with overflow; lower abdomen full and painful.	Pulse Deep and Wiry and without strength.	Cv4 Cv3 B23 B24	Cv6 Sp9 K6 S28 Sp6
2. Blood leakage: blood depressed in bladder.	Blood in urine; urethra painful; incessant urge to micturate.	Pulse Deep and Rough; tongue substance deep red; heart troubled; mouth parched.	Cv4 Cv3 Sp10 B23 B27	K7 B54 Sp9 Sp6
3. Stone leakage: bladder stores Heat.	Urine concentrated and contains gravel; penis painful during micturition	Pulse Wiry and Anxious; micturition incessant	Cv4 Cv3 B23 B22 B27	B28 S28 B54 K1
4. Grease leakage: kidney Empty.	Urine like grease; micturition painful.	Foot Pulse Empty and Pliable.	Cv6 Cv4 Cv3 B23 B22	Sp9 Sp6 B28 Cv5
5. Weariness leakage: great weariness injures spleen.	Slight and painful urinary incontinence, occurring when weary.	Pulse Empty; face yellow; dyspnoea; limbs weak	Cv6 Cv4 Cv3 B20 B23 B22	Sp9 Sp6 K6 Li4 L5

Section 2

NEPHRITIS
K5 B54
B22 B23 B24 B62
Cv3 S36 Sp14
G24 G25

CYSTITIS
B26 B27 B28 B29 B30
B54 Cv2 K12 Sp6 G25
S30 S31 Liv11 Gv1

Section 1

CAUSE OF DISEASE	SYMPTOMS	DIAGNOSTIC FEATURES	MAIN POINTS	SECONDARY POINTS
1. Sovereign and Minister Fires (i.e. heart and kidney) blaze brightly and burn the Yin.	Nocturnal emissions after dreaming.	Inch and Foot Pulses Overflowing or Rapid; mouth dry; urine red.	B15 B23 Cv4 Cv3	H7 Sp6 K12
2. Heart and kidney deficient.	Nocturnal emissions without dreams; associated with palpitation of the heart, vertigo and aching of legs.	Inch and Foot Pulses Deep, Weak and without strength; face appears emaciated.	B15 B23 B38 Cv4	K12 S36 Sp6
3. Mental anxiety injures the spleen.	Nocturnal emissions; palpitation of the heart; insomnia; loss of appetite; general feeling of weakness.	Pulse Empty and Sloweddown; face haggard.	B38 B44 B42 B20 B23	H7 S36 Sp6
4. Accumulated Thoughts (Si: see Introduction) not coordinated.	Intermittent loss of sperm; Shen and Si confused.	Pulse Empty and Floating.	H7 Cv4 B23 B47	B32 Cv3 Sp6
5. Excessive sexual activity; Sperm Barrier weak.	Continuous leakage of sperm which patient cannot control; head dizzy; feet weak; Jing Shen wasted and withered.	Pulse Fine and without strength.	B23 B47 B38 Cv4 Cv3	K12 S36 Sp6
6. Damp and Heat of spleen and stomach remain dormant in the Yin.	Intermittent loss of sperm; mouth greasy; no appetite.	Pulse Deep and Slippery; body fat; tongue thickly furred and greasy.	Cv12 B20 B21	Cv2 Sp9 S36

NOTES
1. *For the Chinese theory of the composition, function etc. of Sperm (Jing), see Introduction.*

Section 2

SPERMATORRHOEA
Sp6
Cv4 Cv3
S36 S25
B31 B32 B33 B34
K23 B47 Sp9

SPERMATORRHOEA—cont.
B67 K12

NYMPHOMANIA
Sp20 S30 S29
Liv2 K3 G43

50. IMPOTENCE   *YANG WEI*

Section 1

CAUSE OF DISEASE	SYMPTOMS	DIAGNOSTIC FEATURES	MAIN POINTS	SECONDARY POINTS
1. Excessive sexual desire.	Penis unable to become erect. Secondary symptoms: loins painful; legs ache.	Foot Pulse Empty and without strength.	B38 B18 B23 Gv3 Cv4	S36 Sp6 G34 Liv3
2. Anxieties depressed and congealed, injure heart and spleen.	As above. Secondary symptoms: Jing Energy exhausted; no appetite; face appears withered and yellow.	Pulse Slowed-down and Weak.	B38 B20 B21 Cv4	Li10
3. Repression injures liver.	As above. Secondary symptoms: Jing Shen upset; chest melancholy and uncomfortable.	(no observations)	Liv13 B18 Cv3	Cv11 Cx6 Liv5 Liv3

CAUSE OF DISEASE	SYMPTOMS	DIAGNOSTIC FEATURES	MAIN POINTS	SECONDARY POINTS
4. Damp overflowing, body flourishing.	As above.	Tongue furred white and greasy; pulse Weak-floating and Slippery.	B20 B23 Cv3	S36 (moxa) S28 Sp9
5. Damp and Heat flow downwards.	As above. Secondary symptoms: testicles cold; emits Yin sweat; urine yellowish-red and foul smelling.	(no observations)	S28 K12 Cv3	Sp9 K7 Liv2

Section 2

IMPOTENCE	LACK OF DESIRE—cont.
K10 K2 Liv4 Liv1	Cv5 Cv6 S28 S45
S30 Sp6 Cv6	
Gv4 K3 L7	FRIGIDITY
K12 Cv2	K7
	Cv4 Cv7
LACK OF DESIRE	Cv1
T4 Gv1 Gv2	S29 Sp6
Liv8 Si5	

51. RED AND WHITE SORES   *CHI BAI YOU FENG*

Section 1

CAUSE OF DISEASE	SYMPTOMS	DIAGNOSTIC FEATURES	MAIN POINTS	SECONDARY POINTS
1. Red sores: spleen and lungs Dry and Hot; caused by struggle between the blood and the Wind Evil which has invaded the blood.	Skin develops red patches which may occur anywhere on the body; the patches are swollen and puffy, inflamed and hot, painful and itching.	Pulse Floating and Rapid.	B12 Li11	B54 Sp10
2. White sores: spleen and lungs Dry and Hot; caused by struggle between Qi and the Wind Evil which has invaded Qi.	Skin develops white patches which may occur anywhere on the body; the patches are swollen and puffy, inflamed and hot, painful and itching.	Pulse Floating.	Li11 T5	B58 G31

52. DAMP RASH   *SHI ZHEN*

Section 1

CAUSE OF DISEASE	SYMPTOMS	DIAGNOSTIC FEATURES	MAIN POINTS	SECONDARY POINTS
Wind Damp, blood Hot	Eruption of small white pustules over whole body.	Itching; sudden rise in temperature; pustules emit yellow fluid when broken.	Li11 B54 Sp10	Li15 T5 Li4

53. RASH (?)   *PEI LEI*

Section 1

Affected by Wind when sweating or by Cold when sleeping uncovered; Wind Evil enters the skin.	At first skin itches, then develops pimples like the two halves of a bean; body slightly hot; body itches; heart troubled.	Pulse Floating.	Li11 T5 B54 B13	Sp10 G31

PURPLISH DISCOLOURATION OF FACE
L9

PRURITIS
Liv8 B54
B13 S15
G41 L7
G37 G31 Gv20

ACNE VULGARIS
L11 H9
Sp2 B54
Liv11 K12

URTICARIA
Liv5 Li14
Sp6 S31

FURUNCULOSIS
L11 H9
plus deep breathing.

WEEPING ECZEMA
B60 B54 Li11
T5 Si3 Sp10

54. SORES IN MOUTH, DEGENERATIVE DISEASES OF MOUTH, THRUSH KOU CHUANG, KOU MI. E KOU CHUANG

Section 1

CAUSE OF DISEASE	SYMPTOMS	DIAGNOSTIC FEATURES	MAIN POINTS	SECONDARY POINTS
1. Empty Fire: excessive mental anxiety; heart and kidney not connected; Empty Fire burns upwards.	Mouth develops pale sores; interior of mouth heavily streaked and mottled white; in severe cases mucosa comes off in patches.	Pulse Empty; no thirst.	B15 B23 Cv24 Li4	B27 S36 K6 B20
2. Full Fire: excessive eating and excessive drinking of alcohol cause the Full Fire of the heart to move wildly.	Mouth develops bright red sores; whole mouth rotten and mottled; in severe cases the jaw and tongue are swollen.	Pulse Full; mouth dry.	Li4 S36 B15 B20	Cv24 H8 Sp2 XM2 (lt.h.side) XM2 (rt.h.side) (let blood)
3. Full Fire: excessive eating of rich foods; Full Heat obstructed and overflowing.	Whole mouth rotten and destroyed; in severe cases spreads to throat; cannot eat or drink; mouth foul smelling; constipation.	Mouth parched; Pulse Full.	Li4 Cv12 S36 Cx7	H8 Cv24 Liv2 S44 XM2 (both sides; let blood)
4. Empty Fire: body may be weak after long illness.	Whole mouth rotten and decayed; face haggard; sleep extremely agitated; Shen Qi diminished.	Pulse Slow and Sloweddown; mouth dry, little thirst.	L:4 S36 B20 B21	Cv12 Cv6 Sp6
5. Spleen Yang Empty and weak: spleen Qi Empty, Yang Qi weary.	Whole mouth rotten and decayed; loose motions; rumblings in abdomen; limbs weak; breathing shallow; face greenish-white.	Pulse Slow and Sloweddown.	Li4 S36 S25	Cv12 Cv6 B20 B21 Sp6
6. Minister Fire (kidney) moves wildly; over indulgence, lack of self-control; kidney Empty; little Jing Energy.	Whole mouth rotten and decayed; throat dry and burning; hands and heart troubled and hot.	Pulse Fine and Rapid.	Li4 K6 B23	Cv24 Cx7 T2
7. Pregnant womb Heat attacks upwards.	Whole mouth develops painful white spots; in severe cases the throat is swollen; difficulty in breast-feeding; patient weeps frequently.	Pulse Rapid; lines on the fingers purple.	Li4 S36	L11 Li1 (let blood) K3

BITTER TASTE IN MOUTH
G38 Liv5 S36

THRUSH
Liv2 Cx8 K6

LIPS CRACKED
S4 Liv3 Li4 T5 G41

PAIN ROOT OF TONGUE
Cv23 G20
H5 Cx7

GLOSSITIS
H9 Cx9 Li4
Cv24 Cv23
K2 Gv12
T5 G41

MOUTH DRY
L5 Gv28 Liv8

55. TOOTHACHE *YA TONG*

Section 1

CAUSE OF DISEASE	SYMPTOMS	DIAGNOSTIC FEATURES	MAIN POINTS	SECONDARY POINTS
1. Fire depressed.	Gums swollen; whole of gums intermittently painful.	Pulse Rapid; tongue furred yellow; constipation.	Li4 S7 S6 S44	Li3 Gv26 Cv24
2. Affected by Wind.	Gums first swollen; if swelling continues then pain begins; pain severe when breathing in through mouth.	Pulse Floating; tongue thinly furred white.	as above	T17
3. Rich foods, Damp and Heat are Transformed into Teeth Worms. (Note 1).	Teeth eaten away by worms and collapse; if one tooth becomes rotten all the teeth will be eaten away; teeth ache continuously.	Tongue furred but appears normal; holes in teeth.	as above	
4. Kidney Empty.	Teeth loose and painful; if severe patient hates cold.	Both Foot Pulses without strength, or Rapid and Fine.	as above	K6

NOTES
1. *Certain diseases are traditionally attributed to 'Chong' i.e. 'worms' or 'insects'. In the past the removal of these Chong from the body was a specialised occupation.*

Section 2

TOOTHACHE (Mainly neuralgia of teeth)
G37 (opposite side to pain) G41
Li4 S44 S6
Li2 T23 T21 Gv26
B60 B62
Cv24 B23 Li3

GINGIVITIS
Gv28 S4 Li19
G16 Si8 L7
Li3 S44 T9 S5
Gv27 T17

56. THROAT SWOLLEN AND PAINFUL *YAN HOU ZHONG TONG*

Section 1

CAUSE OF DISEASE	SYMPTOMS	DIAGNOSTIC FEATURES	MAIN POINTS	SECONDARY POINTS
1. Affected by Seasonal Evil from outside.	Fever, dislikes the cold; throat swollen and painful; eating and drinking difficult; voice croaks.	Pulse Floating, and Rapid; right Inch and Connecting Pulses Abundant.	L11 (let blood) Li4 Gv16 L5	T1 Li1 (let blood) T5 Cv22
2. Full Fire: excessive eating of savoury foods; Hot Poison uneasy and congealed.	Throat swollen and painful; great thirst; constipation; phlegm hot, blocked and overflowing.	Pulse Full and Rapid; throat red and swollen.	L11 XM2 (both sides, let blood) Li4	T2 L10
3. Empty Fire: prone to anger; fond of drinking; likes wine and sex; causes Empty Fire to form obstruction in upper part of body.	Throat dry, tongue parched; heart troubled; mouth parched.	Pulse Empty and Rapid; throat painful but not severe; or pain may be severe where swollen.	K3 Li4 L5	S36 S44 Gv16

TONSILLITIS
K5 Li4 Si17
L3 Li9 B12 Cv22
T10 G38 Si8
Li7 T2
S6 L11 Li5 Cx7
K1 Cv22 S40

PHARYNGITIS
L9 Li6
G20 B17 B18 Si14 S9 S10

PHARYNGITIS—cont.
Cv22 Cv23 T16 T15
S6 S5

LACK OF TASTE
Sp5 Sp4 S44

CERVICAL ADENITIS
B38 Si8 G41 T5
T10 H3 Li14 Li13
S12 Cv17 Cx1 Liv3

57. TINNITUS   *ER MING*

Section 1

CAUSE OF DISEASE	SYMPTOMS	DIAGNOSTIC FEATURES	MAIN POINTS	SECONDARY POINTS
1. Gall-bladder Fire ascends; Wind and Cold restrained outside the body.	Continuous tinnitus.	Pulse Wiry and Rapid; face red; tongue dry; mouth bitter.	G20 Si19 T17	T5 G43 G34
2. Kidney Yin deficient; floating Heat ascends.	Tinnitus variable in intensity.	Pulse Rapid but without strength; mouth and tongue dry; tongue red and not furred.	Si19 K6	H3 K1

Section 2

TINNITUS
K1 G44
G20 B10
G7 G8 G9 G18 Gv16 Gv14
Catarrhal—Liv4 Si16 T17 Si19
L11 Li4 K3 S36
T5 G2 T21 Gv20 Gv19 T18
Si3 Si5 Si19 Si16

TINNITUS—cont.
B62 Cx7

OTITIS EXTERNA
G1 Si19 Li4 Li11

OVER-PRODUCTION OF CERUMEN
T17 T21 Si18 Li4

58. DEAFNESS   *ER LONG*

Section 1

CAUSE OF DISEASE	SYMPTOMS	DIAGNOSTIC FEATURES	MAIN POINTS	SECONDARY POINTS
1. Gall-bladder Fire blazing and abundant, moves upwards into the empty spaces.	Sudden complete deafness.	Pulse Wiry; tongue red; heart troubled; prone to anger.	Si19 T17 B19	T5 G43
2. Kidney Yin deficient, cannot moisten the holes (of the head, i.e. including the ears).	Deafness which begins slowly and increases.	Shen exhausted; loins ache; face dark.	Not suitable for acupuncture	

Section 2

DEAFNESS
Li1 Cx9
T21 T23 T19
K8 K5
T8 T9 G41 G44
G20 B62 B63
G3 G2
G41 Cx9 Liv1

OTITIS MEDIA
T23 G1 Li4
T18 T19 G20
T17 G2
G41 G3
Si19 T21 Si15 S36
Si3 T5

59. DEAFNESS AND DUMBNESS   *LONG YA*

Section 1

CAUSE OF DISEASE	SYMPTOMS	DIAGNOSTIC FEATURES	MAIN POINTS	SECONDARY POINTS
1. Former Heaven (pre-natal)	Cannot hear or speak.	Deaf and dumb from birth.	Gv20 G2 T17 H5 Gv15	Li4 S36 Si19

CAUSE OF DISEASE	SYMPTOMS	DIAGNOSTIC FEATURES	MAIN POINTS	SECONDARY POINTS
2. Latter Heaven (post-natal): prolonged deafness and dumbness resulting from an accident.	As above.	Hearing and speech originally normal; deafness and dumbness occur after illness or accident.	G2 T17 Gv15	T5 H5

Section 2   STUTTERING
Gv4   K5   Cx9

60. SEVERE INFLAMMATION OF THE EYES   *BAO FA HUO YAN*

Section 1

CAUSE OF DISEASE	SYMPTOMS	DIAGNOSTIC FEATURES	MAIN POINTS	SECONDARY POINTS
1. Wind and Heat ascend.	Eye-sockets swollen and painful; eyes shed many tears and are red and itch.	White of the eyes becomes swollen and red; eyes feel rough; photophobia.	G20 B1 Liv2	Li4 G37

Section 2

EYES EASILY BECOME TIRED	CONJUNCTIVITIS
G20 G14 Liv8	T5 Li4 G3
G3 S1 B2 B1	S8 Si3 G20 B10
Cx2 Gv19 B10 Si6	G14 Si18
Gv24a Li4 K1	S44 G15 T3
S8 G16 T23	B1 T23 Liv2 Cx8

PHOTOPHOBIA	BLEPHARITIS
G20 G13 G15	T10 S36 G3
Liv3 B60 Si5	Si4 Li2

STRABISMUS	PTERYGIUM
Circumorbital points	G14 B2 B1 T23
	Or other circumorbital points (A. Chamfrault after
GLAUCOMA	Tsou Lieun)
G20 Li1 Si1	
K1 B62 S43	SPOTS IN FRONT OF EYES
G3 Gv24	Liv2 Liv14 Li4 Si4
	G20 G19 G18
CRIES TOO EASILY	G3 B2
K5 B15	
Cx7 Gv20	STYE
S8 G37 Si3	L11 Si7 B1 (A. Chamfrault)

61. BIRDS EYE (?)   *CHIAO MU*

Section 1

CAUSE OF DISEASE	SYMPTOMS	DIAGNOSTIC FEATURES	MAIN POINTS	SECONDARY POINTS
Liver Wind Evil and Fire rush upwards into the eyes.	Eyes dull in the evening, bright in the morning; eyes feel extremely rough and itch.	At night can only see things directly below the eyes, cannot see anything above.	G20 B1 B18	Li4 S36

Section 2

CATARACT	CATARACT—cont.
Occasionally effective in very early stage	T1 B1 B67 Gv28
Li4 L9 Liv3 G1	S6 G41
G20 B8	B2 G14 S14

62. PURULENT RHINORRHOEA   *BI YUAN*

Section 1

CAUSE OF DISEASE	SYMPTOMS	DIAGNOSTIC FEATURES	MAIN POINTS	SECONDARY POINTS
Wind and Heat in brain.	Thick mucus flows incessantly from nose.	Mucus foul-smelling and yellow.	G20 Gv23 Li20	Li4 G40

NASAL CATARRH
Li4 L7
G1 B2 Li20
G20 Gv14 Gv16 Gv20 Gv28
Cx8 Si2
S3 S45
T17 G15 G19

RHINORRHOEA ASSOCIATED WITH
TENSION
Cx6 Cx7
Gv16 Gv12 Gv24a
T5 K10

HAY FEVER
Liv8 K9 Li4
Li19 Gv23 Gv16
B10 B11 B12
Cv17 Cv20

SNEEZING
L5
G4 S8 B12

SINUSITIS
K8 Liv8
Gv26 S7 S1 S3 G14 B2 Gv28
B64 S45 S40
Si1 Si18
K3 B62
Li11 Li17
Li20 Gv23
B12 G20

ANOSMIA
Sp4 L9
B3 B4 B1
B56 B60
B17 S12
Li20 Li19 Gv25 Gv16 B10

NASAL POLYPS
Li20 Li19
Gv28 Gv26 Gv25 Gv24 Gv14 Gv15 Gv16
K3 L7

63. BREAST ABSCESS *RU YONG*

Section 1

CAUSE OF DISEASE	SYMPTOMS	DIAGNOSTIC FEATURES	MAIN POINTS	SECONDARY POINTS
Liver Qi depressed and congealed; stomach Hot and obstructed.	Breast red, swollen, inflamed and painful; at first alternately hot and cold; swelling hard and painful.	(no observations)	G21 L7 B54	B17 Sp10

Section 2

BREAST ABSCESS
L7 Si1
Sp18 G41
Li8 S34
Cx7 Cv17

64. GOOSE-FOOT WIND (Skin disease of hands only) *E ZHANG FENG*

Section 1

CAUSE OF DISEASE	SYMPTOMS	DIAGNOSTIC FEATURES	MAIN POINTS	SECONDARY POINTS
Blood scorched and affected by Wind which causes it to congeal.	Centre of palm of hand mottled purple and white, changing to white skin; it is hard, thick, dry, withered and cracked; gradually spreads to whole hand.	(no observations)	Cx8	Cx6 Cx7 H8

65. DISEASES OF THE KNEE (Crane-knee Wind) *HAO XI FENG*

Section 1

CAUSE OF DISEASE	SYMPTOMS	DIAGNOSTIC FEATURES	MAIN POINTS	SECONDARY POINTS
1. Affected by Wind and Cold outside; spleen Damp flows downwards.	At first pain inside the patella; after some time it becomes swollen and the thigh becomes increasingly thin.	Colour of swollen skin does not change; Pulse Slowed-down and without strength; tongue pale.	S34 Sp10 Sp9 G34	S36 Sp6
2. Liver and kidney Yin deficient; Damp and Heat flow downwards.	Knee joints red, swollen and painful; Jing Shen does not move; if prolonged the skin and flesh above and below the knee become withered and contracted.	Pulse Fine and Rapid; tongue red, not furred.	S34 Sp9 Sp6	K7 Liv2

Section 2

See No. 35.

66. BERIBERI (Foot Qi) *JIAO QI*

Section 1

CAUSE OF DISEASE	SYMPTOMS	DIAGNOSTIC FEATURES	MAIN POINTS	SECONDARY POINTS
1. Damp: Damp and Heat flow downwards.	Both feet swollen and painful and intensely hot.	Pulse Slippery and Rapid; tongue furred, slippery and greasy.	S28 Sp9 S36	Liv2 G34
2. Dry: affected by Wind and Cold outside.	Alternately hot and cold; both feet painful; no swelling or fever.	Pulse Wiry and Tight; tongue thinly furred white.	T5 Sp9 G34	K7 B60

67. PROLAPSE OF RECTUM *TUO GANG*

Section 1

CAUSE OF DISEASE	SYMPTOMS	DIAGNOSTIC FEATURES	MAIN POINTS	SECONDARY POINTS
1. Qi Empty, sinks downwards.	Prolapse of rectum after defaecation; does not retract.	Pulse Deep and Weak; face white; dyspnoea.	Gv20 Cv8 Gv1	B25 B24 S25 S36
2. Lungs Cold.	Prolapse of rectum, does not retract.	Pulse Empty or Slowed-down; face white; tongue substance pale.	B13 B25 Cv8 Gv1	Cv17 S25 B24 S36
3. Constant diarrhoea: spleen and stomach Empty and Cold.	Prolapse of rectum after diarrhoea; does not retract.	Pulse Deep and Fine; face yellow; tongue pale; prolapse after each bout of diarrhoea.	Gv20 Cv8 B20 B21 Gv1	B25 S25 S36 Sp6
4. Damp and Heat ascend.	Prolapse of rectum, painful.	Pulse Deep and Slippery; tongue furred yellow and greasy; dysuria, urine red; rectum painful.	Gv20 Gv1 B25	S28 S36 Sp6

Section 2

PROLAPSE OF RECTUM	PROLAPSE OF RECTUM—cont.
B58 B57 K5 B62 Gv1 Gv4 Gv20 Sp4 Sp12 S15 S25	Cx6 T7 T3 B31 B32 B33 B34 B35

Diseases of Women

68. IRREGULAR MENSTRUATION   *YUE JING BU TIAO*

Section 1

CAUSE OF DISEASE	SYMPTOMS	DIAGNOSTIC FEATURES	MAIN POINTS	SECONDARY POINTS
1. Blood Hot, Fire brilliant.	Period comes early; large amounts of blood, coloured purple and lumpy; heart troubled and burning; head dizzy; the Five Hearts are troubled and hot.	Pulse Deep and Slippery or Rapid; point of tongue red.	Cv4 Cv3	Cx6 Sp6
2. Blood Hot, Qi Empty.	Period comes early; small amounts of pale blood; dyspnoea; body weary.	Pulse Deep and Slowed-down and without strength; tongue not furred; little saliva.	Cv6 Cv4	Sp10 Sp6
3. Blood Cold and Empty.	Period comes late; small amounts of pale blood; lower abdomen cold and painful.	Pulse Slowed-down and Rough.	Cv4 Cv3 Sp10	S36 Sp6
4. Blood Cold, Qi Empty; both unable to strengthen the lower part of the body.	Period comes late; large amounts of blood which cannot be stopped.	Pulse Deep and Weak.	Gv12 B38 Cv6	Sp10 Sp6
5. Liver and kidney depressed.	Periods irregular, may come early or late.	Pulse Wiry and Rough.	B17 B18 Cv3	Sp8 Sp6

Section 2

IRREGULAR MENSTRUATION
Sp6 Sp10 S25 Cv4 Cv6
Sp4 Cx6
B23

69. DYSMENORRHOEA   *TONG JING*

Section 1

CAUSE OF DISEASE	SYMPTOMS	DIAGNOSTIC FEATURES	MAIN POINTS	SECONDARY POINTS
1. Blood Hot, Qi depressed; dead blood blocked and congealed.	Period comes early; lower abdomen painful; blood purple and lumpy.	Pulse Wiry and Rough.	B17 Cv6 Cv4 Liv13	Sp10 Cx6
2. Qi and blood Empty and deficient; Water does not submerge Wood (Note 1).	Period comes late; lower abdomen painful.	Pulse Slowed-down, Rough and Weak.	Cv6 Cv4	Sp6
3. Blood Empty and Cold.	Lower abdomen painful during period; dragging pain in both sides; limbs and loins aching and tired.	Pulse Deep and Tight.	Cv4 Cv3	S36 Sp6

NOTES
1. *See chapter on The Five Elements in 'Acupuncture'.*

Section 2

DYSMENORRHOEA
Liv8 L7 Sp6 K3
B62 G35 Li4 S28
Liv14 K15

DYSMENORRHOEA—cont.
B31 B32 B33 B34
Gv12

70. AMENORRHOEA   *JING BI*

Section 1

CAUSE OF DISEASE	SYMPTOMS	DIAGNOSTIC FEATURES	MAIN POINTS	SECONDARY POINTS
1. Blood obstructed: caused by Cold Qi lodging in Womb Gate.	Menstruation ceases; lower abdomen swollen and hard; becoming larger daily as though pregnant.	Pulse Deep, Tight and Rough.	Cv4 Cv3 B23	Sp6

CAUSE OF DISEASE	SYMPTOMS	DIAGNOSTIC FEATURES	MAIN POINTS	SECONDARY POINTS
2. Blood deficient: Grief injures heart and spleen.	Menstruation ceases; appetite decreases rapidly; skin and flesh dry and emaciated; Shen tired; body lethargic.	Pulse Weak-floating and Fine and without strength.	B38 B20 B21	Cv4 S36
3. Blood withered: bearing and/or suckling large number of children; excessive sexual intercourse; Jing exhausted. (Note 1).	Menstruation ceases; little appetite; skin dry and withered; incessant coughing.	Pulse Deep, Fine and Rapid; cheekbones red after midday; face dry, white and mat.	B37 B38	Cv4 S36

NOTES

1. *It is important to realise that Jing has a wider meaning than 'sperm', and is present in women. It is the fusion of the male and female Jing which creates life. (See also Introduction.)*

Section 2	AMENORRHOEA	STERILITY
	Li4 Sp6	Sp5 Cv3 (Chamfrault)
	B38 S36 S25	K3 L7
	Liv8	S30 K5
	Cv3 Cv2 S29	
	B60 Cv2 Gv1	

71. MENORRHAGIA   *BENG LOU*

Section 1

CAUSE OF DISEASE	SYMPTOMS	DIAGNOSTIC FEATURES	MAIN POINTS	SECONDARY POINTS
1. Blood excessively Hot; Heat rushes into and injures the Vessel of Conception.	Slight trickle or sudden heavy flow of blood during periods; blood is dark purple, coagulated and lumpy; abdomen swollen and painful.	Pulse Wiry and Rapid or Hollow; tongue substance red.	K14 Cv3	Sp10 Sp6
2. Mental anxiety injures spleen and causes it to be Empty and unable to obtain blood.	Slight trickle or sudden heavy flow of blood which does not cease; whole body weary and lethargic; desires to lie down; little appetite; palpitation of the heart; loins ache.	Pulse Fine and Weak and without strength; face greenish-yellow; lips white; tongue shiny, no saliva.	B20 Cv6 Liv13	Sp6
3. Violent anger injures liver; liver does not store blood; blood Hot and moves wildly.	Slight trickle or sudden heavy flow of blood which does not cease; chest-ribs swollen and full; limbs and loins ache; throat dry; head dizzy.	Pulse Deep and Wiry; face bluish-yellow; lips at first red then white; tongue shiny and slippery.	Liv13 Cv6 Cv3	Liv1 Sp1

Section 2	MENORRHAGIA
	Sp1 Liv3 H5
	Cv6 B55 S18
	H1 B54 Sp2

72. VAGINAL DISCHARGE   *DAI XIA*

Section 1

CAUSE OF DISEASE	SYMPTOMS	DIAGNOSTIC FEATURES	MAIN POINTS	SECONDARY POINTS
1. White discharge: spleen meridian not protected; Damp Evil sinks downwards.	White discharge like saliva or mucus, occurring in middle age; if severe is foul-smelling.	Pulse Slowed-down and Slippery.	B20 G26 B23 Cv3	Sp9 Sp6
2. Green discharge: liver meridian Damp and Hot.	Discharge like green-bean juice, thick and glutinous; foul-smelling.	Pulse Wiry, Slippery, Weak-floating and Slowed-down.	B18 Liv13 Cv3	Sp6 Liv2

573

CAUSE OF DISEASE	SYMPTOMS	DIAGNOSTIC FEATURES	MAIN POINTS	SECONDARY POINTS
3. Black discharge: Fire very Hot and abundant.	Discharge like black-bean juice; foul-smelling; lower abdomen painful; micturition as though pierced with a knife; vagina swollen; face red.	Pulse Slippery and Rapid or Deep and Rapid.	B23 G26 Cv3	Sp6 K6
4. Yellow discharge: Damp Evil in Vessel of Conception.	Discharge like the thick juice of yellow tea and foul-smelling.	Pulse Wiry, Slowed-down and Weak-floating.	B20 B22 G26 Cv4	Sp6 Sp4
5. Red discharge: Damp and Heat injure the blood.	Discharge red like blood but is not blood; slight continuous discharge.	Pulse Deep and Slippery.	B15 B17 B18 Cv3	Sp10 Sp6

Section 2

VAGINAL DISCHARGE	VAGINAL DISCHARGE—cont.
Sp10 Cv2 Cv3	G26 S25 Liv3
Gv1 Gv2 Gv4	Liv11 Sp8 K12
B31 B32 B33 B34	

73. FIBROIDS AND ABDOMINAL TUMOURS (Note 1)   *ZHENG JIA*

Section 1

CAUSE OF DISEASE	SYMPTOMS	DIAGNOSTIC FEATURES	MAIN POINTS	SECONDARY POINTS
1. Food Zheng: poor food after menstruation or confinement produces cold matter.	Hard lump in abdomen which cannot be moved; increases rapidly in size.	Pulse Deep and Slippery.	Cv12 Liv13 B20 B21	S36 Sp4 S25 Cv6
2. Blood Zheng: after menstruation or confinement Zang Qi Empty; affected by cold Wind which contests with the blood.	Hard lump in abdomen which cannot be moved; sides and abdomen swollen and painful; interior of body hot; heart troubled.	Pulse Hard.	Cv12 Liv13 B17 B18 B20	G26 S25 Cv4 Sp10 Sp6
3. Jia: cold Wind invades the body; Qi and blood congealed and obstructed.	Jia Qi attacks upwards and downwards causing pain; moves when pressed.	Pulse Deep and Tight.	Cv12 Cv4 B17 B20 B21	B13 Sp10 Liv3 S36 Sp6

NOTES

1. *Jianshi gives Zheng as a hard and immovable swelling in the abdomen; and Jia as movable when pressed and not constantly present—'sometimes scatters sometimes appears'.*

74. PROLAPSE OF VAGINA   *YIN TING*

Section 1

CAUSE OF DISEASE	SYMPTOMS	DIAGNOSTIC FEATURES	MAIN POINTS	SECONDARY POINTS
1. Qi Empty and descends.	Inside of vagina projects like a snake or a mushroom or a cock's-comb. Secondary symptoms: dragging pain; large quantities of clear urine.	Pulse Weak-floating tongue pale.	Cv6 Cv4 Sp6	Liv1 Liv2
2. Damp and Heat flow downwards.	As above. Secondary symptoms: vagina swollen and painful; urine red.	Pulse Rapid; tongue red.	Cv7 S28 Cv3	Sp6 Liv2

Section 2

PROLAPSUS UTERI
K1 Liv1
H8 K3 Liv8
B31 B32

75. PRURITIS VULVAE *YIN YANG*

Section 1

CAUSE OF DISEASE	SYMPTOMS	DIAGNOSTIC FEATURES	MAIN POINTS	SECONDARY POINTS
Damp and Heat produce Worms, (see Notes to No. 55 Toothache).	Lower part of vagina itches; slight incontinence of urine.	Pulse Wiry and Sloweddown; tongue furred, slippery and greasy.	Cv3 Sp10 Sp6	B54 Liv2

Section 2

PRURITIS VULVAE
S31 S30 Liv11
Cv3 Gv1 Cv1
H8   K10 B60

76. UNPLEASANT SYMPTOMS DURING PREGNANCY *REN ZHEN WU ZU*

Section 1

CAUSE OF DISEASE	SYMPTOMS	DIAGNOSTIC FEATURES	MAIN POINTS	SECONDARY POINTS
1. Spleen and stomach Empty and Weak; Phlegm-fluid stored inside the body.	Vomiting phlegm; heart troubled; head dizzy; limbs tired and lethargic; likes sour foods and dislikes normal food.	Pulse Slippery and without strength or Slowed-down; tongue lightly furred white.	B20 B21 Cx6 Cv12 Liv13 (last 2 only up to 5th month).	Liv2 S36 Sp4
2. Liver Qi depressed and congealed; Qi does not circulate.	Chest-ribs swollen and full; head and eyes dizzy; hates cold, likes heat; chest perturbed; likes sour foods and is particular in choice of food; may be unable to eat; body tired and has no strength; mouth may be dry; may be constipated.	Pulse Deep and Slippery and without strength; both Connecting Pulses Empty and Wiry; tongue furred white.	B18 Liv13 B20 B21	Liv2 Cx6 S36
3. Liver rebels; stomach Hot.	Nausea and vomiting; heart troubled, anxious and annoyed; likes the cold and to drink cool fluids; dislikes food; vomitus sour; head painful; dislikes the heat; constipated; urine red.	Pulse Wiry, Slippery and Rapid; tongue lightly furred yellow.	B18 B19 B21 S36 Cx6	Liv3 S44 G34

Section 2

NAUSEA AND VOMITING OF PREGNANCY
Liv8 G40 S45
Cx6   Sp6 L5 L9

77. ECLAMPSIA (Note 1) *ZI XIAN*

Section 1

CAUSE OF DISEASE	SYMPTOMS	DIAGNOSTIC FEATURES	MAIN POINTS	SECONDARY POINTS
Caused by heart and liver meridians being depressed and Hot.	Sudden collapse in pregnant women; cramp and muscular spasms; becomes unconscious; normal when conscious.	Pulse Wiry and Slippery or Stopped.	Gv26 G20 Gv16 B10	S36 Cx6 G34

NOTES
1. *The Chinese heading is 'Child' plus Xian, one of the three subdivisions of No. 26 Convulsions.*

Section 2

ECLAMPSIA
K2   Cx7
G21 G34
Si14 S36

78. PROLONGED LABOUR   *ZHI CHAN*

Section 1

CAUSE OF DISEASE	SYMPTOMS	DIAGNOSTIC FEATURES	MAIN POINTS	SECONDARY POINTS
Liking for leisure, no physical work, excessive sleeping and resting cause Qi and blood to become obstructed.	Full-term foetus is not born.	Despite labour pains foetus does not turn and move; Pulse Slowed-down.	Li4 Sp6	G21 B67

Section 2

PROLONGED LABOUR
L14 S30 Sp15
Sp6 B67 Gv2
B23 B33

79. RETAINED PLACENTA   *TAI YI BU XIA*

Section 1

CAUSE OF DISEASE	SYMPTOMS	DIAGNOSTIC FEATURES	MAIN POINTS	SECONDARY POINTS
Excessive and prolonged physical toil; Qi weak, blood congealed.	Placenta does not descend; abdomen swollen and painful.	Pulse Empty; face hoary-white; tongue purple.	G21 Cv3 B60	Li4 Sp6

Section 2

RETAINED PLACENTA
G21 Sp6
K3 B67 B47 B32
Cv3 Cv5 Cv6 Cv7

80. POST-NATAL SPASMS   *CHAN HOU JING LÜAN*

Section 1

CAUSE OF DISEASE	SYMPTOMS	DIAGNOSTIC FEATURES	MAIN POINTS	SECONDARY POINTS
1. Blood deficient after confinement; Wind Evil ascends and invades the body.	Muscular spasms and pain; unable to stretch; no sweating.	Pulse Floating and Slowed-down; tongue lightly furred white.	Cx3 T5	Li11 Li4
2. Blood deficient after confinement; unable to use muscles.	Muscular spasms and pain; sweating.	Pulse Empty; tongue pale	Cx3 Si3	Cv6

81. PAIN IN LOWER ABDOMEN AFTER CONFINEMENT
CHAN HOU SHAO FU TONG

Section 1

CAUSE OF DISEASE	SYMPTOMS	DIAGNOSTIC FEATURES	MAIN POINTS	SECONDARY POINTS
1. Dead blood has not been cleansed.	Slight pain in lower abdomen.	Pulse Rough.	S25 Cv4	Sp10 Sp6
2. Water stored up in lower part of body.	Lower abdomen hard and painful; dysuria with slight urinary incontinence; abdomen swollen and painful.	Micturition rough; urinary incontinence; Pulse Deep; tongue furred and slippery.	Cv3 S28	Sp9 K7
3. Dead blood.	Lower abdomen hard, resists pressure; polyuria.	Polyuria; tongue dark purple; Pulse Rough and Blocked.	S25 Cv4 K14	Sp10 Sp6

PAIN IN LOWER ABDOMEN
AFTER CONFINEMENT
Sp6 Cv6

POST PARTUM VAGINAL DISCHARGE
Liv6 Sp6
Cv6 Cv3 Cv2
T7

PUERPERAL FEVER
B25 B31
Li10 S36 Li4 Sp6

82. INSUFFICIENT LACTATION   *RU SHAO*

Section 1

CAUSE OF DISEASE	SYMPTOMS	DIAGNOSTIC FEATURES	MAIN POINTS	SECONDARY POINTS
1. Blood Empty; excessive bleeding during confinement.	Small amount of milk in breast; face very white.	Eats little; Pulse Empty; tongue pale.	Cv17 (moxa) Si1	Li4 S36 Sp6
2. Qi Mai blocked and Cold.	Small amount of milk in breast; heart troubled; agitated and impetuous.	Pulse Large; tongue red.	Cv17 (moxa) Si1 G21	L7

Section 2

INSUFFICIENT LACTATION
Si1 H1 Cv17 S18
B38 (S. de Morant)
G41 Cv3

Diseases of Children

83. ACUTE CONVULSIONS   *JI JING FENG*

Section 1

CAUSE OF DISEASE	SYMPTOMS	DIAGNOSTIC FEATURES	MAIN POINTS	SECONDARY POINTS
1. Heart meridian Hot; eyes see strange things, ears hear strange noises.	Convulsions; easily startled; frequent weeping at night.	Pulse Overflowing and Rapid; face blue-green; tongue red.	Gv14 Gv26	Si4 K1
2. Heart and liver Fire abundant; affected by Wind and Cold from outside.	Body hot but no sweating; convulsions; constipation.	Pulse Floating and Over-flowing, Slippery and Rapid; tongue furred yellowish-white.	Gv13 Si4 Liv3	Li4 L7
3. Phlegm abundant, produces Wind.	Phlegm bubbling; breathing hurried; mouth tightly closed; spasms of limbs.	Pulse Slippery.	Gv12 Cv12	L11 T1
4. Upper Warmer Hot and abundant.	Body hot; heart troubled and anxious; spasms of limbs; face and lips blue-green; small quantities of red urine; mouth parched.	Pulse Overflowing and Rapid.	Gv26 K1	L11 T1

Section 2

SCREAMING FITS	PETIT MAL
K5 L9	B62

84. MILD CONVULSIONS   *MAN JING FENG*

Section 1

CAUSE OF DISEASE	SYMPTOMS	DIAGNOSTIC FEATURES	MAIN POINTS	SECONDARY POINTS
1. Constitution previously weak; spleen Empty; liver abundant and containing Phlegm.	Mild intermittent convulsions; face blue-green and white; body not hot; much phlegm.	Pulse Slowed-down, Minute and Slippery and without strength.	Gv14 Gv12	Cv4 S36
2. Caused by having previously taken Cold Medicine as cure for severe convulsions (see No. 83).	Very mild spasms; eyes slightly open when asleep; not of excitable nature; stools blue-green.	Pulse Empty and Slow; urine blue-green and white.	Gv12 Cv6	G34

Section 2

AFRAID OF DARK
K10 Gv20 Cx9

85. CHRONIC SPLEEN WIND (?)   *MAN PI FENG*

Section 1

CAUSE OF DISEASE	SYMPTOMS	DIAGNOSTIC FEATURES	MAIN POINTS	SECONDARY POINTS
1. Continuous diarrhoea and vomiting all day long; spleen Yang badly injured.	Closes eyes and shakes head; face dark; sweat appears on forehead; troubled sleep; limbs cold.	Pulse Deep and Slow and without strength.	Gv20 Gv12 B20	Sp4
2. Extremely ill all day long; spleen Empty and does not move; muscles are not nourished by the blood; Emptiness produces Wind.	Troubled sleep with eyes partly open; limbs cold; face dull and colourless; spasms almost imperceptible.	Pulse Weak and without strength.	Gv12 B20 Cv6	Liv3

86. PARALYSIS IN CHILDREN, INCLUDING POLIOMYELITIS   *XIAO ER WEI BI*

Section 1

CAUSE OF DISEASE	SYMPTOMS	DIAGNOSTIC FEATURES	MAIN POINTS	SECONDARY POINTS
1. Wei: lungs Hot, bronchi Dry.	Both legs paralysed and weak; unable to walk.	Legs weak and soft to touch; face white.	press points on spine with bamboo needle G20 B11 G34	Li4 T4 Si4 G30 K8 K3 B62
2. Bi: the combined Evils of Wind, Cold and Damp.	Both legs stiff and straight; walking difficult.	Legs stiff and hard when pressed; face blue-green.	Gv12 G20 G30	G34 Sp9

Section 2

See Nos. 35, 37.

87. COUGHING   *KE SOU*

Section 1

CAUSE OF DISEASE	SYMPTOMS	DIAGNOSTIC FEATURES	MAIN POINTS	SECONDARY POINTS
1. Wind and Cold cough: Wind and Cold enter lungs.	Sputum clear and white; coughing; dislikes the cold; nose blocked.	Pulse Floating; tongue lightly furred white.	B12 B13 Cv6	Li4 L7
2. Hot lungs cough: Hot Phlegm in lungs.	Face red; throat dry; sputum yellow and glutinous; coughing.	Pulse Rapid; tongue thickly furred white and fairly dry.	B12 B13	L5 L10
3. Accumulated food cough: accumulation of food produces Phlegm; Heat rebels against the lungs.	Breathing hurried; sputum obstructed; coughing; bad smell of food may remain in mouth; stools foul-smelling.	Pulse Slippery; tongue lightly furred yellow.	B13 B20 B21	L6 Cv12 S36
4. Wind and Heat cough: Wind enters lungs, changes to Heat and causes Phlegm	Face and lips red; mucus from nose concentrated; does not dislike the cold; coughing; sputum slightly concentrated.	Pulse Floating and Rapid.	B12 B13	L5 L9
5. Full Fire cough: Full Fire in lungs; Phlegm thick and turbid.	Face red during coughing bouts; violent vomiting with much noise; sputum concentrated; mouth parched.	Pulse Overflowing and Full; tongue yellow and dry.	Cv22 Cv17 (moxa)	L6 L10
6. Empty lung cough: Wind enters lungs, changes to Heat and is not cured for a long time.	Protracted cough with weak breathing; sweating during coughing bouts; voice low; dyspnoea.	Right Inch Pulse Weak-floating.	B13 Gv12 B38	Cv6 S36
7. Damp and drinking cough: excessive drinking of tea or water may injure the body and produce cold.	Face yellowish-white; large amounts of thin, non-glutinous sputum; stools watery; chest melancholy.	Tongue furred white and greasy; Pulse Slowed-down.	B13 B21	S36 L6

Section 2

See Nos. 3, 5, 6, 9, 12, 13, 14, 15, 16, 18, 19

88. INDIGESTION   *SHANG SHI*

Section 1

CAUSE OF DISEASE	SYMPTOMS	DIAGNOSTIC FEATURES	MAIN POINTS	SECONDARY POINTS
Food and drink injure the spleen. The Classic (Nei Jing?) says: 'If food and drink rebel of their own accord, the intestines and stomach are injured.'	Fever; dislikes food; belches sour breath; dislikes the smell of food; desires to vomit but cannot; dyspnoea; indigestion; swallows sour saliva; abdomen painful and swollen.	Stools sour and foul-smelling; hot at night, cool in morning; feet cold; stomach hot; Pulse Full and has strength.	Cv12 Liv13 B20 B21	Cx6 Sp4 Cv21 S36

89. BLOCKAGE DISEASES   *PI JI*

Section 1

CAUSE OF DISEASE	SYMPTOMS	DIAGNOSTIC FEATURES	MAIN POINTS	SECONDARY POINTS
Eating and drinking irregular; intestines and stomach completely full; semi-digested food obstructed and so overflows; also affected by Cold Qi which congeals.	Hard lump like overturned cup below left ribs; at first like chicken's egg, gradually increasing in size; heavy sweating; emaciated; likes to drink cold water.	Pulse Hard.	XB2 (moxa) Liv13	Sp3

90. *GAN JI* (see Note 1)

Section 1

CAUSE OF DISEASE	SYMPTOMS	DIAGNOSTIC FEATURES	MAIN POINTS	SECONDARY POINTS
1. Spleen Gan: milk and food not properly regulated, forming a blockage and generating Heat which wastes and destroys blood and Qi; Gan Heat injures the spleen.	Face yellow; flesh wasted away; body hot and lethargic; region below heart blocked and full; stomach and abdomen hard; likes to eat mud (?); head large, neck fine; occasional diarrhoea and vomiting; stools smell rotten and are glutinous.	Right Connecting Pulse Deep, Fine and Rapid; face yellow.	XA2 (let yellow fluid.)	S36 Sp4
2. Liver Gan: unlimited food and drink; accumulated Heat becomes Gan; Gan Heat injures the liver.	Face, eyes and fingernails blue-green; eyes diseased and watery; shakes head and rubs eyes; thick fluid flows from ears; large blue-green veins on abdomen; emaciated; thirsty; stools blue-green.	Right Connecting Pulse Wiry and Rapid; face blue-green.	as above	S36 Liv2
3. Heart Gan: food and drink obstructed; accumulated Heat becomes Gan; stored up Heat rises into heart.	Face and eyes red; high fever; sweating; continuously agitated; snaps teeth and moves tongue; mouth and tongue dry and burning; thirsty; sores in mouth; chest-diaphragm full and melancholy; body emaciated.	Pulse Overflowing and Rapid; face red.	as above	S36 H8
4. Lung Gan: food and drink not properly regulated; accumulated Heat becomes Gan; stored up Heat rises to lungs.	Face white; coughing; hair becomes dry and withered; flesh and skin dry and burning; hates the cold; high fever; usually emits blue-green pus from nose; sores develop in nostrils.	Right Inch Pulse Slippery and Rapid.	as above	S36 L10
5. Kidney Gan: food and drink not properly regulated; accumulated Heat becomes Gan; Gan Heat injures kidney.	Face very dark; bleeding from gums; breath foul-smelling; feet very cold; abdomen painful; diarrhoea; associated with incomplete knitting together of fontanel, or late teething and walking.	Pulse Fine and Rapid.	as above	S36 K2
6. Innocent Gan: food and drink not properly regulated; accumulated Heat becomes Gan; Gan Heat becomes Poison.	Sores on neck or hard lump inside back of neck; incessant rectal bleeding with pus; body emaciated; face yellow; fever.	Pulse Wiry and Rapid; tongue deep red.	(press points on spine with bamboo needle)	G40 Liv5

NOTES

1. *Gan seems to be a general term for a large number of complaints common in children below the age of* 15. *Note that whatever the symptoms, food and drink are the cause in each case. The Chinese word Ji in the heading Gan Ji means 'to accumulate'* (*cf. No.* 21 *Qi Accumulation Diseases*).

Section 1

CAUSE OF DISEASE	SYMPTOMS	DIAGNOSTIC FEATURES	MAIN POINTS	SECONDARY POINTS
1. Milk injury vomiting: child takes excess of milk which is stopped in the stomach.	Vomits milk; body hot; face yellow; skin puffy.	Pulse Slippery and Rapid.	Cv12 S36	Cx6 Cv21
2. Food injury vomiting: food and drink not properly regulated; excess of greasy foods; obstruction formed in digestive tract.	Stomach and abdomen swollen and hot; mouth foul-smelling; vomitus sour and glutinous; fever.	Pulse Deep and Floating.	Cv12 Liv13 S36	Cv21 Cx6
3. Cold vomiting: excess of food produces cold.	Food eaten in morning vomited in evening; vomitus neither foul-smelling or sour; limbs cold.	Pulse Deep and Slow; face and lips white.	Gv12 B20 B21	S36
4. Hot vomiting: excess of hot, greasy food; Heat accumulates in middle of body.	Food vomited on entering stomach; mouth parched; body hot; lips red; urine red; vomitus sour and watery.	Pulse Rapid.	Cx6 S36	Sp4 S44
5. Empty vomiting: stomach Qi Empty and weak; cannot digest milk and food.	Jing Shen weary and lethargic; continuous vomiting; micturition and defaecation normal; no thirst; eyes open when asleep.	Pulse Empty and Slow.	Gv12 Cv4 B20 B21	S36
6. Full vomiting: milk and food obstructed; stomach Heat attacks upwards.	Chest and abdomen swollen and painful; hard and painful lump in stomach; micturition and defaecation difficult and rough; thirsty, likes cool fluids; vomitus sour and foul-smelling.	Pulse Deep and Full.	S36	T6 Sp4

Section 2   INTERMITTENT ABDOMINAL PAIN
Liv8

Glossary

A short list of translated terms, with their Chinese equivalents, and brief notes on their meaning.

1. Terms used chiefly in the description of symptoms:

ACCUMULATES, ACCUMULATION:	*ji*	See Notes to No. 21 Qi-Accumulation Diseases.
CONGEAL:	*ning, jie*	Note that as a pulse quality *jie* is translated 'knotted'.
DENSE:	*mi*	Generally refers to stools; close-packed, heavy etc.
DEPRESSED:	*yu*	May refer to an organ or to one of the functional substances.
DISTRESSED:	*fanmen*	Generally refers to heart; a combination of *fan* meaning 'troubled' and *men* meaning 'melancholy'.
HARSH:	*cu*	Coarse, rough etc. Generally refers to breathing.
MELANCHOLY:	*men*	Refers to chest, heart, abdomen etc.
OBSTRUCT, OBSTRUCTION:	*pi, sai, zhi, zu*	No meaningful distinction can be drawn between these four words. Note however that as a pulse quality *zhi* is translated 'blocked'.
THICK:	*chou*	Similar to 'dense'; refers to stools or urine.
TROUBLED:	*fan*	Refers most frequently to the heart.

2. Other terms:

ANIMAL SOUL:	*po*	That aspect of Shen which is controlled by the lungs; see Introduction, part I.
CHEST-DIAPHRAGM:	*xiong ge*	Refers to the inside of the chest above the diaphragm.
CHEST-RIBS:	*xiong xie*	Refers to the outside of the chest, the ribs. Both terms are commonly used in describing the location of pain etc.
CHONG MO:		One of the Eight Extra Meridians, also known as *xue hai*, the Sea of Blood. Traditionally considered as the centre of all blood in the meridians. See 'Acupuncture', chapter X.
COOL MEDICINE:	*liang yao*	One of the categories of Chinese pharmacology.
DORMANT EVIL:	*fu xie*	See Introduction part II.
DORMANT QI:	*fu qi*	,, ,, ,, ,,
EMPTY:	*xu*	Has two meanings; 'hollow' and 'weak', of which the second is the more common.
EXHAUSTED, EXHAUSTION:	*lao*	A whole group of diseases is associated with *lao*; cf. No. 4 in list of Causes of Disease, Introduction part II.
FIRE OF THE FIVE DESIRES:	*wu zhi zhi huo*	The Five Desires (wu zhi) are the same as the Seven Emotions without Mental anxiety and Alarm. The Fire is the motive force of the emotions.
FIVE EXHAUSTIONS:	*wu lao*	May refer to: (a) the Five Zang organs; (b) Qi, Blood, bone (gu), flesh (rou) and sinew or muscle (jin).

582

FULL:	*man*	Most commonly used to describe the state of a particular region of the body, e.g. stomach, abdomen etc.
	shi	Describes the condition of the functional substances of the body, e.g. Qi, Blood, Ying, Wei etc. Also a pulse quality.
GREAT POISON:	*da du*	Large amounts of toxic substances in the body; may also indicate a highly toxic variety of Chinese medicines.
JING ENERGY:	*jing li*	The 'external manifestation' is very similar to 'libido' but see Introduction, part I, under Jing.
LOWER ABDOMEN:	*shao fu*	Defined by the Chinese as the region of the body from the navel downwards.
LOWER WARMER:	*xia jiao*	The region of the body between the navel and the small-intestine, principally the liver and kidney. The lower Triple Warmer.
MIDDLE QI:	*zhong qi*	Qi in the organs of the middle of the body, i.e. stomach and spleen. Also known as Middle Warmer Qi. Qi of the middle Triple Warmer.
MIDDLE WARMER:	*zhong jiao*	The region of the body between diaphragm and navel, principally the stomach and spleen. The middle Triple Warmer.
MINISTER FIRE:	*xiang huo*	The Fire in the kidneys; cf. Sovereign Fire.
PHLEGM:	*tan*	Translated as Phlegm only when it occurs as a 'metaphysical' concept (generally in the first column of the translation) or when the alternative, 'sputum', in unsuitable.
PHLEGM-FLUID	*tan yin*	See Notes to No. 6 Gastritis.

QI DOES NOT TRANSFORM: *qi bu hua*
QI DOES NOT MOVE: *qi bu dong*
QI DOES NOT ACTIVATE: *qi bu xing*

The numerous variations on these lines are essentially the same process. The Qi may be that of a particular organ, and it may fail to act upon another functional substance, e.g. water, blood, etc. See Introduction, part I under Qi.

SEASONAL EVIL:	*shi xie*	The particular Evil, or Qi, appropriate to the time of year. See Introduction, part II.
SEVEN EMOTIONS:	*qi qing*	The emotions are:

xi	Joy (Fire)	bei	Sorrow (Metal)
nu	Anger (Wood)	kong	Fear (Water)
you	Obession (Earth)	jing	Alarm
si	Mental Anxiety		

Abnormality of these emotions cause disease; conversely abnormality may result from a disease. See 'Acupuncture', chapter IX.

SEVEN INJURIES:	*qi shang*	Several explanations exist; the most common are:

(a) Excessive eating injures the spleen, Great anger injures the liver.
Lifting heavy weights or sitting on damp ground

injures the kidneys.

Drinking cold liquids injures the lungs.

Dark thoughts injure the heart.

Wind, rain, cold and heat injure the Form (xing).

Uncontrolled fear injures Desire (zhi)

See 'Acupuncture' chapter IX.

(b) Extreme fear injures Jing.

Worry and anxiety injure Shen.

Excessive joy injures the Animal Soul (po)

Sadness moving inside injures the Spiritual Soul (hun).

Unrestrained melancholy injures Yi (Mind)

Unrestrained rage injures Zhi (Desire).

Excessive weariness injures Qi.

See Introduction, part I.

SOVEREIGN FIRE:	*jun huo*	The Fire in the kidneys; cf. Minister Fire.
SPIRITUAL SOUL:	*hun*	That aspect of Shen controlled by the liver; cf. Animal Soul.
TRUE YIN:	*zhen yin*	Also called True Water (zhen shui); it is the Fluid in the kidneys. See Introduction, part I.
UPPER WARMER:	*shang jiao*	The part of the body above the diaphragm, principally the heart and lungs. Upper Triple Warmer.
WARM POISON:	*wen du*	(a) Extreme Heat changing to Fire and causing diseases characterised by a rash.
		(b) One group of the eighth of the causes of disease; see Introduction, part II. One of the chief conditions caused by Warm Poison is mumps.
WEI YANG:		See Wei in Introduction, part I.
WORMS:	*chong*	The word *chong* embraces insects, reptiles etc. It is one of the nine causes of disease, and may well be the ancient Chinese equivalent of bacteria.

Acupuncture: A New Compilation

(*ZHENJIU XIN BIAN*)

COMPILED BY: YE SIU-TING
PUBLISHED BY: DA XIN PUBLISHING HOUSE, TAIWAN, 1965
Translated by: Frank Liu and Felix Mann

On the whole, I think the sections 'Acupuncture: A New Compilation' and 'Periosteal Acupuncture', are where appropriate, the methods to try first when treating a patient. 'A General Survey of Common Diseases and their Treatment by Acupuncture' (called Section 1 on pages 87 to 164), is also good but less clear due to its traditional classification, and is often therefore only second choice. 'Acupuncture Points used in the Treatment of Specific Diseases or Symptoms' (called Section 2 on pages 87 to 164), is generally not as efficacious as the other three sections.

Strengthening

Tonify CNS. Gv23 Gv22 Gv20 B7 B6 Gv19 Gv16 Gv15 G20 B10 G12
Tonify nose. Gv23 B7
Tonify throat. G20 B10 G21
Tonify lungs and bronchi. Gv12 B13 B37 B38 B16
Prevent influenza. B12 Gv12
Tonify heart. B14 B15 B16 Sp17
Tonify circulation. Cv4 Cv6
Tonify lymphatic circulation. B17 Liv13
Tonify stomach and intestines. B18 B20 B21 B25 B31 S36 S37
Tonify genito-urinary system. Gv4 B23 Gv3 B26 B27 B28 B31/4 Cv4 S28
K13
Tonify endocrine, gonads. Gv20 Gv4 Gv3 Cv4
Tonify muscles. Gv20 Gv13 B11 Gv3 B31
Tonify eye and ear. B18 B23 Gv4 Cv4
Generally tonify body. Cv4 S36 Used for immunization as it strengthens
and increases amount of blood.

Sedating

Inflammation of head or five senses. Si3 Li4 G41 B67
Inflammation of mouth and throat. L11 L10 S44 K3
Heart and lung inflammation. P6 P7 L7 L9
Chest inflammation. H8 P6 G34 G40
Stomach and intestine inflammation. S36 Sp4 P6 Liv2
Liver and gall bladder inflammation. G40 Liv3 T5 Li4
Urinary tract inflammation. L7 K3 Liv8 Sp9
General body auto inflammation. B54 L5 10 commandments of fingers and
toes
Generally for inflammation use distant points
Eructations. Cv22 Cv12 Cv6 L9 P6 S36 Sp4 Liv1 Sp6
Pain and spasms. Same points as for inflammation
Chronic pain and spasms. Use local points and add points as above
Needling: Acute—strong for short period. Chronic—light for long period

Regulating

Constipation. B25 S25 S28 T6 B57
Increase diuresis. Cv3 Sp9 S36 Sp6
Increase perspiration. Gv14 Li4 T5 L8

General Points
Non-tuberculous lymphatic gland swelling. B18 G21
Non-venereal groin and abdominal lymphatic swelling. B57
Spleen swelling. B44 B46 B20
Pulmonary T.B. Gv12 B13 B16
Heart disease. B15 H7 H5 P6
Kidney disease. B22 B23
Bladder. B33 B28 Cv3
Anus. Gv1 P4 B57 Gv20
Stomach. Cv12 P6 S36 B21
Large intestine. B25 S25 S37
Small intestine. Cv6 B26 B27
Uterus. S28 Cv3 Sp6
Eye. G20 XH3 B1 B2 B18
Nose. Gv23 Li20 Li4
Ear. T17 Si19
Mouth. P7 P9
Toothache. S7 Li4
Throat. L11 L10
Arm. Gv13 B11 Li15 Li11
Leg. G33 G30 B54 G34
Mental. Cv15 Cv13 H7 S40
Malaria. Gv14/13
Jaundice. Gv9 Si4

RESPIRATORY SYSTEM

Acute Inflammation of Throat including symptoms such as aphonia,
soreness, cough, headache.
G20 T2 L10
May add B13 Li10 L11
If due to influenza add Gv16 T5 Li4

Chronic Inflammation of Throat
B10 Si14 G21 Cv22 B13 T2 L10
or G20 Si15 Li17 T17 B12 K7 K3

Tuberculosis of Throat
B10 Gv12 B16
May add B13 Cv22 L5 L9 S36 Sp6

or B14 T17 Li17 L10 T2 S40 Sp10
With fever Gv13 P5
Spontaneous perspiration H6 Si3
Anorexia B20 Cv12 S36

Aphonia
G20 S10 B12 T17 Li4 L10
or B10 Li17 G21 Si13 B13 K3 Liv2

Laryngeal Spasm, mainly in male children under 3
Cv12 Cv6 S36 L11 P9 Li4 Sp1 B67

Tracheitis
B11 B13 Cv22 L5 T5 L8 Sp6

Acute Bronchitis
G20 B10 B12 T5 L8
If after treatment headache remains B12 B13 L5 Li4 T5
If after treatment severe cough or tickle in throat remains Cv22 Sp6

Chronic Bronchitis
B13 Cv22 Cv12 K27 L5 S36
or B12 B10 G21 L9 Cv6 S40
Moxa B10 B13 Gv10 Cv22 Cv17 B20 Cv12 S36 S40

Bronchiectasis
B13 B16 B20 S40 Cv12 Cv6 S36

Bronchial Asthma
B13 B16 Cv22 Cv17 G21 Cv12 Cv6 L7 S36 Sp6
Moxa after initial improvement by needles as above B13 B16 Gv12 Gv10
Cv6 S36

Bronchopneumonia Primary treatment by antibiotics. Acupuncture only
of secondary importance.
G20 B11 Gv12 B13 B17 Li11 Li4 S36 S44 T5 Si3 S40 Liv2

Lobar Pneumonia Antibiotics are primary treatment..Acupuncture is only
supportive.
With headache and fever G20 B12 B13 Li11 T5 Li4 B60 S44 Liv2

With fever and thirst Gv14 Gv12 B12 B13 B17 Li11 T5 Li4 Li1 K7 H9 S44 Liv2

With cough and pain in chest L5 L9 Li4 Cv12 Liv13 S36 G34 Sp6

Emphysema
B13 B15 B37 L5 Cv12 S36 Sp6
or B12 B16 B38 Li11 Cv6 S40 L9
Moxa B13 B37 B16 B38 B23 G33

Tuberculosis Drug treatment primary, acupuncture secondary.
Use only 5 acupuncture points, as patients are often weak.
With fever Gv14 Gv12 B14 P5 K7
High fever add Li11 Li5 Li4 Sp6 Liv2 S44
Cough B13 B16 B38 L5 L9
Unproductive cough add Cv22 Sp6
Pain due to cough K27 L1 Cv17 Cv13 Cv11 Cv6 S36
Productive cough B20 Cv12 S40
Spontaneous sweating H6 Si3 May add Sp6 K7
Haemoptysis L5 L7 If severe add B17 Li1 Liv2
Diarrhoea B25 S25 Cv6 S37
Headache, backache, pain in throat. Treat local symptoms.
Anorexia Cv12 S36
When patient is better use Moxa B13 B16 Gv12 Cv4 S36

Pleurisy
Headache and fever G20 B12 Gv13 L5 T5 Li4 G34
Dry pleurisy Gv12 B12 any tender points over ribs L5 L9 G34 G41
Wet pleurisy. Same as dry pleurisy but add B13 B15 B16 B18 Sp9 Sp6
If temperature down but chest still painful—chronic type Gv14 Gv13 Gv10 Gv9 B18 Cv9 G34 Liv13 Sp6

Hydrothorax
B13 B15 B18 B23 B25 B27 Cv6 Sp9 Sp6
Use thin needle on vertebrae T4 to L4 and ribs below T6

CARDIOVASCULAR AND BLOOD DISEASES

Angina Pectoris
G20 B11 G21 B15 B18 L4 L5 P6
If patient has an attack of angina pectoris during treatment use

Acute Endocarditis
L4 Li11 P6 H7 Sp6 K1 Liv3 S42

Valvular Disease
G20 G21 B11 B15 Cv12 Cv6
or B10 B12 B28 B16 Cv11 Cv4
For oedema B23 B32 S36 Sp6 B22 B27 Sp9 K7

Acute Myocarditis
B11 B12 Gv12 B13 Si8 P7

Fatty Heart
G20 G21 B11 B15 Cv12 Cv6 T5 S36
or B10 B12 B38 B16 Cv11 Cv4 S37

Palpitations
G20 G21 B12 B15 P7 S36
or B10 B11 B14 B16 P6 Cv12 Cv6 Sp6

Arteriosclerosis (Liver Yang)
G20 G21 B38 B15 B23 S25 S28 Li15 Li10 G31 S36 Sp6 B60 S41

Shoulder Pain
G20 B11 Si14 Si13 Li15 Li11 Local painful points

Anaemia
B17 B20 B22 B25 Cv4 S36
With tinnitus Si19 T17
With vertigo, headache G20 XH3 S8 T23
With palpitations B15 Cv11
With nausea and vomiting Cv13 Cv12

Chlorosis-Anaemia
Gv20 B10 Gv12 Gv9 B20 B22 Cv4 S36 Sp6

Leukaemia
B20 B18 B17 B22 Gv4 Cv4 S36

Mouth Ulcers and Monilia
XM2 Cv23 S6 S4 Li10 Li4 P7 S44
With fever G20 Gv12 Li11

Aphthous Stomatitis
G20 B10 Gv12 Cv24 Cv23 S4 Li11 Li4 T2

Tonsillitis
Acute G20 B10 B11 L5 L11 Li1
Chronic B10 B11 L10 T2

Mumps
G20 B11 Li11 B10 T5 Li4 T2

Sialorrhea
G20 B10 S6 S4 Cv23

Toothache
S7 Li4
Supplementary points G20 B12

Acute Pharyngitis
G20 B10 B11 Li10 Li4 L11 Li1 K3

Chronic Pharyngitis
B10 B11 Gv12 B17 B18 Li17 Cv23 T2 L10

Oesophagitis
B11 B12 Si15 Gv12 G21 Cv22 Cv17 Cv13 Li10 S36 P6 S44

Stricture of Oesophagus
B11 G21 B14 B17 Cv22 Cv17 Cv13 P6 Li10 S36 S40

Spasm of Oesophagus
G20 B11 B13 Cv17 Cv13 Cv6 Cv3 P3 S36 Sp6
or B10 G21 B14 Cv18 Cv14 Cv4 P6 Sp8

Paralysis of Oesophagus
G20 B10 Si15 G21 B13 B15 B18

Acute Gastritis
B17 B19 B21 Cv22 Cv12 Li10 P6 S36 Sp4

Chronic Gastritis
B18 B21 Cv13 Cv11 S19 S21 P6 S36
or B20 B22 Cv12 S20 S23 S37 Sp4

Gastric Spasm
B18 B20 B22 Cv12 Cv6 S36 S44
or B19 B21 B23 Cv11 S37 Liv2

Dilation of Stomach
B18 B20 B22 Cv14 Cv12 S19 S21 S36
or B19 B21 Cv13 S20 Cv11 S37

Gastric Ulcer
G20 B11 B17 B19 B20 S36
or B10 G21 B18 B21 B22 S37

Gastroptosis
B10 B11 B17 B18 B20 B22 S20 S21

Nervous Dyspepsia
B10 B17 B20 B22 Cv13 Cv11 Cv6 S36
or B11 B18 B21 B44 Cv14 Cv12 S37

Neurogenic Vomiting
G20 B10 B21 K21 Cv12 P3 Cv11 S44 Liv3

Gastric Hyperacidity
B10 B11 B17 B18 B20 Cv12 S25 S36

Atony of Stomach
B18 B20 B22 Cv13 Cv12 Cv10 S19 S21 S36

Acute Entero-Colitis
Duodenitis B16 B17 B18 G24 Cv12 S25 S39 G41
Enteritis B22 B24 B25 Cv11 S25 Cv6 Li11 Li4 S37 S44

Colitis B22 B24 B25 B27 S25 Li10 S36 Li4 S37 S44
Proctitis B25 B27 B29 B30 B32 L5 Li4 S36 S44

Chronic Entero-Colitis
B22 B24 B25 Cv12 S25 Cv6 S28 S36

Appendicitis
Sp10 B54 Sp9 Sp8 Sp6 Liv2 T10 Li11 Li4 Appendix point S36.5

Intestinal Tuberculosis—only early stage
B20 B22 B24 B25 S25 Cv6 S36 Sp6

Intestinal Hernia?
Cv6 S25 S36 Sp6 Liv2
or B20 B22 B24 B25 S25 Cv4 S37 S36 Sp6

Constipation
Atonic B22 B24 B25 S25 Sp16 Cv3 T6 S36 Liv1
Habitual B25 B27 B33 S25 K16 S26 Cv9 T6 S36 B57 Sp3

Duodenal Ulcer
B11 B17 B18 B20 K21 S21 Cv12 P6 S36

Diarrhoea
B22 B25 S34 S25 Cv6 S36

Spastic Colitis
B24 B25 B31 S25 Cv6 S27 S28 S37

Proctitis
B31 B32 B29 Li10 Li4 S36 Sp6 Liv2

Haemorrhoids
Gv1 Gv3 B33 the two whites Sp6

Peritonitis (mediocre results)
Sp10 S36 Sp6 Liv2

Ascites (variable results)
B15 B22 B24 Cv9 Cv4 S28 Sp9 G38 Sp6 Liv2 G41
or B18 B23 B26 S25 Cv6 S27 Sp8 S36 S39 G39 K7 S44 Liv3

Cirrhosis
B16 B18 B20 B23 Liv14 Liv9 Sp9
or B17 B19 B22 B24 Liv13 Sp10 Sp6

Infectious Jaundice
Gv12 Gv9 B20 B43 B45 Li10 Si4 S36 S40 S44

Jaundice
B11 B17 B18 B20 B42 B43 Gv12 Gv9 Sp6

Biliary Colic
B18 B19 Si4 G34 G41 Liv2

Splenomegaly
B18 B20 B44 Cv12 Liv13 Cv6 S36

GENITO-URINARY DISEASES

Acute Nephritis
B10 B12 B23 B25 B31 Liv13 T5 Li4 Sp9 Sp6

Chronic Nephritis
B22 B24 B25 B31 Cv6 S36 Sp9
or B23 B26 B32 S25 Cv4 Sp6

Pyelitis
B23 B25 B54 Sp10 S36 Sp6 K5

Cystitis
B25 B19 B31 B33 S36 Sp10 Sp9 Sp6

Haematuria
B23 B27 Cv6 Cv4 P7 L7 K7

Paralysis of Bladder
G33 B32 B33 Cv4 Cv3 Cv2

Spasm of Bladder
B25 B32 Cv6 Cv4 K10 G37 Liv8 Sp6 Liv3

Bladder Stone
B23 B28 Cv6 Cv4 Cv3 Sp9 Sp6

Nocturnal Enuresis
Gv20 B23 Gv4 Cv4

Stress Incontinence
Gv20 Gv4 B33 Cv4

Urethritis
Cv4 L7 Liv8 Sp6

Impotence
Gv20 B17 B21 B23 Gv4 Gv3 Cv4 Cv3

Nocturnal Emission
B15 B23 Gv3 Cv4 Cv1 Sp6

Orchitis
Li10 Li4 Liv8 Sp6 Liv4 Liv1

Prostatitis
Acute Cv6 Sp10 Sp9 Sp6 L9 K3
Chronic Gv2 Cv3 Gv20 K12 Sp6

Gonorrhoea
Acute B27 Cv6 Liv8 Sp6 Liv2 Li4
Chronic B27 B33 Cv3 Cv2 Sp6

DISEASES OF THE NERVOUS SYSTEM

Cerebral Anaemia
Gv20 G20 B20 Cv4 S36

Hypertensive Encephalopathy
G20 B10 Gv26 Li4 Li1 B60 B67
Mild paralysis of face, hand and leg Gv20 G20 T17 Li15 G34 S6 S7 S4

Cerebral Haemorrhage or Thrombosis
G20 B10 B11 G21 Li15 Li11 Li4 G30 G34 Sp6 B60

Chronic Headache
General points used in all varieties G20 B11 Li4 B62
Summit headache add Gv20 Gv21 Gv19 Si3
Frontal headache add Gv23 G14 S40 S44
Supraorbital headache add B2 G14 XH3
Unilateral headache add S8 XH3 G5 G4 G41

Cerebral Arterio-Sclerosis
Gv20 G21 Gv14 Li15 Li4 G38 B60 Liv2

Migraine
G20 S1 XH3 S7 S40 B60
Supplementary G15 G12 T22 G5 G6 B12 B14 T17 Cv13 Cv12 G41 L7 Liv2

Epilepsy with Fever
Cramps with fever, uraemia, plumbism, eclampsia, pneumonia in children, measles, acute fever, indigestion, intestinal parasites, teething.
G20 B10 Gv12 Cv13 (Cv10 and S25 not in pregnancy) Li11 Li1 S36 S45

Grand and Petit Mal, Violent Madness and Non-Violent Madness
G20 B13 B15 Cv15 Cv12 Cv6 H7 S40 Sp6
Don't exhaust oneself; no smoking; no drinking; restrict meat, especially beef, lamb, chicken; preferably vegetarian diet; reduce sex.

Writer's Cramp and similar conditions
G20 Li11 T5 T4 Li4 Si3

Carpo-Pedal Spasm
Hand Li11 L6 Li4 P7
Foot B60 S41 G41 S43

Chorea
G20 Gv14 Li11 T5 Li4 Si3
or B10 Gv12 Li10 G38 B60 S41

Athetosis
Hand Li11 L5 P7 P8 Si3 Li4
Foot S41 B60 K6 B63 K1

Parkinson's Disease
G20 Gv12 Gv4 Cv12 Cv4 L5 Si3
or B10 B11 Gv9 Cv13 Cv6 L6 B62

Travel Sickness
G20 B10 Cv12 Cv6 S36 S40 S44

Polyneuritis
Hand T5 P7 Li4 Si3 knuckles
Feet S41 B60 K6 toe knuckles

Occipital Neuralgia
G20 B11 G12 T5 Li4 S40 B60

Trigeminal Neuralgia
G20 T17 S7 Li10 Li4
Add for 1st division G14 B2
Add for 2nd   ,,   XH3 S2 S3
Add for 3rd   ,,   S5 S6

*Radial Nerve Neuralgia
B11 Si14 Li12 Li5 B10 Si13 T12 Li10 Li4

Median Nerve Neuralgia
B10 Si13 P2 P4 P6

Ulnar Nerve Neuralgia
B10 Si13 H2 H6 H8

Anterior Thoracic Nerve Neuralgia
B10 Si13 S13 S15 L5 B11 Li15 S14 S16 S36

Long Thoracic Nerve Neuralgia
B11 Si14 L1 Sp19 Sp17 L5

Suprascapular Nerve Neuralgia
B11 Si14 Si12 T10 Si15 Si13 Si10 H3

Upper Subscapular Nerve Neuralgia
Si13 Si10 Si11 Li15

* Neuralgia, paralysis or spasm of a named nerve refers to:
1. Pain in the approximate distribution of this nerve.
2. Muscle weakness of the muscles innervated by this nerve.
3. Muscle spasm or cramps of the muscles innervated by the named nerve. The areas described are only very approximate.

Circumflex Nerve Neuralgia
Li15 Si9 H1 T12

Intercostal Neuralgia
B11 B12 B13 B15 B18 K22 K25 L5 L9

Lumbago
B22 B25 B47 G26 G30 S31
or B23 B27 B46 G28 G29 Liv11

Sciatica (stationary pain)
B23 B25 Sp11 Sp9 Sp6 K4 Sp2

Sciatica (moving pain)
B32 G30 B50 B51 B54 G34 B55 Sp6 B60

Lateral Cutaneous Nerve of the Thigh Neuralgia
G30 G31 G32 G34

Obturator Nerve Neuralgia
Liv10 Sp11 Liv8 Sp6 Liv11 Liv9 K6 Sp9

Pudendal Nerve Neuralgia
B23 B25 B31 B32 Cv1 Sp6 Liv2

Joint Pain without Swelling
Knee XL2 B54 S33 G34 Sp6 B60
Wrist T4 Si5 Li5 Li4 T3 T5

Facial Palsy
S7 S6 S4 Cv24 Li4

Mandibular Nerve Paralysis
Gv20 G20 T17 T21 S6 S7 S4 Li4

Sublingual Nerve Paralysis
G20 B10 G21 Li17 Cv23 P7 H5

Strabismus
G20 B10 T17 XH3 B1 G5 Si6

Torticollis
G12 T16 Si16 G21 Si4 Si8

Radial Nerve Paralysis
G21 Li15 Li11 Li9 T4 L10 Li3
or Li16 T13 Li10 L6 Li5 L11 Li4

Median Nerve Paralysis
B10 Si15 G21 L3 P3 P4 P7 P8

Ulnar Nerve Paralysis
Si15 G21 Si13 T14 T10 Si8 Si7 H7 Si3

Long Thoracic Nerve Paralysis
B10 Si14 L1 Sp19 P1

Rhomboid Nerve Paralysis
B11 Si15 Si13 B13 B36 Li11
or Si14 G21 Si12 Si10 B12 T10

Upper Subscapular Nerve Paralysis
Si13 Si9 Li15 Li11 Si11 Si10 T14 T13

Circumflex Nerve Paralysis
B10 B11 Li15 T14 Li16 Li11

Paralysis of Diaphragm
B17 B18 G25 Liv13 S19 Cv6 S36 Sp6

Anterior Thoracic Nerve Paralysis
B10 B11 Si15 K27 K25 K23 S14 S16

Paralysis of Abdominal Muscles
Gv4 Gv3 B20 B22 B23 B25 Cv12 Cv6 S36 Sp6

Paralysis of Thigh
B23 B25 B31 B20 S33 Liv8 Sp4 Sp9

Obturator Nerve Paralysis
B23 B25 B29 G30 B50 B54 B57 Sp6
or B26 B32 B49 B51 B57 G34 G38 S41

Tibial Nerve Paralysis
B25 B31 B50 Sp11 Sp9 Sp6 K3
or B26 B32 Sp9 Liv8 B57 K6 Sp5

Peroneal Nerve Paralysis
B25 B32 G30 S36 G38 B60 B65
or B26 B31 B49 G34 B59 B62 B67

Facial Tic
G20 B10 T17 Li10 Li4

Sublingual Nerve Spasm
G20 B10 Gv16 Cv23 Li10 P7

Mandibular Nerve Spasm
G20 B10 T17 S7 S6 T5 S45

Spasm of Neck Muscles
G20 B10 G12 Li10 Si4

Spasm of Gastrocnemius
B57 B60

Hiccough
S10 Cv17 Cv14 Cv4

Spasm of Diaphragm
Cv14 Liv14 P6

Polyneuritis
Use local points as in sections on neuralgia and paralysis.
Add Gv14 Gv12 Gv9 B14 B16 Li11 T5 G34 B60

Beri-Beri
G31 S32 S35 XL2 S36 S37 S39 G39 G21 B15 B20 B23 B26 Cv9 Sp9 Sp6

Angio-Neurotic Oedema
Gv12 B17 B18 B25 Li15 Li11 Sp10 Sp6

Neurasthenia
G20 B11 B15 B22 Cv4 P6 S36
or B10 Gv12 B14 B23 Cv6 H5 Sp6

Violent Madness
Cv15 Cv12 Gv26 L11 Sp1 P7 B62 Gv16 S6 Cv24 P8 Gv23 H7 S36 S40

Non-Violent Madness—Singing, crying, happy, sad, senseless talk, cannot distinguish clean from dirty, lives in dream world, likes to sleep, behaves as drunk or crazy.
Cv15 G20 B13 B18 H7 Li4 Cv12 Cv6 S36 S40
or Cv13 B10 B15 B17 Si3 P4 H5 Cv4 S37 Sp6

Hysteria
B13 B15 B22 B32 Cv12 Cv4 Sp6
Treat every 2 or 3 days
If epileptic-like attack during treatment Cv17 Cv12 Cv6 P7

RHEUMATIC DISEASES

Acute and Chronic Rheumatoid Arthritis
Gv14 B11 Li15 Li11 T5 Li4
Plus local points 3 to 6 cm away from pain

Muscular Rheumatism
In loin B22 B24 B46 B31 B54
or B23 B25 B47 B32 S36
In neck G20 B10 Si15 Si14 T10 Si4
In scapular and interscapular area B36 B13 B39 B15 B40 B42
or B37 B12 B38 B14 B41 B18
In shoulders Li16 T15 Li15 Li14 T13 T14
Of pectoralis major and minor S13 S15 Sp20 G23 Li10 G34
or S14 S16 Sp19 Sp21 Li11 S36

Arthritis of Knee
S33 Liv8 Liv7 XL2 G34 Sp6 Sp9

Myositis
Gv14 Gv12 B20 Li11 T5 Li4 S36 Sp6

Gout
B23 B24 B19 Cv4 Sp6
Plus local points

Paget's Disease
Gv12 Gv9 Gv8 B13 B15 B20 B22 Li10 S36 Sp6

Vaginitis and Leucorrhoea
B32 Cv3 K12 Sp10 Sp6 Liv4 B31/4

Pruritis Vulvae
B25 B32 Gv1 Cv3 S30 Sp10 Sp6 B31/4

Acute and Chronic Endometritis
B23 B25 B32 B35 Liv8 Sp7 K4 B24 B27 B33 B30 Sp10 Sp6 Sp5

Acute and Chronic Metritis
B23 B31 Gv2 Cv3 Sp10 S37 Sp8 B24 B33 B35 Cv2 Sp9 S39 Sp6

Perimetritis
B31 B33 Cv6 S36 Sp6 Sp5 Sp3

Cancer of Cervix and Body of Womb (only secondary to radium etc.)
Cv4 Cv3 Cv2 B32 B33 B34 Gv2

Myoma
B32 (deep) Cv3 Liv5 Sp6 Liv2
or B33 (deep) Cv2 Liv6 K8 Liv3
If anaemic B17 B20 Cv4

Spasm of Uterus
B32 B33 S25 Cv6 S29 Cv2 Sp6

Abnormal Uterine Bleeding and Menorrhagia
Sp6 Sp1

Oophoritis
Acute S25 G26 Sp6
Chronic B24 B25 S25 K15 G26 S27 Sp6

Mastitis—particularly due to injury from breast feeding, not abscesses
S16 S18 G21 P3 S37 Liv3

Breast Pain—due to: too much milk, injury, anaemia, sex diseases, hysteria
B18 S14 S16 S18 Cv17 P1 H3

Nausea and Vomiting of Pregnancy
G20 B18 B25 B32 Cv17 S19 K15
or B10 B19 B27 B33 Cv16 S20 G26

Habitual Abortion
Gv4 B23 Gv3 S28 S36 Sp6

Dysmenorrhoea
Cv4 Cv3 S27 S28 Sp10 Sp6

Amenorrhoea
Gv4 B26 B32 Gv4 G26 Sp8 G33
or B23 B33 Gv3 K15 Sp6

DISEASES OF CHILDREN

Epileptic-Like Fits
Gv20 G20 Gv12 Li10 Li4 S36 Liv2

Pertussis
G20 Gv14 B12 Cv22 Cv13 L9 S36
alternate with B10 Gv12 B13 K27 Cv12 L8 S40

Meningitis
G20 Gv14 Gv7 B23 S25 S36
alternate with B10 Gv12 Gv4 B22 Cv6 G34

ENDOCRINE DISEASES

Goitre and Myxoedema
G20 Gv14 B11 Cv22 S10 Gv4 T3
or B10 Gv12 B12 Cv23 S9 Gv3 G26

Addison's Disease
B22 B23 both 2 Chinese inches deep Gv6 Gv5 S25 Sp14

Diabetes—mild
B13 B18 B20 B23 Cv23 Cv12 Cv4 L9 H7 Sp6 K2

Diabetes Insipidus
B22 B24 B23 Cv4

DISEASES OF THE EYES

Conjunctivitis
G20 B2 B1 XH3 Li4 G37

Night Blindness
B18 B19 G20 B1 Li4 S36
or B42 B43 G12 B2 Li10 G37

Blepharitis
B2 B1 S2 G1 Mid dorsal surface of interphalangeal joint of thumb, mid dorsal surface of proximal interphalangeal joint of little finger, prick eyelids till blood flows.

Dacryocystitis
B2 B1 S2 G14 B18 B22 G8

Trachoma
G14 B2 G1 G20 B18 Si19 G37 G42

EAR, NOSE AND THROAT DISEASES

Otitis Media
G20 T17 T21 Li11 Li4
Better result when surgery and acupuncture combined

Sinusitis
G20 Si15 Gv23 Li20 Li10 Li4 B17

Hay Fever, Allergic Rhinorrhoea, Influenza
G20 B10 Gv23 Li20 Li4
In chronic cases add Gv20 B7 Gv23 B12

Epistaxis
G20 Si15 Gv23 Li4 S36 Liv3

Dysentery (only assists medical treatment)
B25 B29 Li4 S37 Gv14 Gv12

Typhoid (before fluid loss only)
XA1 B54 L5 Cv13 Cv12 Cv6 S25 S36 B57

Bubonic Plague (helped in outbreak in Fookin province in Sino-Japanese war 1940)
Pierce skin with three-cornered needle over axillary and groin glands, till blood flows. L5 B54 Li11 Li4 T5 S36 S44 XA1 all till blood flows.

Meningitis (Subsidiary treatment. Reduces intracranial pressure and muscle spasm).
Gv8 Gv8.5 Gv9 G20 B11 to 19 Cv21 Cv17 Cv13 Cv12 Cv10 Li11 Li4 Li1 L11 P9 H9 Si1 T1 K1 B67 Liv1 G44 S45 Sp1 B54 B57 B60 Liv2 S44 all just pricked without leaving needle in place

Malaria (subsidiary treatment)
Gv14 P5 Si3 K7
In chronic cases add B20 B23 Gv4 Cv4

Cold
G20 B13 Gv12 T5
With nasal symptoms add Gv23 Li4
With laryngeal symptoms add T2 L10
With bronchitis add L9 L5
For those who get colds easily B12 B13 S36 daily for one month

Influenza (symptomatic treatment)
Headache G20 G15 B2 S8
Muscular aches Li11 T5 G34 B60
Epistaxis Li4
Nose blocked Gv23
Dry cough L9
Pain in throat L10
Vomits Cv12 S36
Constipation S25
Delirious P5 S44
Body stiff Gv14 Gv12 Gv9
To reduce fever Gv14 Gv12 Li11 Li4 S36 S44

Periosteal Acupuncture

Over the past nine years I have evolved an acupuncture technique which I have christened periosteal acupuncture. It is particularly efficacious in diseases of the joints.

The technique is simple, though in some instances it requires a good knowledge of anatomy. An acupuncture or hypodermic needle is used. The needle at the appropriate place, pierces the soft tissue surrounding the joint and then stimulates the periosteum. The periosteum is 'pecked', much as a woodpecker pecks a tree, till the required degree of stimulation has been achieved.

If mild stimulation is required I use a 30 or 28-gauge stainless steel acupuncture needle and 'peck' only lightly for a short time. When stronger stimulation is appropriate a 25, 23, 21, or even 19-gauge disposable hypodermic needle may be used. The hypodermic needles being hollow are more rigid than acupuncture needles so that the 'pecking' may be done with considerable force, sometimes bending the tip of the needle. If one expects the procedure to be unduly painful (which is rare except with a calcaneal spur or occasionally with the greater trochanter or lateral epicondyle of the humerus) a local anaesthetic may be used. I use 2% xylocaine without adrenaline, injected at the surface of the periosteum. 1 cc or less is sufficient and after a delay of about a minute the more violent type of 'pecking' may commence.

In a patient who has say cervical osteoarthritis with resultant brachial neuralgia, a needle stimulating the transverse process of a lower cervical vertebra, will in the appropriate case alleviate the symptoms. If the needle does not stimulate the periosteum, but instead stimulates the overlying skin or muscles, or hits one of the nerves of the brachial plexus (producing a shooting pain down the arm), the result is in most instances not so good. I have repeatedly stimulated the skin, muscle, or a major nerve trunk over a joint and found it as a rule not as effective as when the periosteum is stimulated in the correct place.

It is well known that there are more nerve fibres and endings in the skin and periosteum than in most other tissues and hence a needle piercing the skin or periosteum hurts more than when passing through the intervening subcutaneous tissue or muscles. I assume there is a local nerve network in the periosteum surrounding the joints and innervating their structures. And I also assume that the nerves in the muscles and skin only communicate with the periosteal nerve network somewhat sparsely. This theory could explain why stimulating the periosteum of joints has a greater effect than pricking the skin. On the other hand, if a disease does not involve a joint, stimulating the skin or periosteum have an equal effect for an equal strength of stimulation.

I would be interested to hear of any histological or physiological research that has been done concerning the above theory.

Whether or not the conditions mentioned below respond, depends mainly on the degree and reversibility of the pathological changes. Although the intra-articular bone rarely regenerates, the positions of the bones relative to one another may be altered by varying the pull of the attached muscles, and hence alleviate temporarily or even permanently the patient's symptoms.

TRANSVERSE PROCESS OF LOWER CERVICAL VERTEBRAE (near Si16)

There are many patients who have pain at the back of the neck, in the occipital area, over the shoulders and down the arms to the fingers. There may be limitation of movement of the neck with crepitus.

A fairly high proportion of these patients may be helped, often even considerably, provided the main symptom is pain. When there are more objective signs, such as paraesthesia, anaesthesia, diminished reflexes, loss of muscular strength and muscle wasting, the chances of success are considerably diminished, though not hopeless—one's clinical judgement being of paramount importance. I imagine the pain is more easily alleviated than the more objective signs, as pain is produced by a milder degree of nerve root compression and hence quite often the pathology is presumably less severe. I would be interested to hear the comments of others on this theory.

The stiffness of the neck may also be alleviated, according to its pathology. Restriction of sideways movement and rotation is easier to alleviate than flexion and extension.

A 30-gauge acupuncture needle is the best. Do not use a hypodermic needle as these are sharpened in such a way as to produce a cutting edge, which cuts its way through the tissues and blood vessels and may thus produce a haematoma. An acupuncture needle is pushed through the tissue like a wedge and hence only rarely causes bleeding.

The transverse processès at the side of the neck are palpated by pressing the overlying muscles firmly against the bone. The greatest tenderness is usually at the level of the 5th or 6th cervical vertebra on the affected side.

The transverse process of maximal tenderness is selected. The needle pierces the overlying skin and muscles going in horizontally and at right angles to the neck. *For this technique, more than any other, the relevant anatomy must first be studied.**

It is often surprisingly difficult to hit the transverse process, the needle passing anteriorly or posteriorly. An accurate assessment should be made of the depth of the tip of the transverse process in each patient, and if this depth is exceeded the needle partially or totally withdrawn and reinserted to find the tip of the transverse process. The vertebra should not be 'pecked' too vigorously.

All the lower cervical vertebrae may be stimulated in the above manner. It is perhaps safer to avoid stimulating the transverse processes of the upper cervical vertebrae considering the more intricate anatomy.

GREATER TROCHANTER (G30)

Mild osteoarthritis of the hip may be alleviated for a few years by needling the greater trochanter. Total replacement of the hip joint is of course the only final answer, but often the degree of pain or limitation of movement does not warrant such a major operation. These mild cases may not too infrequently be helped, but only to a moderate degree. Often the pathology advances and something more drastic has to be done later. There are some patients with pain in the region of the hip joint with a negative X-ray. These patients can be cured, though some of them develop osteoarthritis a few years later.

Although a fine acupuncture needle may be used in the mildest cases or in hypersensitive patients, a thicker hypodermic needle is more often appropriate. Mostly I use a 21-gauge $1\frac{1}{2}''$ needle. In fat patients a 19-gauge $2''$ needle is needed. The greater trochanter apparently moves nearer the surface, thus facilitating needling, with the patient supine. On rare occasions a local anaesthetic is advised.

K5 and G40 on the opposite side may also be used. Also G30 and G26. Liv9 ipsilaterally helps groin pain on abduction.

CORACOID PROCESS (near L1)

The so-called frozen shoulder may be helped or cured by stimulating the coracoid process. If the patient can raise his arm only a few degrees, this method will not help. It is useful though in moderate and mild cases.

* The books I refer to continuously are: J. C. Boileau Grant, 'An Atlas of Anatomy', Williams & Williams, Baltimore. Johannes Sobotta, 'Atlas of Descriptive Human Anatomy', Hafner Publishing Co., New York. (In German: Urban & Schwarzenberg, Munich-Berlin). Eduard Pernkopf, 'Atlas of Topographical and Applied Human Anatomy', W. B. Saunders Co., Philadelphia. (In German: Urban & Schwarzenberg, Munich-Berlin). 'Gray's Anatomy', Longmans, London.

The tip of the coracoid process is 'pecked' with either an acupuncture needle or a 25 or 23-gauge disposable hypodermic. The needle is held horizontally and pierces the skin overlying the tip of the coracoid process.

If the above does not have an immediate effect, needling the transverse process of a tender cervical vertebra may help, for there often seems to be an association. The biceps tendon in the bicipital groove may be palpated for a tender area and needled. Otherwise one may use Li15 Si9 Si10 L5 P3.

It is also important to exercise the shoulder by asking the patient to do those movements he cannot do or finds painful. Swinging the arm in an arc that does not cause pain is in my experience useless. The painful and restricted movements should be forced to such an extent that the patient has tears in his eyes and the movements should be repeated several times a day. The exercise should not be so severe as to cause aching in the shoulder for more than a few minutes after the cessation of the exercise.

LATERAL EPICONDYLE OF HUMERUS (near Li12)

A reasonable, but not too high, proportion of patients with a tennis elbow may be helped or cured by needling the lateral epicondyle of the humerus.

The epicondyle is easiest felt with the elbow at a right angle. A 25-gauge needle is the best size.

If the above procedure does not help, needling Gv14 very strongly may help. Sometimes the neck is also implicated, in which case the appropriate tender transverse process of a cervical vertebra should be stimulated. The following may also be tried: Li4 Li14 Li15 all on the affected side.

A cortisone injection is sometimes more effective. I suspect this is due to its strong irritant properties, for the patient often has severe pain for the following two days, whilst with acupuncture the pain wears off in seconds or minutes. It could be said that cortisone injected at the correct place is no more than powerful acupuncture. It has though the disadvantage that it may cause a small localised area of necrosis, which normal acupuncture does not.

An injection of a local anaesthetic at the appropriate place is of greater benefit whilst the anaesthetic lasts, but afterwards has no greater effect than a dry needle.

If the pain is over the medial epicondyle or the olecranon process, these should instead be needled. As additional stimulation (instead of using large intestine points), one should use in the former instance heart and small intestine and in the latter instance triple warmer acupuncture points.

If the tennis elbow is due to an entrapment lesion, an operation is necessary.

CALCANEAL SPUR

The pain that may be caused by a calcaneal spur or plantar fasciitis may be cured in a high proportion of patients.

The tender area is localised with strong digital pressure on the heel. A 23 or more often 21-gauge needle is used and 1 cc of 2% xylocain is injected down to the bone. The bone is then 'pecked' with considerable strength in the case of a spur and more gently with plantar fasciites. Not infrequently the patient may have some pain for three days afterwards due to the strength of stimulation that is required for this procedure to be effective, and also presumably due to the heel being dependent and walked on. K3 K4 B62 B61 occasionally help.

SACRO-ILIAC JOINT (B26)

A large proportion of patients with low backache or sciatica may be helped by needling the sacro-iliac joint.

Mostly I ask the patient to sit in a chair and lean forwards. A 21-gauge needle is inserted in or near the dimple which overlies the joint. The needle is pushed into the joint between the sacrum and the ileum, which often necessitates touching the bone on either side of the joint till one finds the space between the bones.

This technique works (as with the transverse process of the cervical vertebrae) if the main symptom is pain in the lumbar or sacral area, or is of sciatic distribution. The chances of success are considerably diminished when there is anaesthesia, paraesthesia, muscle weakness or wasting, reduced reflexes, or there are trophic changes.

I assume acupuncture is of benefit in these conditions as it alters the tone of the lumbar muscles, thus altering the alignment of the vertebrae and hence relieves pressure on the nerve roots. I would be interested to hear of readers' comments on this.

In some instances other acupuncture points (acupuncture points do not exist—but one has to describe something) are more effective. My favourite ones at the moment are Liv3 and B62, though there is a choice of about twenty acupuncture points, depending on the distribution of pain or other symptoms and also on the findings of pulse diagnosis.

If a patient has advanced pelvic malignant disease with pain over the sacrum, but anaesthesia of the legs due to involvement of the lumbo-sacral plexus by the tumour, normal acupuncture does not work. Normally with sacral pain one might stimulate B62, but clearly this does not work when the nerve has been interrupted. In this instance an acupuncture point at the opposite end of the body such as B2 works very well.

BELOW MEDIAL CONYLE OF TIBIA (Sp9)

The majority of women have a small, tender oedematous area below the medial condyle of the tibia, a position which could be called Sp9. It is at the insertion of the medial ligament of the knee. Sometimes the tender area is 2 cm in diameter, sometimes there are one or several small areas.

The periosteum at this point may be stimulated gently or strongly according to the case.

This method is surprisingly effective in many painful conditions of the knee. Whether the pain be medial, lateral, anterior or posterior, it is the point of first choice.

Alternative points are G33 B54 peripatella points.

POSTERIOR SPINES OF LOWER LUMBAR VERTEBRAE

Skyrme Rees of Sydney considers that the pain of ordinary low backache and sciatica originates from the lumbar posterior intervertebral joints, the hypophyseal joints—this theory does not include genuine herniated intervertebral discs. The nerve supply to the posterior intervertebral joints arises from the posterior primary division of the segmental nerves, being the first extradural branch. Skyrme Rees divided the above nerves, in the appropriate segments, percutaneously, using a fine scalpel,* a method called rhizolysis.

Norman Shealy of Wisconsin, a neurosurgeon, from whom I first heard of this technique, modified Skyrme Rees' method. Under X-ray control, he inserted, percutaneously, a diathermy probe directly onto the posterior intervertebral joint.

Benjamin Cox of California, likewise a neurosurgeon, modified Norman Shealy's method, which likewise had been a modification of Skyrme Rees'. He inserted, percutaneously, under X-ray control, a dry needle and merely 'pecked' the posterior intervertebral joints.

After the above two doctors told me their methods, I tried to modify them in such a way as to be more easily applicable to the practice of a general practitioner using acupuncture:

Using a 28-gauge 2″ acupuncture needle, I needled, without X-ray control, the posterior intervertebral joint. The result was good, but difficult

---

* *The Treatment of Pain as the Major Disability* by W. Skyrme Rees 1975. Visual Abstracts (Australia) Pty., Sydney.

to perform, except in the thinnest of patients. I was also not too sure that the needle was always in the correct position.

Later I stimulated instead the lamina of the lower lumbar vertebrae: a simpler technique with equally good results.

Most recently I have merely stimulated the posterior spinous process. I ask the patient to sit on a chair, leaning forward, to produce a slight kyphosis in the lumbar area. The posterior spine is palpated and a 28-gauge 2″ acupuncture needle is inserted about one inch laterally. The needle is angled in such a way that the lateral side of the spine is stimulated, rather nearer the lamina than the tip of the spinous process. As the spinal cord terminates at L2, I only use the above technique for the lower three lumbar vertebrae. Above this level I use a modification—see below.

A comparison of the results obtained by Skyrme Rees, with the modifications of Norman Shealy, Benjamin Cox and myself is difficult, as all four methods depend to a considerable extent on the skill of the individual doctor. The experience of my own practice and the heresay of colleagues suggests the results are similar, though I know several doctors prefer one method to another.

G. S. Hackett has for many years used a related technique in which a sclerosing solution is injected into, and around, various ligaments in the lumbar and sacral area, a method called prolotherapy. Some doctors who used these sclerosing solutions for several years, have since tried my periosteal needling techniques, and have found that both methods produce similar results.

POSTERIOR SPINES OF THORACIC VERTEBRAE AND UPPER LUMBAR VERTEBRAE

The posterior spines of the above vertebrae may be stimulated by a slight modification of the technique described for the lower lumbar vertebrae. Due to the proximity of the spinal cord, I needle the lateral side of the spinous process somewhat nearer the tip of the spinous process (whilst for the lower lumbar vertebrae it was somewhat nearer the lamina). In the upper lumbar and lower thoracic region I still use a 28-gauge 2″ needle. In the upper thoracic area, where the spinous processes are nearer the surface I use a 30-gauge 1″ needle, piercing the skin only ½″ lateral to the midline.

The needle may also be inserted in the midline so that the tip of the spinous process is stimulated. At the moment I am inclined to think that the results of this method are not quite as good as when the lateral side of the spinous process is needled.

The upper lumbar and thoracic vertebrae may be stimulated in painful conditions, which one thinks are of vertebral origin and of a partially reversible nature.

Stimulating the transverse processes of the cervical vertebrae may often be used for treating pain in the head, neck and even interscapular area down to a level of T6 or 7. Treatment of the sacro-iliac joint, the ischial tuberosity or the lumbar vertebrae often helps in the ordinary types of lumbago or sciatica. Neither of the above methods though, help pain in the lower half of the thoracic area, which is best treated by stimulating the tender vertebrae. Interscapular pain, as mentioned above, is often referred from the cervical area, and should then of course be treated via the cervical vertebrae. Sometimes interscapular pain is of upper thoracic origin, in which case the appropriate thoracic vertebrae should be treated.

ISCHIAL TUBEROSITY

The patient is asked to sit on a chair and lean as far foward as possible. A second chair may be placed in front of him so that the patient may lean his arms or head on it. The ischial tuberosity is palpated and 'pecked' with a 28-gauge 2″ needle.

This method helps selected patients with low backache and suprisingly enough patients with pain in the knee. On a few ocassions it helps coccydynia, though at the time of writing I still do not have a satisfactory answer for most cases.

TEMPERO-MANDIBULAR JOINT

The patient is asked to open and close his mouth several times, so that the head of the mandible may be palpated, and most particularly the joint space above it identified. A 30-gauge 1″ needle is inserted into the joint space.

This technique may be used in patients with mild pain in the tempero-mandibular joint. Sometimes orthodontic treatment is more satisfactory.

Catarrh of the eustachian tube occasionally responds.

There are some patients who have pain below the eye, along or just below the inferior orbital margin. This may respond to needling the tempero-mandibular joint, suggesting it is pain referred from this joint. On a few occasions even pain anywhere in the cheek, or mandible may respond, possibly even supraorbital pain.

FIRST METACARPO-PHALANGEAL JOINT

Osteoarthritis may develop in the joint, with a tender nodule over its lateral aspect. Sometimes local needling helps.

LIVER AND ABDOMINAL SYMPTOMS

One of the commonest symptoms I treat are patients who are 'livery'. I use the word in its French rather than in the Anglo-Saxon sense, which is described in detail in my book *Meridians of Acupuncture*.

This may not infrequently be helped by needling the periosteum or perichondrium of the lower ribs. I usually stimulate in the mid-nipple line between the inferior margin of the breast and the lower costal margin. The nearest, non-existent acupuncture point, would be liver 14.

If the patient's symptoms involve the lower abdomen, the anterior superior iliac spine may be pecked. Sometimes the rib point mentioned above as well as the anterior superior iliac spine are needled.

STERNUM, MANUBRIUM, ANTERIOR RIBS

The above may be stimulated in mild conditions of the chest involving bronchospasm.

Usually I needle the sternum or manubrium anywhere in the midline. Sometimes I needle in the region of the costo-chondral junction of the 2nd and 3rd ribs.

The needling of ribs may easily be performed in thin patients whose ribs can be palpated. Unless one is completely sure that one has been able to isolate a rib between two fingers, the procedure should not be performed.

APPENDIX

Atlas of Acupuncture

Points and meridians in relation to
Surface Anatomy

The Atlas is reproduced here in much reduced
format. The full size version printed in two
colours can be obtained from the publishers.

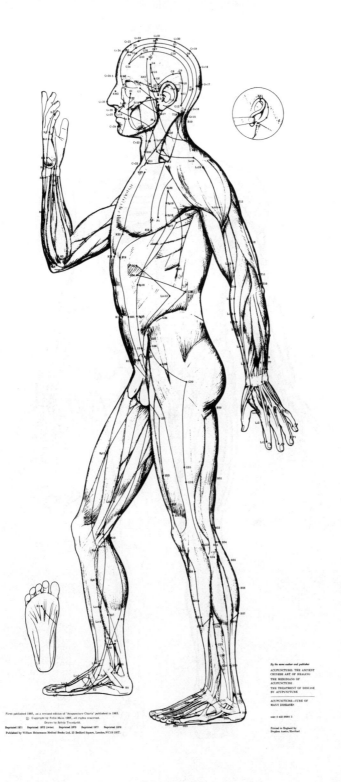

First published 1965, as a revised edition of 'Acupuncture Charts' published in 1962.
© Copyright by Felix Mann 1965, all rights reserved.
Drawn by Sylvia Treadgold.

Reprinted 1971   Reprinted 1972 (twice)   Reprinted 1972   Reprinted 1977   Reprinted 1979

Published by William Heinemann Medical Books Ltd, 23 Bedford Square, London, WC1B 3HT.

By the same author and publisher

ACUPUNCTURE: THE ANCIENT
CHINESE ART OF HEALING

THE MERIDIANS OF
ACUPUNCTURE

THE TREATMENT OF DISEASE
BY ACUPUNCTURE

ACUPUNCTURE—CURE OF
MANY DISEASES

ISBN 0 433 20301 3

Printed in England by
Stephen Austin/Hertford

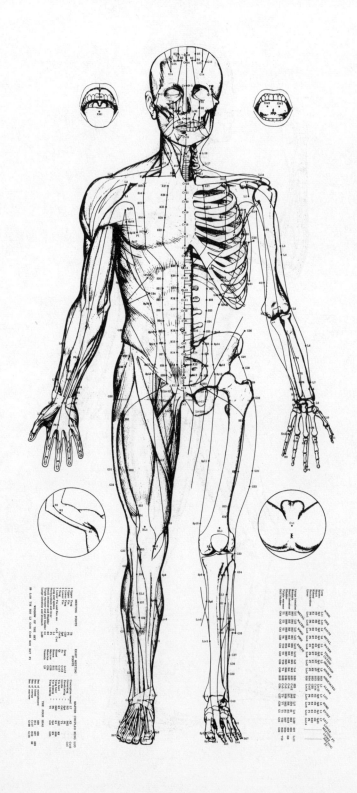

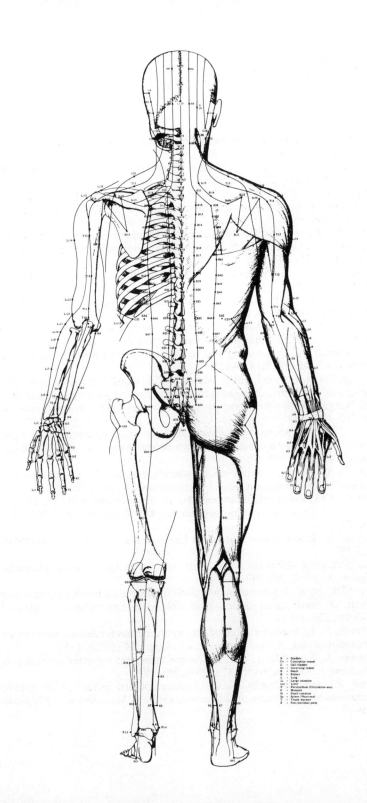

B   = Bladder
Cv = Conception vessel
G   = Gall bladder
Gv = Governing vessel
H   = Heart
K   = Kidney
L   = Lung
Li = Large intestine
Liv = Liver
P   = Pericardium (Circulation-sex)
S   = Stomach
Si = Small intestine
Sp = Spleen (Pancreas)
T   = Triple warmer
X   = Non-meridian point

REFERENCES
compiled by Alexander Macdonald

Acupuncture and Myofascial Pain

Arroyo, P. Jr. Electromyography in the evaluation of reflex muscle spasm, *J. Florida M.A.*, **53** (1966), 29–31.

Awad, E. A. Interstitial myofibrositis: hypothesis of the mechanism, *Arch. Phys. Med.*, **54** (1973), 449–453.

Dimitrijevic, M. R. and Nathan, P. W. Studies of spasticity in man, 3. Analysis of reflex activity evoked by noxious cutaneous stimulation, *Brain*, **91** (1968), 349–368.

Dorigo, B., Bartoli, V. *et al*. Fibrositic myofascial pain in intermittent claudication, effect of anaesthetic block of trigger points on exercise tolerance, *Pain*, **6** (1979) 183–190.

Dorrington, K. L. Skin turgor: do we understand the clinical sign? *Lancet*, i (1981), 264–266.

Edeiken, J., Wolferth, C. C. Persistent pain in shoulder region following myocardial infarction, *Am. J. Med. Sci.*, **191** (1936), 201–210.

Francini, Fabio, Zoppi, Massimo, Maresca, Marco and Procacci, Paolo. Skin potential and EMG changes induced by cutaneous electrical stimulation. I. Normal nan in arousing and non-arousing environment, *Appl. Neurophysiol.*, **42** (1979), 113–124.

Procacci, Paolo, Francini, Fabio, Maresca, Marco and Zoppi, Massimo. Skin potential and EMG changes induced by cutaneous electrical stimulation. II. Subjects with reflex sympathetic dystrophies, *Appl. Neurophysiol.*, **42** (1979), 125–134.

Gunn, C. C., Ditchburn, F. G., King, M. H. *et al*. Acupuncture loci: a proposal for their relationship to known neural structures, *Am. J. Chinese Med.*, **4** (1976), 183–195.

Gunn, C. C. Transcutaneous neural stimulation. Needle acupuncture and 'Teh Ch'i' phenomenon, *Am. J. Acupuncture*, **4** (1976), 317–321.

Gunn, C. C. Utilizing trigger points, *Am. J. Acupuncture*, **5** (1977), 29–34.

Gunn, C. C. Type IV acupuncture points, *Am. J. Acupuncture*, **5** (1977), 51–52.

Gunn, C. C. Motor points and motor lines, *Am. J. Acupuncture*, **6** (1978), 55–58.

Gunn, C. C. and Milbrandt, W. E. Early and subtle signs in low-back sprain, *Spine*, **3** (1978), 267–281.

Gunn, C. C. *et. al*. Dry needling of muscle motor points for chronic low-back pain. A randomized clinical trial with long-term follow-up, *Spine*, **5** (1980), 279–281.

Hagbarth, K. E. Excitatory and inhibitory skin areas for flexor and extensor motorneurones, *Acta. Physiol. Scand. Suppl.* 94 (1952), 1–54.

Hagbarth, K. E. and Kerr, D. I. B. Central influences on spinal afferent conduction, *J. Neurophysiol.*, **17** (1954), 295–307.

Eldred, E. and Hagbarth, K. E. Facilitation and inhibition of gamma efferents by stimulation of certain skin areas, *J. Neurophysiol.*, **17** (1954), 59–65.

Kukelberg, E. and Hagbarth, K. E. Spinal mechanism of the abdominal and erector spinae skin reflexes, *Brain*, **81** (1958) 280–304.

Hagbarth K. E. Spinal withdrawal reflexes in the human lower limbs, *J. Neurol. Neurosurg. Psychiat.*, **23** (1960), 222–227.

Eble, J. N. Reflex relationships of paravertebral muscles, *Am. J. Physiol.*, **200** (1961), 939–943.

Hay, K. M. The treatment of pain trigger areas in migraine, *J. Roy. Coll. Gen. Pract.*, **26** (1976), 372–376.

Kraft, G. H., Johnson, E. W. and LaBan, M. M. The fibrositis syndrome, *Arch. Phys. Med.*, **49** (1968), 155–162.

MacConnaill, M. A. The movements of bones and joints. 2. Function of the musculature, *J. Bone Jnt. Surg.*, **31–B** (1949), 100–104.

Macdonald, A. J. R. Abnormally tender muscle regions and associated painful movements, *Pain*, **8** (1980), 197–205.

McCloskey, D. I. Kinesthetic sensibility, *Phys. Rev.*, **58, 4** (1978), 763–820.

Melzack, R., Stillwell, D. M., Fox, E. J. Trigger points and acupuncture points for pain: correlations and implications, *Pain*, **3** (1977), 3–23.

Mennet, P., Ulrych, I., Ulrych, J. *et al. Muscle Relaxant Therapy in Fibrositis Syndrome*, Proc. Int. Symp. 'Spasticity—a Topical Survey' (ed. W. Birkmayer) Vienna, 6th April, 1971.

Mense, S. Muscular nociceptors, *J. Physiol. Paris*, **73** (1977), 233–240.

Moldofsky, H., Scarisbrick P., England, R. and Smythe, H. Musculoskeletal symptoms and non-REM sleep disturbance in patients with 'fibrositis syndrome' and healthy subjects, *Psychosomatic Med.*, **37** (1975), 341–351.

Moldofsky, H. and Scarisbrick, P. Induction of neurasthenic musculoskeletal pain syndrome by selective sleep stage deprivation, *Psychosomatic Med.*, **38, No. 1** (January–February 1976), 35.

Moldofsky, H. *Rheumatic Pain Modulation Syndrome: The Inter-Relationships between Sleep, Central Nervous System Serotonin and Pain.* Proc. Int. Cong. Florence, 1980. F. Sicutari, S. Gurini, A. Friedman, Raven Press.

Smythe, H. A. 'Fibrositis' as a disorder of pain modulation, *Clin. Rheum. Dis.*, **5, No. 3** (December 1979), 823.

Scott, D. S., Lundeen, T. F. Myofascial pain involving the masticatory muscles: an experimental model, *Pain*, **8** (1980), 207–215.

Simons, D. G. Muscle pain syndromes—Part I (Special Review), *Am. J. Phys. Med.*, **Vol. 54, Pt. 6** (1975), 289–311.

Simons, D. G. Muscle pain syndromes—Part II (Special Review), *Am. J. Phys. Med.*, **Vol. 55, Pt. 1** (1976), 15–42.

Simons, D. G. Electrogenic nature of palpable bands and 'jump sign' associated with myofascial trigger points, *Adv. Pain Res. Therapy*, **Vol. I** (1976).

Taverner, D. Muscle spasm as a cause of somatic pain, *Ann.Rheum. Dis.*, **13** (1954), 331–335.

Travell, J., Berry, C. and Bigelow, N. Effects of referred somatic pain on structures in the reference zone. *Am. Physiol. Soc., Fed. Proc.*, **3** (1944), 49.

Travell, J. Basis for the multiple uses of local block of somatic trigger areas (procaine infiltration and ethyl chloride spray), *Miss. Valley Med. J.*, **71** (1949), 13–21.

Travell, J., Rinzler, S. H. The myofascial genesis of pain, *Postgrad. Med.*, **Vol. II, No. 5** (1952), 425–434.

Travell, J. Ethyl chloride spray for painful muscle spasm, *Arch. Phys. Med.*, **May** (1952), 291–298.

Travell, J. Assessment of drugs for therapeutic efficacy, *A. J. Phys. Med.*, **34** (1955), 129–140.

Travell, J. Factors affecting pain of injection, *J. Am. Med. Assoc.*, **158** (1955), 368–371.

Weeks, V. D., Travell, J. Postural vertigo due to trigger areas in the sterno-cleidomastoid muscle, *J. Paediat.*, **47** (1955), 315–327.

Travell, J. *Symposium on Mechanism and Management of Pain Syndromes*, Proc. Rudolf Virchow Medical Soc., **16** (1957), 1–8.

Weeks, V. D., Travell, J. How to give painless injections. *A.M.A. Scientific Exhibits* (1957), 318–322.

Travell, J. Mechanical headache, *Headache*, **7** (1967), 23–29.

Travell, J. Myofascial trigger points: clinical view. *Adv. Pain Res. Ther.*, **1** (1976), 919–926.

Wyant, G. M. Chronic pain syndromes and their treatment. II Trigger points. *Can. Anaesth. Soc. J.*, **26, No. 3, May** (1979).

Segmental Acupuncture and Referred Pain.

Bahr, R., Blumberg, H., Jänig, W. Do dichotomizing afferent fibers exist which supply visceral organs as well as somatic structures? A contribution to the problem of referred pain, *Neurosci. Lett.*, **24** (1981), 25–28.

Bogduk, N. Headaches mediated by C3 dorsal ramus. Proceedings of the National Meeting of the Australasian Chapter of the International Association for the Study of Pain 1983. In Press.

Bowsher, D. Termination of the central pain pathway in man: The conscious appreciation of pain, *Brain*, **80** (1957), 606–622.

Brain Research, **87** (1975) complete issue.

Copeman, W. S. G., Ackerman, W. L. Edema or herniations of fat lobules as a cause of lumbar and gluteal fibrosis, *Arch. Intern. Med.*, **79** (1947), 22–35.

Cushing, H. The sensory distribution of the fifth nerve, *Bull. Johns Hopkins Hosp.*, **15** (1904), 213–232.

Cyriax, J. *Textbook of Orthopaedic Medicine Vol. 1*, 5th Edn., Bailliere, Tindall & Cassell (1970), 34–58.

Denny–Brown, D., Kirk, E. J., Yanagisawa, N. The tract of Lissauer in relation to sensory transmission in the dorsal horn of spinal cord in the Macaque monkey, *J. Comp. Neurol.*, **151** (1973), 175–200.

Denny–Brown, D., Yanagisawa, N. The function of the descending root of the fifth nerve, *Brain*, **96** (1973), 783–814.

Denslow, J. S., Hassett, C. C. The central excitatory state associated with postural abnormalities, *J. Neurophysiol.*, **5** (1944), 393–402.

Edeiken, J., Wolferth, C. C. Persistent pain in the shoulder region following myocardial infarction, *Am. J. Med. Sci.*, **191** (1936), 201–210.

Elliot, F. A. Tender muscles in sciatica, *Lancet*, **i** (1944), 47–48.

Feinstein, B. Referred pain from paravertebral structures. In: *Approaches to the Validation of Manipulative Therapy* (Eds. Buerger, A. A., Tobis, J. S.) Charles C. Thomas (1977), 139–167.

Fender, F. A. Foerster's scheme of dermatomes, *Arch. Neurol. Psychiat.*, **41** (1939), 688–693.

Foerster, O. The dermatomes in man, *Brain*, **56** (1933), 1–39.

Gobel, S., Falls, W. M., Bennett, G. J., Abdelmoumene, M., Hayashi, H., Humphrey, E. An EM analysis of the synaptic connections of horseradish peroxidase-filled stalked cells and islet cells in the substantia gelatinosa of adult cat spinal cord, *J. Comp. Neurol.*, **194** (1980), 781–807.

Grant, J. C. B. *Grant's Atlas of Anatomy*. Williams & Wilkins (1972), 664–665.

Harman, J. R. Angina in the analgesic lamb, *Brit. Med. J.*, **2** (1951), 521–522.

Hay, K. M. The treatment of pain in trigger areas in migraine, *J.Roy. Coll. Gen. Pract.*, **26** (1976), 372–376.

Head, H. On disturbances of sensation with especial reference to the pain of visceral disease, *Brain*, **16** (1893), 1–133.

Hodge, C. J., King, R. B. Medical modification of sensation, *J. Neurosurg.*, **44** (1976), 21–28.

Holmes, T. H., Wolff, H. G. Life situations, emotions and backache. *Res. Publ. Assoc. Res. Nerv. Ment. Dis.*, **29** (1950), 750–772.

Hou, Zonglian. A study of the histologic structure of acupuncture points in types of fibres conveying needling sensation, *Chinese Med. J. (Engl.)*, **92** (1979), 233–234.

Inman, V. T., Saunders, J. B. de C. M. Referred pain from skeletal structures, *J. Nerv. Ment. Dis.*, **99** (1944), 660–667.

Keegan, J. J., Garrett, F. D. The segmental distribution of the cutaneous nerves in the limbs of man, *Anat. Rec.*, **102** (1948), 409–437.

Kellgren, J. H. Observation on referred pain arising from muscle, *Clin. Sci.*, **3** (1938), 175–190.

Kellgren, J. H. On the distribution of pain arising from deep somatic structures with charts of segmental pain areas, *Clin.Sci.*, **4** (1939), 35–46.

Kellgren, J. H. Pain. In: *Copeman's Textbook of Rheumatic Diseases* (Ed. Scott, J. T.) 5th Edn, Churchill Livingstone (1978), 62–77.

Kellgren, J. H. Somatic structures simulating visceral pain, *Clin. Sci.* (1939–42), 303–309.

Kellgren, J. H. Some painful joint conditions and their relation to osteoarthritis, *Clin. Sci.*, **4** (1939), 193–201.

Kerr, F. W. L. Evidence for a peripheral etiology of trigeminal neuralgia. *J. Neurosurg.*, **26** (1967), 168–174.

Kerr, F. W. L. Trigeminal and cervical volleys, *Arch. Neurol.*, **5** (1961), 171–179.

Kirk, E. J., Denny–Brown, D. Functional variation in dermatomes in the Macaque monkey following dorsal root lesions, *J.Comp. Neurol.*, **139** (1970), 307–320.

Korr, I. M. Sustained sympathicotonia as a factor in disease. In: *The Neuro-biologic Mechanisms in Manipulative Therapy* (Ed. Korr, I. M.) Plenum Press (1977), 229–268.

Lange, M. *Die Muskelhärten (Myogelosen)*. München, J. F. Lehmann's Verlag (1931).

Lewis, T., Kellgren, J. H. Observations relating to referred pain, viscero motor reflexes and other associated phenomena, *Clin. Sci.*, **4** (1939), 47–71.

Lewit, K. The needle effect in the relief of myofascial pain, *Pain*, **6** (1979), 83–90.

Lu Gwei–Djen and Needham, J. *Celestial Lancets, a History and Rationale of Acupuncture and Moxa*. Cambridge University Press (198?) 204–213.

Lu Gwei–Djen and Needham, J. op. cit., 117–119, 192–193.

Macdonald, A. J. R. Abnormally tender muscle regions and associated painful movements, *Pain*, **8** (1980), 197–205.

Macdonald, A. J. R., Macrae, K. D., Master, B. R., Rubin, A. P. Superficial acupuncture in the relief of chronic low back pain: a placebo-controlled randomised trial, *Ann. Roy. Coll. Surg. Engl.*, **65** (1983), 44–46.

Medical Research Council. Aids to the investigation of peripheral nerve injuries. Medical Research Council War Memorandum No. 7. Her Majesty's Stationery Office; 2nd Edn. (1943) 47–48.

Melzack, R., Stillwell, D. M., Fox, E. J. Trigger points and acupuncture points for pain: correlations and implications, *Pain*, **3** (1977), 3–23.

Pflug, E., Bonica, J. J. Physiopathology and control of postoperative pain, *Arch. Surg.*, **112** (1977), 773–781.

Ruch, T. C. Mechanisms of referred pain. In: *Physiology and Biophysics. Vol. 1: The Brain and Neural Function* (Eds. Ruch, T. C., Patton, W. D.) W. B. Saunders (1979), 312–316.

Sato, A., Brooks Chandler, McC., Koizumi, K., *Integrative Functions of the Autonomic Nervous System*. University of Tokyo Press and Elsevier/North Holland Biomedical Press (1979).

Sainsbury, P., Gibson, J. G. Symptoms of anxiety and tension and the accompanying physiological changes in the muscular system, *J.Neurol. Neurosurg. Psychiat.*, **17** (1954), 216–224.

Selzer, M., Spencer, W. A. Interactions between visceral and cutaneous afferents in the spinal cord: reciprocal primary afferent depolarization, *Brain Res.*, **14** (1969), 349–366.

Selzer M., Spencer, W. A. Convergence of visceral and cutaneous pathways in the lumbar spinal cord, *Brain Res.*, **14** (1969), 331–348.

Shanghai College of Traditional Medicine. *Acupuncture: a Comprehensive Text*. Eastland Press (1981), 218–219.

Sherrington, C. S. Experiments in examination of the peripheral distribution of the fibres of the posterior roots of some spinal nerves—Part II. *Phil. Trans. Roy. Soc.*, **190** (1898), 45–193.

Simons, D. G. Muscle pain syndromes: Part 1, *Am. J. Phys. Med.*, **54** (1975), 289–311; Part 2, *Am. J. Phys. Med.*, **55** (1976), 15–42.

Smythe, H. A. 'Fibrositis' as a disorder of pain modulation, *Clin. Rheum. Dis.*, **5** (1979), 823–832.

Szentagothai, J. Neuronal and synaptic arrangement in the substantia gelatinosa Rolandi, *J. Comp. Neurol.*, **122** (1964), 219–239.

Taverner, D. Muscle spasm as a cause of somatic pain, *Ann. Rheum. Dis.*, **13** (1954), 331–335.

Tfelt–Hansen, P., Lous, I., Olesen, J. Prevalence and significance of muscle tenderness during common migraine attacks, *J. Headache*, **21** (1981), 49–54.

Travell, J. Myofascial trigger points: Clinical view. In: *Advances in Pain Research and Therapy. Vol 1.* (Eds. Bonica, J. J., Albe-Fessard, D.) Raven Press (1976), 919–926.

Travell, J. Temporomandibular joint pain referred from muscles of the head and neck, *J. Prosth. Dent.*, **10** (1960), 745–763.

Travell, J., Rinzler, S. H. The myofascial genesis of pain, *Postgrad. Med.*, **11** (1952), 425–434.

In Chinese

Zhenjiuxue Jiangyi (Lectures in Acupuncture and Moxibustion); compiled by the Acupuncture Research Section of the Shanghai Academy of Chinese Medicine; published by the Shanghai Scientific and Technical Publishing House, Shanghai, 1960.

Zhongyixue Gailun (A Summary of Chinese Medicine); compiled by the Nanking Academy of Chinese Medicine; published by the People's Hygiene Publishing House, Peking, 1959.

Zhenjiuxue (The Study of Acupuncture); compiled by the Acupuncture Research Section of the Nanking Academy of Chinese Medicine; published by the Jiangsu People's Publishing House, Nanking, 1959.

Changjian Jibing Zhenjiu Zhiliao Bianlan (A General Survey of Common Diseases and their Treatment by Acupuncture in Tabular Form); compiled by the Peking School of Chinese Medicine; published by the People's Hygiene Publishing House, Peking, 1960.

Jingluoxue Tushuo (An Illustrated Survey of Meridians); compiled by Hiujan and Zhu Ru-gong assisted by Wu Shao-de, Wu Guo-zhang and Zhang Shi-yi; published by the Shanghai Scientific and Technical Publishing House, Shanghai, 1959.

Yuxuexue Gailun (A General Survey of Acupuncture Points); compiled by Hiu-jan and Zhu Ru-gong, assisted by Wu Shao-de and Zhang Shi-yi; published by the Shanghai Scientific and Technical Publishing House, Shanghai, 1961.

Zhengiufa Huilun (General Thesis of Acupuncture Treatment); compiled by Lu Hiu-jan; published by the Shanghai Scientific and Technical Publishing House, Shanghai, 1962.

Zhengiu Yhyetupu (Description of Acupuncture Points in Tabular Form); compiled by Lu Hiu-jan; published by the Hong Kong Hong Yei Publishing Co., Hong Kong, 1967.

Zhengiu Dacheng (Summary of Famous Ancient Works on Acupuncture—

Ming); by Jang Gi-zhou; published by The People's Hygiene Publishing House, Peking, 1963.

Zhengiuhye Shouce (Handbook of Acupuncture); compiled by Wang Hye-tai; published by The People's Hygiene Publishing House, Peking, 1962.

Huangdi Neiging Suwen Gizhu (The Yellow Emperors Classic of Medicine in Dialogue Form with Annotations—Ching); by Zhang Jin-an; published by The Shanghai Scientific and Technical Publishing House, Shanghai, 1963.

Zhengiu Giajibing (A Classic Thesis on Acupuncture—Gin); by Huang Pu-mi; published by The People's Hygiene Publishing House, Peking, 1964.

Zhengiu Gefu Hyangie (Selection of Songs and Rhymes on Acupuncture with Explanations); by Chen Bi-liu and Zhen Zhuo-ren; published by The People's Hygiene Publishing House, Peking, 1962.

Zhungguo Jihye Dacidian (The Encyclopaedia of Chinese Medical Science in 4 volumes); edited by Shai Kwan.

In Other Languages

L'Acupuncture Chinoise; by Georges Soulié de Morant; published by Jacques Lafitte, Paris, 1957.

Essai sur l'Acupuncture Chinoise Pratique; by J. E. H. Niboyet; published by Dominique Wapler, Paris, 1951.

Complements d'Acupuncture; by J. E. H. Niboyet; published by Dominique Wapler, Paris, 1955.

Traité de Médicine Chinoise—several volumes; by A. Chamfrault; published by Coquemard, Angoulême, 1954 and later.

La Voie Rationalle de la Médicine Chinoise; by Jean Choain; published by Editions, S.L.E.L. Lille, 1957.

L'Acupuncture Chinoise; by P. Ferreyrolles; published by Editions S.L.E.L., Lille, 1953.

L'Acupuncture; by Yosio Manaka, Odawara, Japan, 1960.

Acupuncture; by Henri Goux; published by Maloine, Paris, 1955.

Acupuncture; by H. Voisin; published by Maloine, Paris, 1959.

Einführung in die Akupunktur; by Johannes Bischko; published by Haug, Heidelberg, 1970.

Die Akupunktur eine Ordnungstherapie; by Gerhard Bachmann; published by Haug, Ulm, 1959.

Die Chinesisehe Medizin; by Fr. Hübotter; published by Asia Major, Leipzig, 1929.

The Yellow Emperors Classic of Internal Medicine; by Ilza Veith—translated from classic Chinese; published by Williams and Wilkins, Baltimore, 1949.

INDEX

The entries in the index relate to Sections 1 to 3 only.